T0263833

Vascular Anomalies

Guest Editors

ARIN K. GREENE, MD, MMSc
CHAD A. PERLYN, MD, PhD

CLINICS IN PLASTIC SURGERY

www.plasticsurgery.theclinics.com

January 2011 • Volume 38 • Number 1

SAUNDERS an imprint of ELSEVIER, Inc.

W.B. SAUNDERS COMPANY
A Division of Elsevier Inc.

1600 John F. Kennedy Boulevard • Suite 1800 • Philadelphia, Pennsylvania 19103-2899

http://www.theclinics.com

CLINICS IN PLASTIC SURGERY Volume 38, Number 1
January 2011 ISSN 0094-1298, ISBN-13: 978-1-4557-0492-7

Editor: Joanne Husovski
Developmental Editor: Jessica Demetriou

Clinics in Plastic Surgery (ISSN 0094-1298) is published quarterly by Elsevier Inc., 360 Park Avenue South, New York, NY 10010-1710. Months of issue are January, April, July, and October. Business and Editorial Offices: 1600 John F. Kennedy Blvd., Suite 1800, Philadelphia, PA 19103-2899. Periodicals postage paid at New York, NY and additional mailing offices. Subscription prices are $411.00 per year for US individuals, $617.00 per year for US institutions, $203.00 per year for US students and residents, $467.00 per year for Canadian individuals, $721.00 per year for Canadian institutions, $530.00 per year for international individuals, $721.00 per year for international institutions, and $256.00 per year for Canadian and foreign students/residents. To receive student/resident rate, orders must be accompanied by name of affiliated institution, date of term, and the *signature* of program/residency coordinator on institution letterhead. Orders will be billed at individual rate until proof of status is received. Foreign air speed delivery is included in all *Clinics* subscription prices. All prices are subject to change without notice. **POSTMASTER:** Send address changes to *Clinics in Plastic Surgery*, Elsevier Health Sciences Division, Subscription Customer Service, 3251 Riverport Lane, Maryland Heights, MO 63043. **Customer Service: 1-800-654-2452 (US and Canada). From outside of the United States and Canada, call 314-447-8871. Fax: 314-447-8029. E-mail: JournalsCustomerService-usa@elsevier.com (for print support); JournalsOnlineSupport-usa@elsevier.com (for online support).**

Reprints. For copies of 100 or more of articles in this publication, please contact the Commercial Reprints Department, Elsevier Inc., 360 Park Avenue South, New York, New York 10010-1710. Tel.: (+1) 212-633-3812; Fax: (+1) 212-462-1935; E-mail: reprints@elsevier.com.

Clinics in Plastic Surgery is covered in *Current Contents, EMBASE/Excerpta Medica, Science Citation Index, MEDLINE/PubMed (Index Medicus), ASCA, and ISI/BIOMED*.

Printed and bound by CPI Group (UK) Ltd, Croydon, CR0 4YY

Transferred to Digital Print 2011

Contributors

GUEST EDITORS

ARIN K. GREENE, MD, MMSc
Assistant Professor of Surgery, Department of Plastic and Oral Surgery, Vascular Anomalies Center, Children's Hospital Boston, Harvard Medical School, Boston, Massachusetts

CHAD A. PERLYN, MD, PhD
Clinical Assistant Professor of Surgery, Florida International University College of Medicine, Miami Children's Hospital, Miami, Florida

AUTHORS

DENISE M. ADAMS, MD
Professor of Clinical Medicine, Division of Hematology/Oncology; Medical Director, Hemangioma and Vascular Malformation Center, Cincinnati Children's Hospital Medical Center, University of Cincinnati, Cincinnati, Ohio

AHMAD I. ALOMARI, MD, MSc
Assistant Professor of Radiology, Department of Radiology, Vascular Anomalies Center, Children's Hospital Boston, Harvard Medical School, Boston, Massachusetts

RYAN ARNOLD, MD
Fellow in Pediatric Interventional Radiology, Division of Vascular and Interventional Radiology and Vascular Anomalies Center, Children's Hospital Boston; Harvard Medical School, Boston, Massachusetts

FANNY BALLIEUX, BSc
Center for Vascular Anomalies, Division of Plastic Surgery, Cliniques Universitaires St Luc, Brussels, Belgium

LAURENCE M. BOON, MD, PhD
Center for Vascular Anomalies, Division of Plastic Surgery, Cliniques Universitaires St Luc; Laboratory of Human Molecular Genetics, de Duve Institute, Université Catholique de Louvain, Brussels, Belgium

RENEE M. BURKE, MD
Division of Plastic Surgery, Miami Children's Hospital, Miami, Florida

ANNE MARIE CAHILL, MD
Chief, Interventional Radiology Division, Department of Radiology, The Children's Hospital of Philadelphia, Philadelphia, Pennsylvania

GULRAIZ CHAUDRY, MB, ChB
Assistant Professor of Radiology, Division of Vascular and Interventional Radiology and Vascular Anomalies Center, Children's Hospital Boston, Harvard Medical School, Boston, Massachusetts

STEVEN J. FISHMAN, MD
Associate Professor of Surgery, Department of Surgery, Vascular Anomalies Center, Children's Hospital Boston, Harvard Medical School, Boston, Massachusetts

ARIN K. GREENE, MD, MMSc
Assistant Professor of Surgery, Department of Plastic and Oral Surgery, Vascular Anomalies Center, Children's Hospital Boston, Harvard Medical School, Boston, Massachusetts

ANITA GUPTA, MD
Department of Pathology, Cincinnati Children's Hospital, Cincinnati, Ohio

IAN N. JACOBS, MD
Associate Professor of Otorhinolaryngology-Head and Neck Surgery, University of Pennsylvania School of Medicine; Medical Director, Division of Otolaryngology, The Center for Pediatric Airway Disorders, The Children's Hospital of Philadelphia, University of Pennsylvania School of Medicine, Philadelphia, Pennsylvania

HARRY KOZAKEWICH, MD
Department of Pathology, Children's Hospital Boston, Boston, Massachusetts

ANN M. KULUNGOWSKI, MD
Department of Surgery, Vascular Anomalies Center, Children's Hospital Boston, Harvard Medical School, Boston, Massachusetts

BORIS LAURE, MD
Department of Maxillofacial Surgery, Trousseau Hospital, Tours, France

MARILYN G. LIANG, MD
Department of Dermatology, Harvard Medical School, Children's Hospital Boston, Boston, Massachusetts

SHEILAGH M. MAGUINESS, MD
Department of Dermatology, Harvard Medical School, Children's Hospital Boston, Boston, Massachusetts

ROBERT J. MORIN, MD
Division of Plastic Surgery, Miami Children's Hospital, Miami, Florida

DARREN B. ORBACH, MD, PhD
Assistant Professor of Radiology, Department of Radiology, Vascular Anomalies Center, Children's Hospital Boston, Harvard Medical School, Boston, Massachusetts

CHAD A. PERLYN, MD, PhD
Clinical Assistant Professor of Surgery, Florida International University College of Medicine, Miami Children's Hospital, Miami, Florida

AMIR TAGHINIA, MD
Instructor in Surgery, Department of Plastic and Oral Surgery, Children's Hospital Boston, Harvard Medical School, Boston, Massachusetts

JOSEPH UPTON, MD
Professor of Surgery, Department of Plastic and Oral Surgery, Children's Hospital Boston, Harvard Medical School, Boston, Massachusetts

MIIKKA VIKKULA, MD, PhD
Laboratory of Human Molecular Genetics, de Duve Institute, Université Catholique de Louvain, Brussels, Belgium

S. ANTHONY WOLFE, MD
Chief, Division of Plastic Surgery, Miami Children's Hospital, Miami, Florida

Contents

Preface: Vascular Anomalies ix

Arin K. Greene and Chad A. Perlyn

Vascular Anomalies: Current Overview of the Field 1

Arin K. Greene

Vascular anomalies are disorders of the endothelium that can affect each part of the vasculature (capillaries, arteries, veins, or lymphatics). Although nearly always benign, vascular anomalies can involve any anatomic structure. Significant progress in understanding and treating patients with vascular anomalies has been made during the past quarter century since the introduction of a biologic classification for these lesions.

Pathogenesis of Vascular Anomalies 7

Laurence M. Boon, Fanny Ballieux, and Miikka Vikkula

Vascular anomalies are localized defects of vascular development. Most of them occur sporadically (ie, there is no familial history of lesions, yet in a few cases clear inheritance is observed). These inherited forms are often characterized by multifocal lesions that are mainly small in size and increase in number with patients' age. The authors review the known (genetic) causes of vascular anomalies and call attention to the concept of Knudson's double-hit mechanism to explain incomplete penetrance and large clinical variation in expressivity observed in inherited vascular anomalies. The authors also discuss the identified pathophysiological pathways involved in vascular anomalies and how it has opened the doors toward a more refined classification of vascular anomalies and the development of animal models that can be tested for specific molecular therapies.

Diagnostic Imaging of Vascular Anomalies 21

Ryan Arnold and Gulraiz Chaudry

Medical imaging has become critically important in the diagnosis and treatment planning of vascular anomalies. The classification of lesions into fast-flow and slow-flow categories, the identification of a soft tissue mass, and the determination of the extent of the lesions are all facilitated by the use of magnetic resonance imaging, ultrasonography, catheter angiography, and other imaging studies. The use of these imaging techniques in the diagnosis and assessment of vascular tumors, malformations, and combined malformation syndromes is discussed in this article.

Histopathology of Vascular Anomalies 31

Anita Gupta and Harry Kozakewich

Over the past decade, many changes and updates have occurred in the world of vascular anomalies, including their histopathology. An appreciation has developed that a combined team approach is optimal in arriving at a correct diagnosis. Technical advances such as immunohistochemical stains for GLUT1, an excellent marker for infantile hemangioma, and vascular immunostains such as D2-40, PROX1, and vascular endothelial growth factor receptor 3, which distinguish lymphatics from arteries and veins, have been of immense help in daily practice.

Management of Hemangiomas and Other Vascular Tumors 45

Arin K. Greene

Vascular tumors of childhood are typically benign. The 4 most common types are infantile hemangioma (IH), congenital hemangioma (CH), kaposiform hemangioendothelioma (KHE), and pyogenic granuloma (PG). Vascular tumors must be differentiated from vascular malformations. Although tumors and malformations may appear as raised, blue, red, or purple lesions, their management differs significantly.

Management of Capillary Malformations 65

Sheilagh M. Maguiness and Marilyn G. Liang

Capillary malformations (CMs) are the most common vascular malformations. They are comprised of the small vessels of the capillary network in skin and mucous membranes. In the vast majority of affected individuals, CMs are isolated and not associated with any underlying abnormalities. Depending on size and location, however, they may cause significant morbidity due to disfigurement or stigmatization and, rarely, herald the presence of an underlying syndrome.

Management of Lymphatic Malformations 75

Arin K. Greene, Chad A. Perlyn, and Ahmad I. Alomari

Lymphatic malformation results from an error in the embryonic development of the lymphatic system. Clinically, lymphatic malformation is characterized by the size of the malformed channels: microcystic, macrocystic, or combined (microcystic/macrocystic).This article describes the clinical features, diagnosis, and management of lymphatic malformations.

Management of Venous Malformations 83

Arin K. Greene and Ahmad I. Alomari

Venous malformation results from an error in vascular morphogenesis. Although this condition is present at birth, it may not become evident until childhood or adolescence when it has grown large enough to cause a visible deformity or symptoms. This article discusses the types, diagnosis, and the nonoperative and operative management of venous malformations.

Management of Arteriovenous Malformations 95

Arin K. Greene and Darren B. Orbach

This article describes the clinical features, diagnosis, and management of arteriovenous malformation, capillary malformation–arteriovenous malformation, and PTEN-associated vascular anomaly.

Management of Combined Vascular Malformations 107

Ann M. Kulungowski and Steven J. Fishman

Like single-channel–type vascular malformations, combined lesions are categorized as slow-flow and fast-flow lesions. Many of the combined vascular malformations are associated with soft tissue and skeletal hypertrophy. This article discusses the diagnosis, management, and treatment of patients with capillary lymphaticovenous malformation, capillary-arteriovenous malformation, and capillary-arteriovenous fistulas and congenital lipomatous overgrowth, vascular malformations, epidermal nevi, and skeletal anomalies syndrome.

Special Considerations in Vascular Anomalies: Airway Management 121

Ian N. Jacobs and Anne Marie Cahill

Vascular anomalies are disorders of abnormal vasculogenesis or lymphogenesis. All types of vascular anomalies may involve the airway, causing varying degrees of upper airway obstruction as well as dysphagia and bleeding. Certain signs and symptoms may implicate airway involvement with a hemangioma or vascular malformation. It is necessary to distinguish a vascular anomaly from other airway lesions such as a congenital cyst. This is accomplished with imaging and endoscopy.

Special Considerations in Vascular Anomalies: Operative Management of Craniofacial Osseous Lesions 133

Renee M. Burke, Robert J. Morin, Chad A. Perlyn, Boris Laure, and S. Anthony Wolfe

The treatment of vascular anomalies of the head and neck typically focuses on restoration of abnormal structures of the soft tissues. However, vascular anomalies can affect the craniofacial skeleton, and osseous reconstruction may be indicated. Osseous involvement occurs as either a primary or secondary phenomenon. In primary osseous involvement, the vascular anomaly expands the bone from within. Secondary osseous involvement occurs when bony hypertrophy develops because of increased flow of the surrounding soft tissue. This article focuses on the management of the osseous deformities associated with vascular anomalies.

Special Considerations in Vascular Anomalies: Operative Management of Upper Extremity Lesions 143

Joseph Upton and Amir Taghinia

The past 3 decades has seen a steady, almost exponential, increase in knowledge of vascular anomalies. A useful biologic classification system has evolved. A careful physical examination augmented with refined imaging will yield an accurate diagnosis and set the stage for treatment. A multidisciplinary team can offer treatment options with some degree of predictability. One option is surgery, which can be fraught with numerous complications. This article focuses on surgical principles and technical pearls in the treatment of these unique problems involving the upper limb. If incorporated into routine management, these suggestions will improve surgical outcomes.

Special Considerations in Vascular Anomalies: Hematologic Management 153

Denise M. Adams

Proper care of the patient with a vascular anomaly requires the expertise of multiple specialists. Because of the need for an interdisciplinary approach, several vascular anomalies centers have now been developed across the world. A hematologist/oncologist provides clinical acumen in establishing a correct diagnosis and guiding the medical management of these patients. These patients can have complicated coagulopathies and need medical therapy. This article emphasizes the hematologic complications and management of these patients.

Index 161

Clinics in Plastic Surgery

FORTHCOMING ISSUES

April 2011

Cosmetic Medicine and Minimally Invasive Surgery/State of the Art
Malcolm D. Paul, MD, FACS,
Raffi Hovsepian, MD, and
Adam Rotunda, MD, *Guest Editors*

July 2011

Toolbox for Autologous Breast Reconstruction
Maurice Nahabedian, MD,
Guest Editor

October 2011

Functional Hand Reconstruction
Michael W. Neumeister, MD, FRCSC, FACS,
Guest Editor

RECENT ISSUES

October 2010

Perforator Flaps
Peter C. Neligan, MB, BCh, FRCS(I), FRCS(C), FACS,
Guest Editor

July 2010

Abdominoplasty
Al Aly, MD, FACS,
Guest Editor

April 2010

Rhinoplasty: Current Concepts
Ronald P. Gruber, MD, and
David Stepnick, MD, FACS,
Guest Editors

RELATED INTEREST

Birthmarks of Medical Significance
Pediatric Clinics - October 2010
Guest Editors: Beth A. Drolet, Maria C. Garzon

THE CLINICS ARE NOW AVAILABLE ONLINE!

Access your subscription at:
www.theclinics.com

Preface
Vascular Anomalies

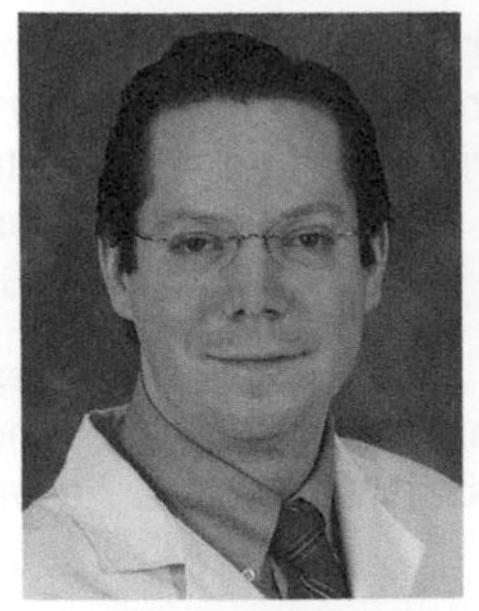
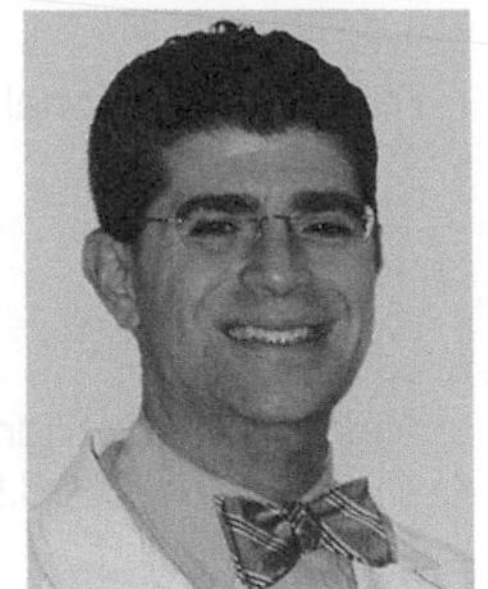

Arin K. Greene, MD, MMSc   Chad A. Perlyn, MD, PhD
Guest Editors

"Disease is very old and nothing about it has changed. It is we who change as we learn to recognize what was formerly imperceptible."
—From John Martin Charcot,
De l'Expectation en Medecine

For decades, *Clinics in Plastic Surgery* has provided plastic surgeons with outstanding clinical guidelines on a variety of relevant topics. This issue is unique because it is the first volume devoted solely to vascular anomalies. Compared to other areas of plastic surgery, the field of vascular anomalies is relatively young and has rapidly expanded since 1982 when Mulliken and Glowacki proposed the biological classification of these lesions.

The purpose of this volume is to improve the care of patients with vascular anomalies by providing an up-to-date manual for management. The issue is focused on diagnosis and treatment, not on history, basic science, or current research. Experts in several disciplines contributed to this volume, because patients with vascular anomalies often require multidisciplinary care.

This issue of *Clinics in Plastic Surgery* was designed to recapitulate the thought process we go through when managing a patient with a vascular anomaly. The initial article outlines terminology and classification; any physician treating these patients must have mastered this nosologic framework. Pathogenesis then is presented, followed by the imaging and histopathological characteristics of these lesions. With this background, the diagnosis and current management of each major type of vascular anomaly are described. Finally, four articles are included that focus on particularly challenging problems caused by vascular anomalies.

Although patients with vascular anomalies usually require the expertise of more than one specialist, plastic surgeons will continue to be primary caretakers of these patients. Most lesions involve the integument, and management often requires the reconstructive surgeon's creativity, surgical problem-solving skills, and a mastery of operative principles. Although great progress has been made over the past quarter century, vascular anomalies continue to cause significant morbidity, and many of our current therapies are inadequate. The field is rapidly evolving and some of the treatments presented in this issue soon will become obsolete as newer and more effective therapies become available.

We thank all of the contributors to this issue of *Clinics in Plastic Surgery*. We also would like to recognize Dr John B. Mulliken, who has trained many of the authors in this issue and has been an inspiration to a generation of physicians who are focused on these patients. If there is one theme that the reader should retain, it is that terminology is critically important. This field is complicated because different types of vascular anomalies

Clin Plastic Surg 38 (2011) ix–x
doi:10.1016/j.cps.2010.09.001

often look similar and their nomenclature can be confusing. We hope that this *Clinics in Plastic Surgery* issue will improve patient care by serving as a reference for any specialist managing an individual with a vascular anomaly.

Arin K. Greene, MD, MMSc
Department of Plastic and Oral Surgery
Vascular Anomalies Center
Children's Hospital Boston
Harvard Medical School
300 Longwood Avenue
Boston, MA 02115, USA

Chad A. Perlyn, MD, PhD
Florida International University College of Medicine
Miami Children's Hospital
13400 SW 120th Street
Miami, FL 33186, USA

E-mail addresses:
arin.greene@childrens.harvard.edu (A.K. Greene)
Chad.Perlyn@mch.com (C.A. Perlyn)

Vascular Anomalies: Current Overview of the Field

Arin K. Greene, MD, MMSc

KEYWORDS

• Classification • Hemangioma • History
• Vascular anomalies • Vascular malformations

Vascular anomalies are disorders of the endothelium that can affect each part of the vasculature (capillaries, arteries, veins, or lymphatics). Lesions are usually diagnosed during infancy or childhood and are common; the estimated prevalence is 4.5%.[1] Although nearly always benign, vascular anomalies can involve any anatomic structure. The most common problem is psychological morbidity caused by disfigurement; many lesions affect the head and neck. Local complications include bleeding, destruction of anatomic structures, infection, obstruction, pain, thrombosis, and ulceration. Vascular anomalies can also cause congestive heart failure, disseminated intravascular coagulation, pulmonary embolism, thrombocytopenia, and sepsis.

The field of vascular anomalies is confusing because (1) numerous types of vascular anomalies exist, (2) different lesions often look similar, and (3) many practitioners use imprecise terminology. Because vascular anomalies most commonly involve the integument, patients are often referred to a plastic surgeon. Although the reconstructive surgeon can manage many lesions independently, several types of anomalies require the care of additional specialists.

Significant progress in understanding and treating patients with vascular anomalies has been made during the past quarter century since a biologic classification for these lesions was introduced. For example, imaging instead of biopsy is now the standard for diagnostic confirmation, antiangiogenic drug treatment is available for problematic vascular tumors, sclerotherapy has replaced resection of vascular malformations in many instances, and techniques for excision have been improved. Several multidisciplinary vascular anomalies centers now serve as regional, national, or international referral sites. However, despite improvements in the management of vascular anomalies, these disorders continue to cause significant morbidity and their etiopathogenesis remains poorly understood.

TERMINOLOGY

The field of vascular anomalies has been impeded by imprecise terminology that has created diagnostic confusion, blocked communication between physicians, inhibited research, and caused incorrect treatment. Historically, vascular anomalies were labeled descriptively, according to the type of food they resembled (cherry, strawberry, port wine).[2] Vascular anomalies were later divided histopathologically into angioma simplex, angioma cavernosum, or angioma racemosum; these terms became synonymous with superficial hemangioma, deep hemangioma or venous malformation (VM), and arteriovenous malformation (AVM), respectively.[2] Lymphatic malformation (LM) was separated into lymphangioma or cystic hygroma.[2]

Capillary or strawberry hemangioma became associated with hemangioma affecting the dermis, which appears red. Hemangioma located below the skin is blue and was often called cavernous

Disclosures: none.
Department of Plastic and Oral Surgery, Vascular Anomalies Center, Children's Hospital Boston, Harvard Medical School, 300 Longwood Avenue, Boston, MA 02115, USA
E-mail address: arin.greene@childrens.harvard.edu

Clin Plastic Surg 38 (2011) 1–5
doi:10.1016/j.cps.2010.08.004

hemangioma. The terms capillary and cavernous were also used to describe capillary malformation (CM) and VM, respectively. Another label for CM was port-wine stain. Cystic hygroma and lymphangioma became common terms for macrocystic and microcystic lymphatic malformations, respectively. To add to the confusing terminology, hemangioma continued to be used to describe any type of vascular anomaly, including both tumors and malformations.

CLASSIFICATION

A biologic classification clarified the field of vascular anomalies by categorizing lesions based on their clinical behavior and cellular characteristics (**Table 1**).[3] Vascular tumors rapidly enlarged postnatally and demonstrated endothelial proliferation. Malformations were errors in vascular development and had stable endothelial turnover; lesions were named based on the primary vessel that was malformed (capillary, arterial, venous, lymphatic).[3] The terminology was further clarified because the suffix "-oma", meaning upregulated cellular growth, was reserved for vascular tumors. Thus, terms such as lymphangioma (microcystic lymphatic malformation), cystic hygroma (macrocystic lymphatic malformation), and cavernous hemangioma (VM), which describe nonproliferating malformations, were abandoned.[3] Using this classification, 90% of vascular anomalies could be correctly diagnosed by history and physical examination.[4] This classification was accepted by the International Society for the Study of Vascular Anomalies (ISSVA) in 1996 (**Table 2**).[5]

The most common vascular tumors consist of infantile hemangioma (IH), congenital hemangioma (CH), pyogenic granuloma, and kaposiform hemangioendothelioma (KHE) (**Fig. 1**). Malformations are divided into rheologically slow-flow lesions (CM, VM, LM) or fast-flow anomalies (AVM, arterial aneurysm/atresia/ectasia/stenosis) (**Fig. 2**).[6] Combined vascular anomalies, most commonly lymphatic venous malformation, can also occur. Eponymous syndromes that include vascular anomalies exist; one example is Klippel-Trénaunay syndrome, a capillary lymphatic venous malformation of an extremity with overgrowth.

The classification of vascular anomalies continues to expand and has become more precise as the knowledge of these lesions evolves (**Table 3**). For example, CHs and KHE have been differentiated from IH. Genetic studies have identified subtypes of VMs (cutaneomucosal, glomuvenous). New vascular anomalies have recently been characterized (ie, capillary malformation–arteriovenous malformation, phosphatase and tensin homolog–associated vascular anomaly).

Table 1
Classification of vascular lesions in infants and children (1982)

Hemangiomas	Malformations
Proliferating phase	Capillary
Involuting phase	Venous
	Arterial
	Lymphatic
	Fistulae

Data from Mulliken JB, Glowacki J. Hemangiomas and vascular malformations in infants and children: a classification based on endothelial characteristics. Plast Reconstr Surg 1982;69:412–22.

Table 2
ISSVA classification (1996)

	Malformations	
Tumors	Simple	Combined
Hemangioma	Capillary (C)	AVF, AVM, CVM, CLVM LVM, CAVM, CLAVM
Others	Lymphatic (L)	
	Venous (V)	
	Arterial (A)	

Abbreviations: AVM, arteriovenous malformation; AVF, arteriovenous fistula; CAVM, capillary arterial venous malformation; CLAVM, capillary lymphatic arteriovenous malformation; CLVM, capillary lymphatic venous malformation; CVM, capillary venous malformation; LVM, lymphatic venous malformation.

Data from Enjolras O, Mulliken JB. Vascular tumors and vascular malformations (new issues). Adv Dermatol 1997;13:375–423.

VASCULAR ANOMALIES CENTER

Since the biologic classification of vascular anomalies was introduced, vascular anomalies centers now exist to manage patients who previously had been medical nomads. The most common specialties involved in these programs include plastic surgery, dermatology, interventional/diagnostic radiology, general/pediatric surgery, hematology/oncology, and orthopedic surgery. Although many noncomplicated hemangiomas and CMs can be treated by a single physician, most lesions, particularly malformations, require interdisciplinary care. For example, two-thirds of

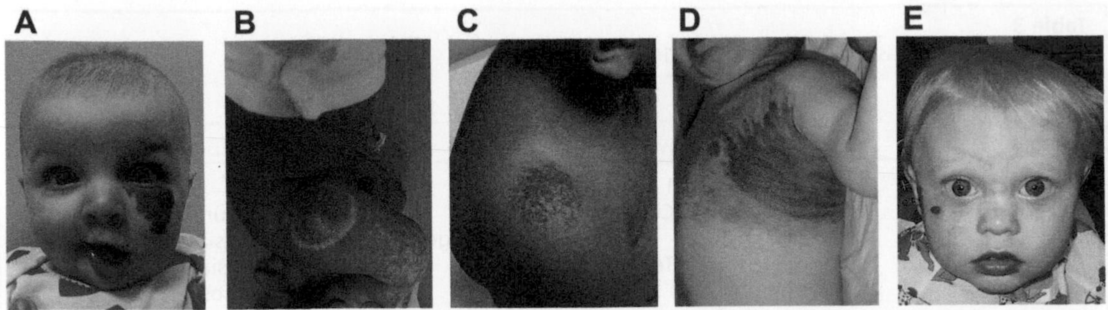

Fig. 1. Vascular tumors of infancy and childhood. (*A*) A 3-month-old girl with an enlarging IH of the left cheek first noted at 2 weeks of age. (*B*) A 2-week-old boy with a rapidly involuting CH of the lower extremity that was fully grown at birth. (*C*) A 6-year-old boy with a noninvoluting CH of the shoulder that has not changed since birth. (*D*) An 11-month-old boy with KHE and significant thrombocytopenia. (*E*) A 7-month-old boy with a 4-week history of a bleeding pyogenic granuloma of the right cheek.

patients referred to the author's center have a vascular malformation, despite being much less common than vascular tumors (**Table 4**).

Patients with problematic vascular anomalies should be referred to an interdisciplinary vascular anomalies center. The field is complicated, and patients are more likely to be diagnosed and treated correctly when managed in a program specializing in these conditions. For example, 47% of patients evaluated in the author's center have an incorrect referral diagnosis; malformations are more likely to be misdiagnosed (54.4%) than tumors (29.6%). Collecting patients in referral centers facilitates clinical and basic research, further improving the care for these patients.

FUTURE DIRECTIONS

Although significant progress has been made in the field of vascular anomalies, many challenges exist. Incorrect terminology continues to pervade the medical community; it remains difficult to conduct clinical research and communicate with other physicians (**Table 5**). The use of imprecise terminology also increases the likelihood that a patient will be treated incorrectly. In a review of the most recent 1-year literature of articles containing the term hemangioma, 71.3% of investigators used hemangioma erroneously to describe another vascular anomaly.[7] Patients whose lesions were mislabeled were more likely to be managed incorrectly (20.6%) when compared with patients whose anomalies were correctly designated using standardized ISSVA terminology (0.0%) ($P<.001$).[7] Continuing education will increase the use of accepted biologic terms to describe these lesions.

Research in the field of vascular anomalies continues to improve. Basic studies have been limited by the lack of animal models that

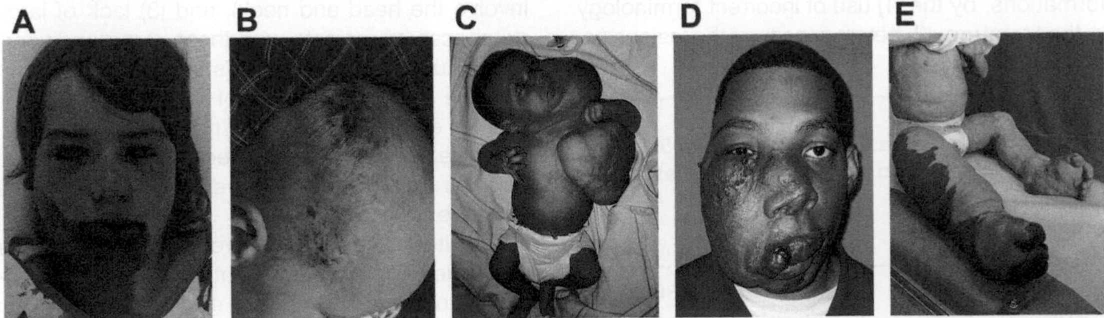

Fig. 2. Vascular malformations. (*A*) A 13-year-old boy with a CM of the face and neck; note overgrowth of lower lip. (*B*) An 18-month-old girl with a VM of the scalp. (*C*) An infant boy with a lymphatic malformation of the neck and trunk. (*D*) A 25-year-old man with an arteriovenous malformation on the right side of the face. (*E*) A 20-month-old girl with Klippel-Trénaunay syndrome (capillary lymphatic venous malformation of an extremity with overgrowth).

Table 3
Classification of vascular anomalies (2010)

Tumors	Malformations: Slow Flow	Malformations: Fast-Flow
IH	CM Cutis marmorata telangiectatica congenita Telangiectasias	AM Aneurysm Atresia Ectasia Stenosis
CH Rapidly involuting congenital hemangioma Noninvoluting congenital hemangioma	LM Microcystic Macrocystic Primary lymphedema	AVM CM-AVM Hereditary hemorrhagic telangiectasia PTEN-AVA
Hemangioendotheliomas KHE Others	VM Cerebral cavernous malformation Cutaneomucosal venous malformation Glomuvenous malformation Verrucous hemangioma	Combined malformations Capillary arteriovenous malformation Capillary lymphatic arteriovenous malformation
Pyogenic granuloma	Combined malformations Capillary venous malformation Capillary lymphatic malformation Capillary lymphatic venous malformation Lymphatic venous malformation	

Abbreviations: AM, arterial malformation; AVM, arteriovenous malformation; CM-AVM, capillary malformation arteriovenous malformation; LM, lymphatic malformation; PTEN-AVA, phosphatase and tensin homolog–associated vascular anomaly.

recapitulate human disease. Clinical investigation has been impeded, particularly for vascular malformations, by the (1) use of incorrect terminology in the literature, (2) heterogeneity of the lesions (ie, one lymphatic malformation may be small and located on an extremity, whereas another could involve the head and neck), and (3) lack of large databases of patients with these rare conditions. In the future, animal models will provide insight into the etiopathogenesis of vascular anomalies and will enable the testing of novel therapies. Clinical research will be facilitated as the numbers of patients being treated in well-organized centers continue to increase.

Despite improvement in treatments of vascular anomalies, many lesions continue to cause significant morbidity and are not curable. As research continues to evolve, new management strategies will be developed. Pharmacotherapy may become available to treat vascular malformations, preventing their expansion or reducing their recurrence after embolization, sclerotherapy, or resection.

Table 4
Epidemiology of vascular anomalies in 5620 patients referred to a vascular anomalies center

Tumors (35.2%)		Malformations (64.8%)	
IH	85.9%	Venous	36.8%
KHE	6.3%	Lymphatic	28.3%
CH	5.4%	Arteriovenous	14.3%
Others	2.4%	Capillary	11.0%
		Combined	9.6%

Table 5
Incorrect terminology commonly used to describe vascular anomalies

Tumors		Malformations	
Correct Biologic Term	**Incorrect Descriptive Term**	**Correct Biologic Term**	**Incorrect Descriptive Term**
Hemangioma	Capillary hemangioma Cavernous hemangioma Strawberry hemangioma	Capillary malformation	Capillary hemangioma Port-wine stain
Kaposiform hemangioendothelioma	Hemangioma	Lymphatic malformation	Lymphangioma Cystic hygroma
Pyogenic granuloma	Hemangioma	Venous malformation	Cavernous hemangioma
		Arteriovenous malformation	Arteriovenous hemangioma

As the etiopathogenesis of vascular anomalies becomes better understood, prevention of these lesions may become possible. New vascular anomalies will be identified as larger numbers of patients with these rare lesions are studied. For example, 5.2% of patients referred to the author's center are unable to be diagnosed; they have vascular anomalies that have not yet been characterized.

The future of the field of vascular anomalies is exciting because a significant opportunity exists to improve the lives of these patients. Plastic surgeons are well positioned to make progress because of their training; management of vascular anomalies requires creativity, surgical problem-solving skills, and a mastery of operative principles. Plastic surgeons who treat these patients are at the interface of translational medicine; knowledge of basic vascular biology is often translated to clinical management. Plastic surgeons, in collaboration with other medical and surgical specialists, continue to be the primary caretakers of patients with vascular anomalies.

REFERENCES

1. Greene AK, Kim S, Rogers GF, et al. The risk of vascular anomalies with Down syndrome. Pediatrics 2008;121:e135–40.
2. Young AE, Mulliken JB. Arteriovenous malformations. In: Mulliken JB, editor. Vascular birthmarks: hemangiomas and malformations. Philadelphia: Saunders; 1988. p. 24–37.
3. Mulliken JB, Glowacki J. Hemangiomas and vascular malformations in infants and children: a classification based on endothelial characteristics. Plast Reconstr Surg 1982;69:412–22.
4. Finn MC, Glowacki J, Mulliken JB. Congenital vascular lesions: clinical application of a new classification. J Pediatr Surg 1983;18:894–900.
5. Enjolras O, Mulliken JB. Vascular tumors and vascular malformations (new issues). Adv Dermatol 1997;13:375–423.
6. Mulliken JB. Cutaneous vascular anomalies. Semin Vasc Surg 1993;6:204–18.
7. Hassanein A, Mulliken JB, Fishman SJ, et al. Evaluation of terminology for vascular anomalies in current literature. Plast Reconstr Surg, in press.

Pathogenesis of Vascular Anomalies

Laurence M. Boon, MD, PhD[a,b], Fanny Ballieux, BSc[a], Miikka Vikkula, MD, PhD[b,*]

KEYWORDS

• Angiogenesis • Pathogenesis • Mutation • Somatic
• Genetic • Gene • Hemangioma • Vascular malformation

Vascular anomalies are localized defects of vascular development. Most of them occur sporadically (ie, there is no familial history of lesions, yet in a few cases clear inheritance is observed). These inherited forms are often characterized by multifocal lesions that are mainly small in size and increase in number with patients' age. On the basis of these inherited forms, molecular genetic studies have unraveled a number of inherited mutations giving direct insight into the pathophysiological cause and the molecular pathways that are implicated. Genetic defects have been identified for hereditary haemorrhagic telangiectasia (HHT), inherited cutaneomucosal venous malformation (VMCM), glomuvenous malformation (GVM), capillary malformation-arteriovenous malformation (CM-AVM), cerebral cavernous malformation (CCM), and some isolated and syndromic forms of primary lymphedema. The authors focus on these disorders, the implicated mutated genes, and the underlying pathogenic mechanisms. The authors also call attention to the concept of Knudson's double-hit mechanism to explain incomplete penetrance and the large clinical variation in expressivity of inherited vascular anomalies. This variability renders the making of correct diagnosis of the rare inherited forms difficult. Yet, the identification of the pathophysiological causes and pathways involved in them has had an unprecedented impact on our thinking of their etiopathogenesis, and has opened the doors toward a more refined classification of vascular anomalies. It has also made it possible to develop animal models that can be tested for specific molecular therapies, aimed at alleviating the dysfunctions caused by the aberrant genes and proteins.

Vascular anomalies are histopathologically characterized by a focal increase in the number of vessels that are abnormally tortuous and enlarged. This phenomenon is likely caused by localized defects in vascular development during vasculogenesis and especially during angiogenesis.[1] Vasculogenesis is defined as vessel growth from embryonic cells: hemangioblasts (mesoderm derived precursors) that give rise to angioblasts (endothelial precursors) and hemocytoblasts (blood cell precursors). Angioblast fusion takes place in vascular islets inducing the formation of the primary capillary plexus. During angiogenesis, this primary capillary system extends and matures. It involves both endothelial cell proliferation and mural cell recruitment to generate the fully

The authors have nothing to disclose.
Conflict of interest statement: none declared.
These studies were partially supported by the Interuniversity Attraction Poles initiated by the Belgian Federal Science Policy, network 6/05; Concerted Research Actions (A.R.C.), Convention No 07/12-005 of the Belgian French Community Ministry; the National Institute of Health, Program Project P01 AR048564; EU FW6 Integrated project LYMPHANGIOGENOMICS, LSHG-CT-2004-503,573; the F.R.S.-FNRS (Fonds de la Recherche Scientifique); and la Communauté française de Wallonie-Bruxelles et de la Lotterie nationale, Belgium (all to M.V.).
[a] Division of Plastic Surgery, Center for Vascular Anomalies, Cliniques Universitaires St Luc, Avenue Hippocrate 10, B-1200 Brussels, Belgium
[b] Laboratory of Human Molecular Genetics, de Duve Institute, Université Catholique de Louvain, Avenue Hippocrate 74, BP 75.39, B-1200 Brussels, Belgium
* Corresponding author.
E-mail address: miikka.vikkula@uclouvain.be

Clin Plastic Surg 38 (2011) 7–19
doi:10.1016/j.cps.2010.08.012

developed and functional vascular and lymphatic trees.[2] The pathophysiological studies of vascular anomalies have been helped by the astounding parallel progress made in understanding the factors and regulation of the development of the lymphatic and vascular systems.[1,2]

Several angiogenic factors, such as vascular endothelial growth factors (VEGFs), fibroblast growth factors, platelet derived growth factor beta (PDGF-beta), and angiopoietins (ANGPT-1 and ANGPT-2) regulate angiogenesis. They activate precursor cells, and lead to migration, proliferation, and differentiation of the primary capillary plexus. Vascular endothelial growth factors, angiopoietins, and their endothelial tyrosine kinase receptors are central regulators of vasculogenesis, angiogenesis, and lymphangiogenesis.[2]

Most vascular anomalies are sporadic, yet rare familial cases have been recorded. These forms have allowed to use molecular genetics for the identification of the underlying causes (**Table 1**).[3] This molecular characterization of the inherited forms has subsequently led to hypothesize on the causes of the more common sporadic forms. In the first such extrapolation, this was shown to be true.[4] Thus, there is hope that in the near future, the molecular basis of vascular anomalies will be deciphered, allowing a precise classification of all of them. Moreover, some inherited forms have been proven to follow paradominant inheritance, which may be a general rule.[1] Thus, inhibition of second hits may play a role in prevention of lesions in the familial forms. Finally, the data have laid the ground to develop specific in vitro and in vivo models of vascular anomalies. These can be used to characterize in detail the pathophysiological mechanisms and to develop novel specific treatments.

HEMANGIOMA

The etiopathogenesis of hemangioma of infancy still remains a mystery (see **Table 1**). Different hypotheses have been proposed, such as human papillomavirus virus-8 infection, abnormal hormonal influence, and chorionic villus sampling.[5] Local hypoxia has also been suggested as an initiating factor for proliferation.[6]

Many angiogenic factors are highly expressed in proliferating hemangiomas.[7,8] In contrast, the vascular endothelial growth factor receptor 1 (VEGFR1; *FLT1)* is regularly downregulated.[7] The lack of this decoy receptor results in persistent activation of VEGFR2 by VEGF. The VEGFR1 downregulation seems to be caused by amino acid substitutions in VEGFR2 and in the tumor endothelial marker-8 (TEM8), an integrinlike receptor, at least in some cases, although these changes are not specific to patients with hemangioma. Normalization of VEGFR2 signaling with soluble VEGFR1, or by other means, may become an effective treatment.[7]

To date, we know that endothelial cells from proliferating hemangiomas show patterns of X chromosome inactivation suggestive of clonal origin.[8,9] Bischoff and coworkers reported that hemangioma endothelial cells (HemECs) and hemangioma endothelial progenitor cells, both present in hemangiomas, are immature and share features with cord blood ECs, and are able to recapitulate hemangiomas in nude mice.[10–13] HemECs express genes that are expressed by placenta, umbilical cord, and bone marrow stem cells. One of them, the glucose transporter protein GLUT-1, has become a marker for histopathological diagnosis of hemangiomas.[14] Thus, it could be that hemangiomas are the result of a localized abnormal proliferation of progenitor cells, which preferentially occurs in children with predisposing genetic variants. Yet, the triggering factors for such growth remain unknown. New clues may come from hemangiomas being part of a polymalformative syndrome, such as PHACES (posterior fossa malformation, facial hemangioma, arterial anomalies, cardiovascular anomalies, eye anomalies, and sternal anomalies).[15]

VENOUS MALFORMATIONS

Venous malformations are classified into sporadic venous malformations (VM), dominantly VMCM, and dominantly inherited GVM (see **Table 1**). They account for 94%, 1%, and 5% of venous anomalies, respectively. No sex preponderance has been observed.[3,16]

Sporadic venous malformation is the most common referral to specialized centers for vascular anomalies because they often cause functional impairment, organ dysfunction, esthetic disfigurement, and can sometimes threaten life.[3,4,16] They are present at birth, never regress, and grow proportionately with the child. VMs tend to enlarge during puberty and pregnancy, and can become symptomatic.[17] Pain at awakening, after activity, or with temperature variation are commonly experienced.[17]

Local intravascular coagulation (LIC), characterized by elevated D-dimer level with normal fibrinogen level, is present in almost 50% of patients with a venous malformation.[18,19] This coagulopathy can cause acute pain and the formation of thrombi, which often calcify and form pathognomonic phleboliths.[18,19] Severe LIC (elevated D-dimer level with low fibrinogen level) is often

Table 1
Vascular anomalies with known genetic mutations, loci, or predisposing factors

Vascular Anomaly	Clinical Signs	Linked Locus/Loci	Mutated/Predisposing Gene
Hemangioma	Erythematous macular patch, blanched spot or telangiectasia with rapid postnatal growth	—	VEGFR2/TEM8, predisposing variants
Venous malformation (VM)	Bluish lesion compressible on palpation	—	*TIE2, 40%–50%*
Cutaneo-mucosal venous malformation (VMCM)	Multiple small punctate bluish spots	9p21-22	*TIE2*
Glomuvenous malformation (GVM)	Small, multifocal bluish-purple, cobblestone and hyperkeratotic lesions	1p21-22	*Glomulin*
Capillary malformation-Arteriovenous malformation (CM-AVM)	Multifocal capillary malformation with pale halo, AVM, AVF, Vein of Galen, aneurysmal malformation, Parkes Weber syndrome	5q13-22	*RASA1*
Hereditary hemorrhagic telangiectasia (HHT1/HHT2/HHT3/HHT4)	Epistaxis, telangiectasia, AVM (lung, liver, brain, gastrointestinal tract)	9q33-34/12q11-14/5q/7p14	*ENG/ ACVRL1/?/?*
HHT juvenile polyposis (JPHT)	HHT with juvenile polyposis	18q21	*SMAD4*
Angioma serpiginosum	Patchy capillary malformation with dilated capillaries following Blaschko's lines, mild nail, hair dystrophy, papillomatosis	Xp11.3-Xq12	*PORCN ?*
Cerebral cavernous malformation (CCM1/CCM2/CCM3)	Cerebral capillaro-venous malformations, and sometimes cutaneous lesions (HCCVM)	7q21-Q22/7p15-p13/3q25.2-27	*KRIT1/malcavernin/PDCD10*
Nonne-Milroy syndrome	Lymphedema, hydrocele, large caliber leg veins, cellulitis, curled toenails, papillomatosis	5q34-35	*VEGFR3*
Lymphedema-distichiasis	Lymphedema, distichiasis, ptosis, yellow nails, syndactyly, cleft palate, and cardiac septal defects	16q24.3	*FOXC2*
Hypotrichosis-lymphedema-telangiectasia (HLT)	Sparse hair, lymphedema, and cutaneous telangiectasias	20q13.33	*SOX18*
Hennekam syndrome	Peripheral lymphedema, with visceral involvement, mental retardation and unusual, flat face, hypertelorism, and broad nasal bridge	18q21.32	*CCBE1*
OLEDAID	Osteoporosis lymphedema anhidrotic ectodermal dysplasia with immunodeficiency	Xq28	*NEMO*
Primary congenital resolving lymphedema	Early onset lymphedema with papillomatosis resolving at 30 to 40 year of age	6q16.2-q22.1	?
Aagenaes syndrome or hereditary lymphedema cholestasis (HLC)	Extended lymphedema of lower extremities, malabsorption, growth retardation, rickets, cholestatic jaundice, and hepatomegaly	15q	?

Abbreviations: AVF, arteriovenous fistula; HCCVM, hyperkeratotic cutaneous capillary-venous malformation.

associated with extensive VM of the extremities.[19] This coagulopathy can decompensate into disseminated intravascular coagulopathy during surgery and cause severe hemorrhage, if not treated with low molecular weight heparin. Therefore, measurement of this specific biomarker should be done as a routine test for every VM. Moreover, it can help to differentiate VM from GVM and other vascular anomalies with normal D-dimer level.

VMCMs are clinically characterized by small (<5 cm in diameter), multifocal, and hemispherical bluish lesions. They mainly involve skin and oral mucosa, but can also invade superficial muscle, gastrointestinal tract, lungs, and brain.[17,20–22] VMCMs are often asymptomatic and family members can be unaware of their lesions. They are inherited as an autosomal dominant trait with high penetrance. Genome-wide scans permitted to identify the mutated gene, *TIE2/TEK,* located on 9p21-22.[20,21] The most common mutation causes an Arg849-to-Trp substitution (R849 W) in the intracellular kinase domain of the membrane-bound tyrosine kinase receptor (see **Table 1**).[21,22]

Expression analysis of the R849 W mutant receptor showed that this mutation causes a 6- to 10-fold increase in autophosphorylation of the receptor.[21] So far, 8 hyperphosphorylating mutations have been identified, R849 W being the most common with an incidence of 60%.[16,20,22,23] *TIE2* signaling pathway is crucial for angiogenesis and vascular maturation.[4,20] The receptor substitutions affect intracellular signaling thereby altering endothelial migration, vascular sprouting, maturation, and stability.[16,20] Because VMCMs are localized, but caused by an inherited predisposition, modifying factors must exist. The authors hypothesized that this could be a somatic second-hit mutation in the same gene.[21] In one resected VMCM, the authors identified a somatic second hit in the normal allele of *TIE2,* in addition to the inherited *TIE2* mutation.[16] This finding is analogous to the Knudson's double-hit hypothesis for retinoblastoma[24] and suggests that the inherited form of venous malformation needs a somatic alteration to eliminate the protective wild-type *TIE2* allele before the inherited mutation can induce the development of a VMCM lesion (**Fig. 1**).[16]

Encouraged by this finding, the authors decided to look for implication of somatic TIE2 mutations in sporadic VMs, and identified them in 50% of lesions.[4] These mutations differ somewhat from the inherited ones that cause VMCM. The most common one, L914F, accounts for 85% of lesions, and has not been observed as an inherited mutation, suggesting that it causes lethality, when germline.[4,16] The other 20% are caused by pairs of double mutations that always occur together on the same allele.[4] All the mutations cause hyperphosphorylation of the TIE2 receptor and render *TIE2* an interesting target for future therapies.[4,16]

Glomuvenous malformations clinically resemble VMs (**Fig. 2**A,B,C).[17] Most of them (at least 70%) are inherited as an autosomal dominant disorder.[3,17,25–29] Like most inherited lesions, they are multifocal, small, and new lesions can occur with time. In contrast to VMCMs, GVMs are more bluish purple, hyperkeratotic, and with a cobblestone appearance.[17] Classically, GVMs involve skin and subcutis, and rarely mucosa. Extremities are often affected. Pain on palpation is pathognomonic.[3,17] No sex preponderance is noted.

Similar to VMCM, there is a large interfamilial and intrafamilial variability in size, color, and location of lesions, suggesting that the inherited mutation alone is not sufficient for the phenotype to occur. This clinical variability may hinder diagnosis because some patients may have a single, small lesion that does not suggest GVM to the physician (see **Fig. 2**B). Moreover, another family member may have a large lesion covering a whole extremity or, for example, the thorax, which the patient does not necessarily think of being expression of the same disorder as the tiny blue spot of a relative. Thus, when physicians ask about familial history of the disease, the patients' likely answer is, "none." In addition, GVM can also present as a large, plaquelike lesion in childhood, reminiscent of a capillary malformation.[25] Thus, identification of GVM, as all other rare inherited vascular anomalies, needs detailed questioning of family history and evaluation of lesions.

Histologically, GVMs have a variable number of pathognomonic, abnormally differentiated vascular smooth muscle cells, known as *glomus cells*.[26,28] GVM is linked to 1p21-22 and is caused by loss of function of glomulin (see **Table 1**).[27,29] Interestingly, 75% of patients with GVM can be genetically diagnosed by screening 1 of the 8 common glomulin mutations.[27–29] Similar to VMCM, a somatic second-hit mutation has been identified in a GVM tissue of a patient, who also carried an inherited glomulin mutation.[21] Therefore, GVM follows paradominant transmission, and a complete localized loss of glomulin needs to occur for GVMs to develop.[16,20,21]

Little is known about glomulin function. *Glomulin* (FAP68) seems to alter vascular smooth muscle cell phenotype, probably via the transforming growth factor beta (TGFβ) or hepatocyte growth factor signaling pathways, as glomulin has been demonstrated to bind the HGF receptor and one of the TGFβ receptor binding proteins.[30,31] In the

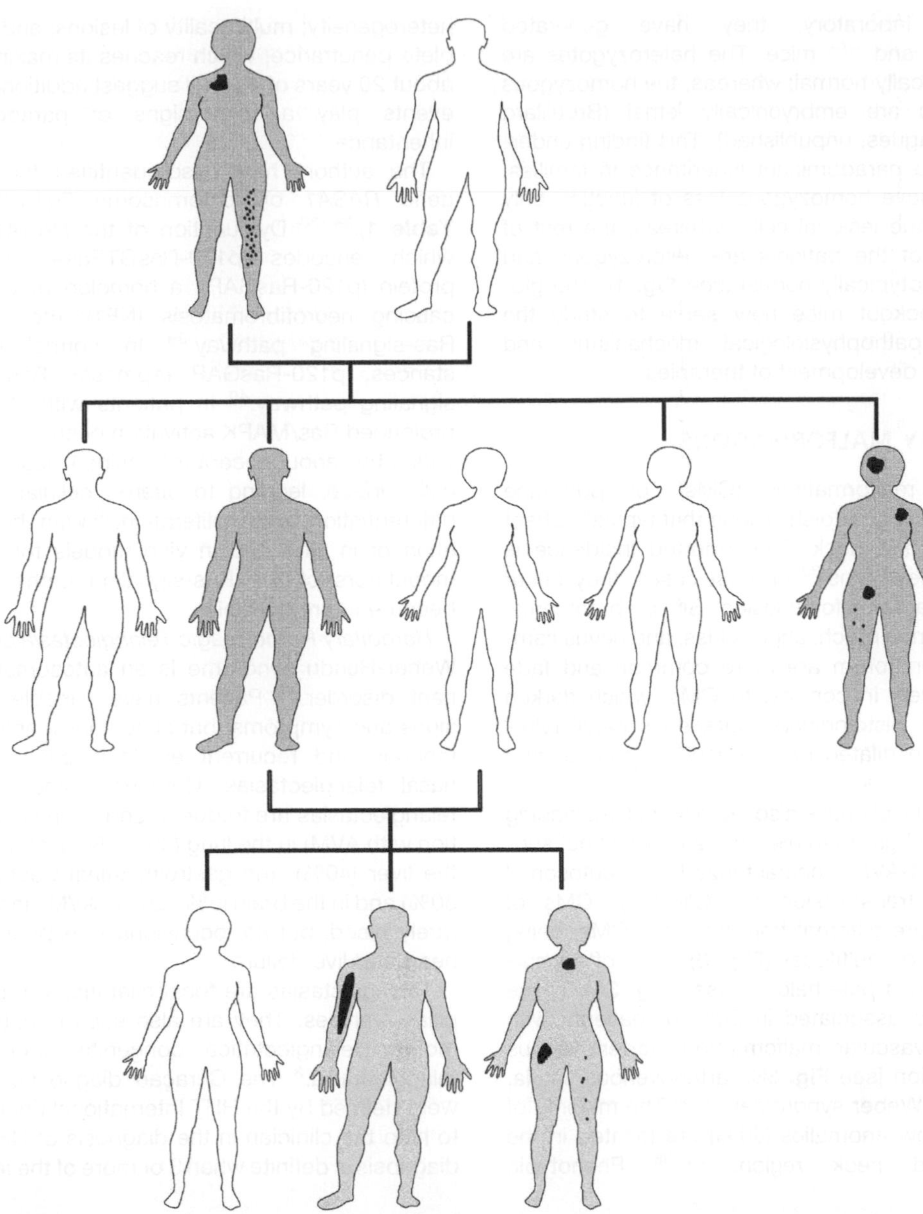

Fig. 1. Scheme of paradominant inheritance. White individual signifies no mutation, unaffected; gray individual signifies carrier of an inherited mutation that predisposes to lesions; irregular black spots of different size and form signifies localized vascular anomalies caused by somatic second-hit mutations in the same gene.

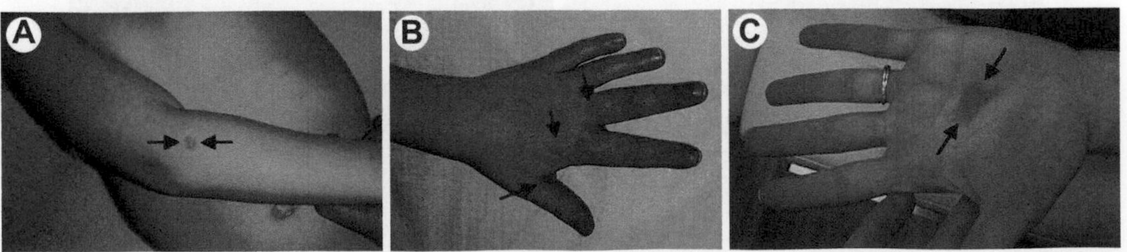

Fig. 2. Clinical variability of CM-AVM within the same family. (*A*) a CM with a white halo on the arm, (*B*) an AVM of the hand of the same patient, and (*C*) a CM without a halo on the palm of the mother (*arrows*).

authors' laboratory, they have generated glomulin$^{\pm}$ and $^{-/-}$ mice. The heterozygotes are phenotypically normal; whereas, the homozygous knockouts are embryonically lethal (Brouillard and colleagues, unpublished). This finding underscores the paradominant inheritance in families. Patients have homozygous loss of function only locally in the lesional cells; whereas, the rest of the cells of the patients are heterozygous and thus phenotypically normal (see **Fig. 1**). The glomulin knockout mice now serve to study the detailed pathophysiological mechanisms and eventually development of therapies.

CAPILLARY MALFORMATIONS

Capillary malformations (CMs), or port-wine stains, are flat, reddish lesions that typically affect the head and neck. The reported incidence is 0.3% of newborns.[32] In most cases, they occur as a sporadic unifocal lesion. Similar birthmarks, called salmon patch, angel's kiss, and nevus flammeus neonatorum are more common and fade progressively in contrast to CMs, which darken with age.[3] Histologically, cutaneous capillarylike vessels are dilated or increased in number and size.[33]

Inherited CMs have also been identified, leading the authors' group to discover a new distinct subentity: CM-AVM, characterized by autosomal dominant transmission.[34,35] Clinically, CMs of CM-AVM are different from common CMs, being smaller and multifocal (**Fig. 3**), and often surrounded by a pale halo[35–37](see **Fig. 3**A). These lesions are associated in 30% of patients with fast-flow vascular malformations (arteriovenous malformation [see **Fig. 3**B], arteriovenous fistula, or Parkes Weber syndrome).[35–38] The majority of the fast-flow anomalies (80%) are located in the head and neck region.[16,35–38] Phenotypic heterogeneity; multifocality of lesions; and incomplete penetrance, which reaches its maximum by about 20 years of age, all suggest additional, local events play a role: signs of paradominant inheritance.

The authors have also identified the causal gene *RASA1* on chromosome 5q13-22 (see **Table 1**).[34–38] Dysfunction of the *RASA1* gene, which encodes p120-RasGTPase activating protein (p120-RasGAP), a homolog of the gene causing neurofibromatosis (NF1), modifies the Ras-signaling pathway.[39] In normal circumstances, p120-RasGAP represses Ras/MAPK-signaling pathway.[40] In patients with CM-AVM, prolonged Ras/MAPK activation occurs after activation by various receptor tyrosine kinases on the cell surface, leading to altered cellular growth, differentiation, and proliferation.[40] With the generation of in vitro and in vivo models for testing, modulators of the Ras-signaling pathway may become future therapies.

Hereditary Hemorrhagic Telangiectasia or Osler-Weber-Rendu syndrome is an autosomal dominant disorder.[41] Patients have variable clinical signs and symptoms, but almost invariably spontaneous and recurrent epistaxis secondary to nasal telangiectasias. Cutaneous and mucosal telangiectasias are frequent, and seen in association with AVM) in the lung (30%–50% of patients), the liver (40%), the gastrointestinal tract (15%–30%) and in the brain (5%–20%). AVMs in the liver rarely bleed, but are occasionally responsible for heart and liver failure.

Telangiectasias are focal dilatations of postcapillary venules. They are also seen in cutis marmorata telangiectatica congenita, and ataxia telangiectasia.[3] The Curaçao diagnostic criteria were defined by the HHT International Foundation to help the clinician in the diagnosis of HHT. The diagnosis is definite when 3 or more of the features

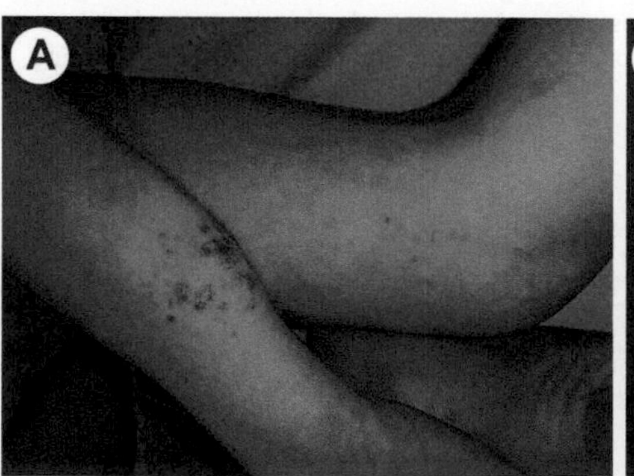

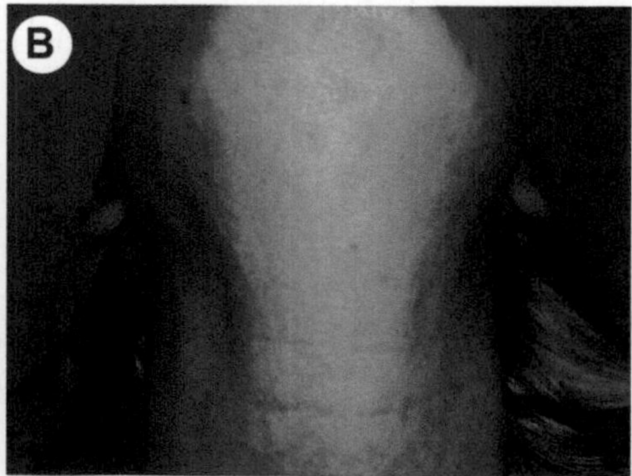

Fig. 3. Clinical variability of GVM within the same family. (*A*) A painful GVM of the arm and the leg of a boy, and (*B*) a small asymptomatic GVM on the neck of the mother.

are present, possible or suspected when 2 findings are present, and unlikely with fewer than 2 findings. Genetic diagnostic tests can also be helpful.[41] Mutations in 3 genes have been identified: *endoglin* (*ENG*) (HHT1 on 9q33-34);[42–44] *activin receptor-like kinase1* (*ACVRL1*) (HHT2 on 12q11-14);[45,46] and *SMAD4*, localized on chromosome 5 (JPHT; HHT associated with juvenile polyposis) (see **Table 1**).[47,48] Two additional chromosomal loci are known, but the genes have not yet been identified (HHT3 on 5q and HHT4 on 7p14).[41] More than 150 *ENG* mutations and 120 *ACVRL1* mutations have been identified.[3,41] A useful genotype-phenotype correlation exists. HHT1 is more commonly associated with AVMs in the lung; whereas, patients with HHT2 likely have hepatic AVMs.[41] However, because genes for HHT3 and HHT4 have not yet been identified, a negative genetic result does not rule out the diagnosis. Moreover, paradominant inheritance, in which the subject inherits a germline mutation from an affected parent, which becomes significant only when a second mutation affects the other allele, may also apply to the multifocal, localized telangiectasias and fast-flow lesions of HHT (**Fig. 1**).

Angioma Serpiginosum

Angioma serpiginosum is a progressive, patchy CM[49] characterized by dilated capillaries following Blaschko's lines, associated with mild nail and hair dystrophy.[50] Typical lesions begin in childhood, involve extremities, and are often asymmetric.[51] Clinically, only incomplete blanching is obtained on pressure. In several cases, papillomatosis of the esophagus is found.[50] This rare congenital cutaneous disorder results from X-linked dominant transmission, localized on Xp11.3-Xq12 (see **Table 1**).[50] This locus includes 5 genes, *PORCN* being one of them.[52] Dysfunction in this gene causes Goltz-Gorlin syndrome, characterized by focal dermal hypoplasia, esophageal papillomas, and eye and skeletal anomalies.[53] The resemblance suggests that angioma serpiginosum, in association with papillomatosis of esophagus, is a variant of Goltz-Gorlin syndrome.

Cerebral Cavernous Malformation

Cerebral cavernous malformations or cerebral capillary malformations involve the brain, the eye, and the spinal cord.[54] Histologically, CCMs are composed of capillarylike vessels and large saccular vessels with fibrotic walls.[55] Clinically, patients can be asymptomatic or complain about headaches and epilepsy, and cerebral bleeding can occur.[54,55] CCMs can be inherited as an autosomal dominant disorder (20% of patients), although the majority are sporadic.[55] Four chromosomal loci have been identified[55]: CCM1 (7q21-q22), with mutations in *KRIT-1* (KREV1 interaction trapped 1);[56–58] CCM2 (7p15-p13), with mutations in *malcavernin*;[59,60] and CCM3 (3q25.2-27), with mutations in *PDCD10* (see **Table 1**).[61] A fourth gene has been suggested to exist on the same 3q26.3-27.2 locus (CCM4).[62] CCM1 represents almost 40% of inherited cerebral cavernous malformations and more than 100 mutations have been identified in *KRIT-1*.[55,63] The vast majority of all CCM mutations lead to a premature termination codon, suggesting loss of function of the respective protein. Only 4 missense mutations have been reported in CCM1.[63]

Cutaneous vascular malformations are seen in 9% of patients with CCM.[64–67] There are 3 distinct phenotypes: hyperkeratotic cutaneous capillary-venous malformation (HCCVM)(39%), capillary malformation (34%), and venous malformation (21%).[64–67] The high frequency of KRIT1 mutations (87%) in patients with CCM with cutaneous vascular malformations suggests that *KRIT1* has an important function also in cutaneous angiogenesis.[65–67] No HCCVM, CM, or VM were detected in patients with CCM2 mutation; whereas, VMs were sometimes observed in patients with both CCM1 and CCM3.[65–67] Therefore, the presence of a cutaneous vascular malformation may be a clue for detecting CCMs, with the specific molecular diagnosis.

CCMs, like VMCMs and GVMs, are likely caused by paradominant inheritance. Somatic second hits have been identified in a small number of lesions for the 3 CCM genes,[68–70] suggesting localized, complete loss of function of one of the CCM proteins to take place. Thus, the authors' hypothesis that the clinical variability in patients with inherited vascular malformations may be explained by Knudson's double-hit theory[22] seems to be true for several of them. The difficulty encountered in the identification of the second hits in CCM is likely caused by high tissular heterogeneity, as observed for sporadic venous malformations.[4]

In vitro and in vivo studies have helped to unravel the function of CCM proteins. CCM1 is expressed in astrocytes, neurons, epithelial, and endothelial cells;[71] whereas, CCM2 is expressed in mesenchymal and parenchymal vessels.[72] CCM proteins act as a scaffold and function in a complex.[72–76] *KRIT1* also interacts with the β1 integrin cytoplasmic domain associated protein 1 (ICAP-1α), which is implicated in the regulation of cell adhesion and migration.[72] In return, ICAP-1α is able to sequester *KRIT1* into the nucleus.[72] In contrast, the phosphotyrosine-binding domain of CCM2 is able to sequester *KRIT1* in the cytoplasm.[73] Thus, ICAP-1α and CCM2 are implied in the same signaling pathway and both are able to sequester KRIT1.[55,76]

KRIT $1^{-/-}$ embryos die during gestation because of defective vascular development.[77] Conditional endothelial deletion of CCM2 affects angiogenesis leading to massive heart and blood vessel defects, and to embryonic death.[73] In contrast, neuroglial-specific deletion does not lead to cerebrovascular defects.[73] This underscores the endothelial function of the CCM proteins, and the paradominant effect in CCM patients. CCM2 is the human ortholog of OSM, a osmosensing scaffold for MEKK3.[75] OSM interacts with the p38 mitogen activated kinase pathway (p38MAPK) in response to osmolarity stress, which is a crucial mediator of cellular survival. As CCM3 interacts with CCM1 and CCM2, a multifaceted signaling complex is constituted by the 3 CCM proteins and seems to be involved in several cellular functions, including homeostasis of cell-cell junctions and cytoskeletal remodeling.[76]

Whitehead and Li suggested statins for treatment of CCMs to stabilize blood vessels. They based their hypothesis on the observation that without CCM2, vascular endothelium is malformed and leads to dilated, leaky blood vessels. This malformation coincides with increased Rho activity, which regulates endothelial formation. Because simvastatin injection is an inhibitor of Rho activity, it may become a potential treatment for CCMs.[78]

Lymphatic Malformations

Lymphatic malformations (LMs) are also focal lesions. Genetic approach has not been possible, because LMs occur sporadically, with no evidence for inheritance. This sporadic occurrence suggests that the potential genetic causes may be somatic events, which when in germline, are incompatible with life.[3] The etiology remains unknown. In contrast, genetic analysis of inherited primary lymphedema has unraveled key regulators and molecular pathways involved in lymphangiogenesis.[3,16]

LYMPHEDEMA

Lymphedema is a defect of lymphatic drainage, characterized by the accumulation of lymphatic fluid in the interstitial space, classically involving the lower extremities. It is divided into primary (from an unknown cause) and secondary (from a known cause, such as infection and surgery). Primary lymphedema is further subdivided according to age at onset, into congenital, pubertal, and late-onset lymphedema.[79] Five aberrant genes have been identified (see **Table 1**).[16,80–84]

Familial congenital lymphedema, Nonne-Milroy syndrome, is inherited as an autosomal dominant trait and maps on 5q34-35 (see **Table 1**). It is caused by dominant missense mutations in the tyrosine kinase domain of the vascular endothelial growth factor receptor 3 (VEGFR3; also known as FLT-4), a crucial regulator of lymphatic development.[2,80] Lymphedema in this syndrome is principally present on lower extremities, from toes upwards to the hips. Most patients have lymphedema limited below the knees and less than 30% have associated hydrocele, large caliber leg veins (23%), cellulitis (20%), curled toenails (10%), or papillomatosis (10%).[85] This congenital lymphedema seems to evolve slowly.

Interestingly, de novo dominant VEGFR3 mutations have also been identified in patients with congenital lymphedema without family history.[86,87] Thus, clinically the diagnostic criteria of Nonne-Milroy syndrome are not fulfilled. Yet, the molecular cause is the same, demonstrating how molecular classification can help in identifying patients with the same etiopathogenic underpinning, even if clinical criteria are different. Furthermore, dominant VEGFR3 mutations have been identified in patients with sporadic *hydrops fetalis*/generalized fetal edema.[87] Although associated with a high risk of mortality, the presence of a VEGFR3 mutation appears to be a good sign for prognosis, because most of the few reported to date had in utero resorption of the lymphedema, leading to a limited lower extremity lymphedema present at birth.[87]

In addition to Nonne-Milroy syndrome, with dominant transmission, a specific VEGFR3 amino-acid mutation has been found in a family with recessive inheritance of lymphedema.[88] Consanguinity between the healthy parents of the affected child was the clue to the discovery. The large clinical variability in patients with proven *VEGFR3* mutations illustrates how important it is for the clinician to be alert of various signs that may lead to the precise, molecular diagnosis, which will likely be the basis for therapeutic choices in the future.

Puberty-onset lymphedema, Meige's disease, becomes evident around puberty and represents 80% of primary lymphedema. One-third of the patients have a familial predisposition.[89] Genetic analysis revealed mutations in the FOXC2 gene, located on chromosome 16q24.3 (see **Table 1**).[81] These mutations cause lymphedema often associated with distichiasis (presence of an extra row of eyelashes), and sometimes with ptosis, yellow nails, syndactyly, cleft palate, and cardiac septal defects.[3,81]

FOXC2, a transcription factor, has several functions. One of them is to regulate angiogenesis by controlling the expression of target genes, such as Ang-2,[90] integrin β 3,[91] D114, and Hey-2, via interaction with VEGF-Notch signaling pathway in endothelial cells.[92] FOXC2 also inhibits secretion of PDGFβ, which is overproduced by lymphatic collecting ducts in Meige's disease. This overproduction increases vascular smooth muscle cell recruitment, abnormal mural tone, and lymphatic dysfunction.[93]

Hypotrichosis-Lymphedema-Telangiectasia (HLT) is a rare condition characterized by sparse hair, lymphedema, and cutaneous telangiectasias. Both recessive and dominant transmission is possible. This syndrome is caused by mutations in the *SOX18* gene, in 20q13.33 (see **Table 1**).[83] The dominant nonsense mutation is located in the transactivation domain; whereas, the homozygous recessive substitutions are in the DNA-binding domain.[83] Arrival to the diagnosis is not easy because the lack of hair is not evident at birth, the age at onset of lymphedema is variable, and the telangiectasias may be mild and localized.

Hennekam syndrome is another rare form of lymphedema, characterized by extensive peripheral lymphedema with visceral involvement; mental retardation; and unusual flat face, hypertelorism, and broad nasal bridge.[94] Hydrops fetalis can also been seen. This phenotype is severe, causing significant morbidity and mortality. Both autosomal recessive and dominant transmission of the Hennekam syndrome are possible.[84]

Genetic analysis in zebrafish identified the *Ccbe1* gene (Collagen and calcium-binding EGF domain) to be required for lymphangiogenesis.[95] The zebrafish Ccbe1 mutants are devoid of parachordal lymphangioblasts and lymphatic vessels. Zebrafish Ccbe1 is expressed along the migration routes of endothelial cells, suggesting a role in cellular guidance. Patients with Hennekam syndrome have either homozygous or a combination of two different heterozygous recessive mutations in *CCBE1*, localized on 18q21.32 (see **Table 1**).[84,96]

Other rare forms of familial lymphedema include osteoporosis lymphedema anhidrotic ectodermal dysplasia with immunodeficiency (OLEDAID), which becomes evident during childhood and results from a premature termination codon mutation in the NFκB essential modulator (*NEMO*). The gene on Xq28, encodes NEMO, which moderates NFκB activation. So far, only 2 patients have been reported (see **Table 1**).[82]

Another type of *Primary congenital resolving lymphedema* was reported in one Pakistani family. This autosomal dominant form of congenital lymphedema with reduced penetrance maps to 6q16.2-q22.1 (see **Table 1**).[97] Although the gene has not been unraveled, it is clearly a novel regulator of lymphatic function.

Aagenaes Syndrome or Hereditary Lymphedema Cholestasis (HLC) is a recessive disorder that occurs in families with consanguinity (see **Table 1**).[98,99] It typically appears during childhood. Extended lymphedema of the lower extremities is associated with malabsorption, growth retardation, rickets, cholestatic jaundice, and hepatomegaly. Lymphedema may be complicated by infections. The implicated gene is unknown, but mapped to 15q. Like the one for primary congenital resolving lymphedema, it is likely an important regulator of lymphatic development or function.[99]

CONCLUDING REMARKS

Vascular malformations classically present autosomal dominant transmission. However, it is necessary to perform careful clinical questioning of familial history and examination of patients and their parents for detecting this. There is large clinical variation in signs and symptoms, and lesions can be small enough to be overlooked, hindering identification of familial inheritance.[17,21,22,35,36,55,86] Classically, the index patient, the one that seeks medical advice, is the most severely affected, and thus, family members' insignificant lesions are not even thought to be of the same pathology, which is an important reason for patients to deny familial history of their disorder.

Though dominant inheritance by pedigree analysis, the molecular mechanism often seems to involve paradominance. This paradominance means that the inherited mutation is accompanied at various time points of development of the fetus and the child by secondary mutations on the second allele of the same gene in the dividing cells. Such somatic mutations are common; nonhereditary; and lead to localized, complete abolishment of normal gene function. This phenomenon logically explains why inherited vascular malformations are localized, multifocal, of variable size, and increase in number by age.[3,4,22,29,68–70] This discovery has also opened the door for unraveling the causes of the nonhereditary vascular malformations.

The identification of the underlying genetic mutations in different families and disorders are crucial starting points to better understand the pathophysiologic mechanisms that play a role in the development of vascular anomalies. This identification also enables more accurate diagnosis, which in time, will lead to a more precise evaluation of prognosis and development of treatments. Moreover, unraveling the pathophysiological mechanisms of vascular anomalies allows the unraveling of key regulators and pathways implicated in angiogenesis.

ACKNOWLEDGMENTS

The authors thank Liliana Niculescu for expert secretarial assistance.

REFERENCES

1. Brouillard P, Vikkula M. Vascular malformations: localized defects in vascular morphogenesis. Clin Genet 2003;63:340.
2. Lohela M, Bry M, Tammela T, et al. VEGFs and receptors involved in angiogenesis versus lymphangiogenesis. Curr Opin Cell Biol 2009;21:154.
3. Brouillard P, Vikkula M. Genetic causes of vascular malformations. Hum Mol Genet 2007;16(Spec No. 2): R140.
4. Limaye N, Wouters V, Uebelhoer M, et al. Somatic mutations in angiopoietin receptor gene TEK cause solitary and multiple sporadic venous malformations. Nat Genet 2009;41:118.
5. Holmes LB. Chorionic villus sampling and hemangiomas. J Craniofac Surg 2009;1(20 Suppl):675.
6. Pocock B, Boon LM, Vikkula M. Molecular basis of vascular birthmarks. Sem Plast Surg 2006;20:149.
7. Jinnin M, Medici D, Park L, et al. Suppressed NFAT-dependent VEGFR1 expression and constitutive VEGFR2 signaling in infantile hemangioma. Nat Med 2008;14:1236.
8. Bischoff J. Progenitor cells in infantile hemangioma. J Craniofac Surg 2009;20(Suppl 1):695.
9. Boye E, Yu Y, Paranya G, et al. Clonality and altered behavior of endothelial cells from hemangiomas. J Clin Invest 2001;107:745.
10. Yu Y, Flint AF, Mulliken JB, et al. Endothelial progenitor cells in infantile hemangioma. Blood 2004;103: 1373.
11. Yu Y, Fuhr J, Boye E, et al. Mesenchymal stem cells and adipogenesis in hemangioma involution. Stem Cells 2006;24:1605.
12. Khan ZA, Melero-Martin JM, Wu X, et al. Endothelial progenitor cells from infantile hemangioma and umbilical cord blood display unique cellular responses to endostatin. Blood 2006;108:915.
13. Khan ZA, Boscolo E, Picard A, et al. Multipotential stem cells recapitulate human infantile hemangioma in immunodeficient mice. J Clin Invest 2008;118: 2592.
14. North PE, Waner M, Mizeracki A, et al. GLUT1: a newly discovered immunohistochemical marker for juvenile hemangiomas. Hum Pathol 2000;31:11.
15. Frieden IJ, Reese V, Cohen D. PHACE syndrome. The association of posterior fossa brain malformations, hemangiomas, arterial anomalies, coarctation of the aorta and cardiac defects, and eye abnormalities. Arch Dermatol 1996;132:307.
16. Limaye N, Boon LM, Vikkula M. From germline towards somatic mutations in the pathophysiology of vascular anomalies. Hum Mol Genet 2009;18:R65.
17. Boon LM, Mulliken JB, Enjolras O, et al. Glomuvenous malformation (glomangioma) and venous malformation: distinct clinicopathologic and genetic entities. Arch Dermatol 2004;140:971.
18. Dompmartin A, Acher A, Thibon P, et al. Association of localized intravascular coagulopathy with venous malformations. Arch Dermatol 2008;144:873.
19. Dompmartin A, Bailleux F, Thibon P, et al. Elevated D-dimer level is diagnostic for venous malformations. Arch Dermatol 2009;145:1239–44.
20. Wouters V, Limaye N, Uebelhoer M, et al. Hereditary cutaneomucosal venous malformations are caused by TIE2 mutations with widely variable hyper-phosphorylating effects. Eur J Hum Genet 2010; 18(4):414–20.
21. Boon LM, Mulliken JB, Vikkula M, et al. Assignment of a locus for dominantly inherited venous malformations to chromosome 9p. Hum Mol Genet 1994;3: 1583.
22. Vikkula M, Boon LM, Carraway KL 3rd, et al. Vascular dysmorphogenesis caused by an activating mutation in the receptor tyrosine kinase TIE2. Cell 1996;87:1181.
23. Calvert JT, Riney TJ, Kontos CD, et al. Allelic and locus heterogeneity in inherited venous malformations. Hum Mol Genet 1999;8:1279.
24. Knudson AG Jr. Mutation and cancer: statistical study of retinoblastoma. Proc Natl Acad Sci U S A 1971;68:820.
25. Mallory SB, Enjolras O, Boon LM, et al. Congenital plaque-type glomuvenous malformations presenting in childhood. Arch Dermatol 2006;142:892.
26. Goodman TF, Abele DC. Multiple glomus tumors. A clinical and electron microscopic study. Arch Dermatol 1971;103:11.
27. Brouillard P, Enjolras O, Boon LM, et al. Glomulin and glomuvenous malformation. In: Epstein CJ, Erickson RP, Wynshaw-Boris A, editors. Inborn errors of development. 2nd edition. New York: Oxford University Press; 2008. p. 1561.
28. Brouillard P, Boon LM, Mulliken JB, et al. Mutations in a novel factor, glomulin, are responsible for glomuvenous malformations ("glomangiomas"). Am J Hum Genet 2002;70:866.
29. Boon LM, Brouillard P, Irrthum A, et al. A gene for inherited cutaneous venous anomalies ("glomangiomas")

localizes to chromosome 1p21-22. Am J Hum Genet 1999;65:125.

30. Chambraud B, Radanyi C, Camonis JH, et al. FAP48, a new protein that forms specific complexes with both immunophilins FKBP59 and FKBP12. Prevention by the immunosuppressant drugs FK506 and rapamycin. J Biol Chem 1996;271:32923.
31. Grisendi S, Chambraud B, Gout I, et al. Ligand-regulated binding of FAP68 to the hepatocyte growth factor receptor. J Biol Chem 2001;276:46632.
32. Jacobs AH, Walton RG. The incidence of birthmarks in the neonate. Pediatrics 1976;58:218.
33. Mulliken JB, Young AE. Vascular birthmarks: hemangiomas and malformations. Philadelphia: WB Saunders; 1988.
34. Eerola I, Boon LM, Watanabe S, et al. Locus for susceptibility for familial capillary malformation ('port-wine stain') maps to 5q. Eur J Hum Genet 2002;10:375.
35. Eerola I, Boon LM, Mulliken JB, et al. Capillary malformation-arteriovenous malformation, a new clinical and genetic disorder caused by RASA1 mutations. Am J Hum Genet 2003;73:1240.
36. Revencu N, Boon LM, Mulliken JB, et al. Parkes Weber syndrome, vein of Galen aneurysmal malformation, and other fast-flow vascular anomalies are caused by RASA1 mutations. Hum Mutat 2008;29: 959.
37. Boon LM, Mulliken JB, Vikkula M. RASA1: variable phenotype with capillary and arteriovenous malformations. Curr Opin Genet Dev 2005;15:265.
38. Thiex R, Mulliken JB, Revencu N, et al. A novel association between RASA1 mutations and spinal arteriovenous anomalies. Am J Neuroradiol 2010;31: 775–9.
39. Ballester R, Marchuk D, Boguski M, et al. The NF1 locus encodes a protein functionally related to mammalian GAP and yeast IRA proteins. Cell 1990;63:851.
40. Kulkarni SV, Gish G, van der Geer P, et al. Role of p120 Ras-GAP in directed cell movement. J Cell Biol 2000;149:457.
41. Govani FS, Shovlin CL. Hereditary haemorrhagic telangiectasia: a clinical and scientific review. Eur J Hum Genet 2009;17:860.
42. McAllister KA, Grogg KM, Johnson DW, et al. Endoglin, a TGF-beta binding protein of endothelial cells, is the gene for hereditary haemorrhagic telangiectasia type 1. Nat Genet 1994;8:345.
43. Shovlin CL, Hughes JM, Scott J, et al. Characterization of endoglin and identification of novel mutations in hereditary hemorrhagic telangiectasia. Am J Hum Genet 1997;61:68.
44. Cymerman U, Vera S, Karabegovic A, et al. Characterization of 17 novel endoglin mutations associated with hereditary hemorrhagic telangiectasia. Hum Mutat 2003;21:482.
45. Johnson DW, Berg JN, Gallione CJ, et al. A second locus for hereditary hemorrhagic telangiectasia maps to chromosome 12. Genome Res 1995;5:21.
46. Johnson DW, Berg JN, Baldwin MA, et al. Mutations in the activin receptor-like kinase 1 gene in hereditary haemorrhagic telangiectasia type 2. Nat Genet 1996;13:189.
47. Gallione CJ, Repetto GM, Legius E, et al. A combined syndrome of juvenile polyposis and hereditary haemorrhagic telangiectasia associated with mutations in MADH4 (SMAD4). Lancet 2004; 363:852.
48. Cole SG, Begbie ME, Wallace GM, et al. A new locus for hereditary haemorrhagic telangiectasia (HHT3) maps to chromosome 5. J Med Genet 2005;42:577.
49. Vikkula M. Vascular Pathologies: angiogenomics: towards a genetic nosology and understanding of vascular anomalies. Eur J Hum Genet 2007.
50. Blinkenberg EO, Brendehaug A, Sandvik AK, et al. Angioma serpiginosum with oesophageal papillomatosis is an X-linked dominant condition that maps to Xp11.3-Xq12. Eur J Hum Genet 2007;15: 543.
51. Katta R, Wagner A. Angioma serpiginosum with extensive cutaneous involvement. J Am Acad Dermatol 2000;42:384.
52. Houge G, Oeffner F, Grzeschik KH. An Xp11.23 deletion containing PORCN may also cause angioma serpiginosum, a cosmetic skin disease associated with extreme skewing of X-inactivation. Eur J Hum Genet 2008;16:1027.
53. Grzeschik KH, Bornholdt D, Oeffner F, et al. Deficiency of PORCN, a regulator of Wnt signaling, is associated with focal dermal hypoplasia. Nat Genet 2007;39:833.
54. Rigamonti D, Hadley MN, Drayer BP, et al. Cerebral cavernous malformations. Incidence and familial occurrence. N Engl J Med 1988;319:343.
55. Revencu N, Vikkula M. Cerebral cavernous malformation: new molecular and clinical insights. J Med Genet 2006;43:716.
56. Laberge-le Couteulx S, Jung HH, Labauge P, et al. Truncating mutations in CCM1, encoding KRIT1, cause hereditary cavernous angiomas. Nat Genet 1999;23:189.
57. Sahoo T, Johnson EW, Thomas JW, et al. Mutations in the gene encoding KRIT1, a Krev-1/rap1a binding protein, cause cerebral cavernous malformations (CCM1). Hum Mol Genet 1999;8:2325.
58. Serebriiskii I, Estojak J, Sonoda G, et al. Association of Krev-1/rap1a with Krit1, a novel ankyrin repeat-containing protein encoded by a gene mapping to 7q21-22. Oncogene 1997;15:1043.
59. Denier C, Goutagny S, Labauge P, et al. Mutations within the MGC4607 gene cause cerebral cavernous malformations. Am J Hum Genet 2004; 74:326.

60. Liquori CL, Berg MJ, Siegel AM, et al. Mutations in a gene encoding a novel protein containing a phosphotyrosine-binding domain cause type 2 cerebral cavernous malformations. Am J Hum Genet 2003; 73:1459.
61. Bergametti F, Denier C, Labauge P, et al. Mutations within the programmed cell death 10 gene cause cerebral cavernous malformations. Am J Hum Genet 2005;76:42.
62. Liquori CL, Berg MJ, Squitieri F, et al. Low frequency of PDCD10 mutations in a panel of CCM3 probands: potential for a fourth CCM locus. Hum Mutat 2006; 27:118.
63. Riant F, Bergametti F, Ayrignac X, et al. Recent insights into cerebral cavernous malformations: the molecular genetics of CCM. Febs J. 2010;277(5): 1070–5.
64. Labauge P, Enjolras O, Bonerandi JJ, et al. An association between autosomal dominant cerebral cavernomas and a distinctive hyperkeratotic cutaneous vascular malformation in 4 families. Ann Neurol 1999;45:250.
65. Eerola I, Plate KH, Spiegel R, et al. KRIT1 is mutated in hyperkeratotic cutaneous capillary-venous malformation associated with cerebral capillary malformation. Hum Mol Genet 2000;9:1351.
66. Toll A, Parera E, Gimenez-Arnau AM, et al. Cutaneous venous malformations in familial cerebral cavernomatosis caused by KRIT1 gene mutations. Dermatology 2009;218:307.
67. Sirvente J, Enjolras O, Wassef M, et al. Frequency and phenotypes of cutaneous vascular malformations in a consecutive series of 417 patients with familial cerebral cavernous malformations. J Eur Acad Dermatol Venereol 2009;23:1066.
68. Gault J, Shenkar R, Recksiek P, et al. Biallelic somatic and germ line CCM1 truncating mutations in a cerebral cavernous malformation lesion. Stroke 2005;36:872.
69. Akers AL, Johnson E, Steinberg GK, et al. Biallelic somatic and germline mutations in cerebral cavernous malformations (CCMs): evidence for a two-hit mechanism of CCM pathogenesis. Hum Mol Genet 2009;18:919.
70. Pagenstecher A, Stahl S, Sure U, et al. A two-hit mechanism causes cerebral cavernous malformations: complete inactivation of CCM1, CCM2 or CCM3 in affected endothelial cells. Hum Mol Genet 2009;18:911.
71. Denier C, Gasc JM, Chapon F, et al. Krit1/cerebral cavernous malformation 1 mRNA is preferentially expressed in neurons and epithelial cells in embryo and adult. Mech Dev 2002;117:363.
72. Zawistowski JS, Stalheim L, Uhlik MT, et al. CCM1 and CCM2 protein interactions in cell signaling: implications for cerebral cavernous malformations pathogenesis. Hum Mol Genet 2005;14:2521.
73. Boulday G, Blecon A, Petit N, et al. Tissue-specific conditional CCM2 knockout mice establish the essential role of endothelial CCM2 in angiogenesis: implications for human cerebral cavernous malformations. Dis Model Mech 2009;2:168.
74. Plummer NW, Gallione CJ, Srinivasan S, et al. Loss of p53 sensitizes mice with a mutation in Ccm1 (KRIT1) to development of cerebral vascular malformations. Am J Pathol 2004;165:1509.
75. Uhlik MT, Abell AN, Johnson NL, et al. Rac-MEKK3-MKK3 scaffolding for p38 MAPK activation during hyperosmotic shock. Nat Cell Biol 2003;5: 1104.
76. Hilder TL, Malone MH, Bencharit S, et al. Proteomic identification of the cerebral cavernous malformation signaling complex. J Proteome Res 2007;6:4343.
77. Whitehead KJ, Plummer NW, Adams JA, et al. Ccm1 is required for arterial morphogenesis: implications for the etiology of human cavernous malformations. Development 2004;131:1437.
78. Whitehead KJ, Chan AC, Navankasattusas S, et al. The cerebral cavernous malformation signaling pathway promotes vascular integrity via Rho GTPases. Nat Med 2009;15:177.
79. Lazareth I. Classification of lymphedema. Rev Med Interne 2002;23(Suppl 3):375s.
80. Irrthum A, Karkkainen MJ, Devriendt K, et al. Congenital hereditary lymphedema caused by a mutation that inactivates VEGFR3 tyrosine kinase. Am J Hum Genet 2000;67:295.
81. Finegold DN, Kimak MA, Lawrence EC, et al. Truncating mutations in FOXC2 cause multiple lymphedema syndromes. Hum Mol Genet 2001; 10:1185.
82. Doffinger R, Smahi A, Bessia C, et al. X-linked anhidrotic ectodermal dysplasia with immunodeficiency is caused by impaired NF-kappaB signaling. Nat Genet 2001;27:277.
83. Irrthum A, Devriendt K, Chitayat D, et al. Mutations in the transcription factor gene SOX18 underlie recessive and dominant forms of hypotrichosis-lymphedema-telangiectasia. Am J Hum Genet 2003;72: 1470.
84. Alders M, Hogan BM, Gjini E, et al. Mutations in CCBE1 cause generalized lymph vessel dysplasia in humans. Nat Genet 2009.
85. Brice G, Child AH, Evans A, et al. Milroy disease and the VEGFR-3 mutation phenotype. J Med Genet 2005;42:98.
86. Ghalamkarpour A, Morlot S, Raas-Rothschild A, et al. Hereditary lymphedema type I associated with VEGFR3 mutation: the first de novo case and atypical presentations. Clin Genet 2006;70:330.
87. Ghalamkarpour A, Debauche C, Haan E, et al. Sporadic in utero generalized edema caused by mutations in the lymphangiogenic genes VEGFR3 and FOXC2. J Pediatr 2009;155:90.

88. Ghalamkarpour A, Holnthoner W, Saharinen P, et al. Recessive primary congenital lymphoedema caused by a VEGFR3 mutation. J Med Genet 2009;46:399.
89. Dale RF. The inheritance of primary lymphoedema. J Med Genet 1985;22:274.
90. Xue Y, Cao R, Nilsson D, et al. FOXC2 controls Ang-2 expression and modulates angiogenesis, vascular patterning, remodeling, and functions in adipose tissue. Proc Natl Acad Sci U S A 2008;105:10167.
91. Hayashi H, Sano H, Seo S, et al. The Foxc2 transcription factor regulates angiogenesis via induction of integrin beta3 expression. J Biol Chem 2008;283: 23791.
92. Hayashi H, Kume T. Foxc transcription factors directly regulate Dll4 and Hey2 expression by interacting with the VEGF-Notch signaling pathways in endothelial cells. PLoS One 2008;3:e2401.
93. Petrova TV, Karpanen T, Norrmen C, et al. Defective valves and abnormal mural cell recruitment underlie lymphatic vascular failure in lymphedema distichiasis. Nat Med 2004;10:974.
94. Hennekam RC, Geerdink RA, Hamel BC, et al. Autosomal recessive intestinal lymphangiectasia and lymphedema, with facial anomalies and mental retardation. Am J Med Genet 1989;34: 593.
95. Hogan BM, Bos FL, Bussmann J, et al. Ccbe1 is required for embryonic lymphangiogenesis and venous sprouting. Nat Genet 2009;41:396.
96. Connell F, Kalidas K, Ostergaard P, et al. Linkage and sequence analysis indicate that CCBE1 is mutated in recessively inherited generalised lymphatic dysplasia. Hum Genet 127:231
97. Malik S, Grzeschik KH. Congenital, low penetrance lymphedema of lower limbs maps to chromosome 6q16.2-q22.1 in an inbred Pakistani family. Hum Genet 2008;123:197.
98. Sigstad H, Aagenaes O, Bjorn-Hansen RW, et al. Primary lymphoedema combined with hereditary recurrent intrahepatic cholestasis. Acta Med Scand 1970;188:213.
99. Bull LN, Roche E, Song EJ, et al. Mapping of the locus for cholestasis-lymphedema syndrome (Aagenaes syndrome) to a 6.6-cM interval on chromosome 15q. Am J Hum Genet 2000;67: 994.

Diagnostic Imaging of Vascular Anomalies

Ryan Arnold, MD[a], Gulraiz Chaudry, MB, ChB[a,b,*]

KEYWORDS

- Vascular anomaly • Vascular malformation • Imaging
- Radiology

Medical imaging has become critically important in the diagnosis and treatment planning of vascular anomalies. The classification of lesions into fast-flow and slow-flow categories, the identification of a soft tissue mass, and the determination of the extent of the lesions are all facilitated by the use of magnetic resonance imaging (MRI), ultrasonography, catheter angiography, and other imaging studies.[1–3] Ultrasonography is typically the first-line imaging study for the evaluation of vascular anomalies in children because sedation is not required. MRI may be indicated for diagnostic confirmation or to better define the anatomy of the lesion. Computed tomography (CT) gives superior resolution for osseous lesions.

VASCULAR TUMORS

Infantile Hemangioma

Infantile hemangiomas are benign tumors composed of endothelial cells. These lesions follow a predictable clinical course of proliferation in infancy followed by involution, usually within the first 5 to 7 years of life. Most cases do not require imaging. If clinical features are atypical or the anatomic extent of the lesion must be determined, ultrasonography and MRI can be of use.

Typical ultrasonographic appearance of an infantile hemangioma, both in the proliferating stage as well as the involuting stage, is a well-circumscribed hypervascular mass showing low-resistance arterial waveforms (**Fig. 1**). Most hemangiomas are hypoechoic, although up to 18% have been reported to be hyperechoic.[4] Hemangioma can be differentiated from arteriovenous malformations (AVMs) by the presence of solid parenchymal tissue.

Proliferating infantile hemangiomas are lobulated hypervascular masses. On MRI studies, the lesions are isointense to muscle on T1-weighted sequences and hyperintense on T2-weighted sequences. High-flow central and peripheral vessels, seen as flow voids, are evident on T2-weighted sequences.[5] After contrast administration, these masses enhance intensely and diffusely (**Fig. 2**). In contrast to AVMs, arteriovenous shunting is not typically seen in infantile hemangioma.[6]

During involution, infantile hemangiomas become more heterogeneous in appearance. MRI of involuting infantile hemangiomas demonstrates regions of fibrofatty deposition, manifested by areas of increased signal on T1-weighted sequences. Contrast enhancement diminishes and becomes inhomogeneous.[6]

Rapidly Involuting Congenital Hemangioma and Noninvoluting Congenital Hemangioma

Congenital hemangiomas are tumors that have reached their maximal size at birth. Two variant forms of congenital hemangioma have been described: rapidly involuting congenital hemangioma (RICH) and noninvoluting congenital hemangioma (NICH). These lesions are distinguishable from infantile hemangioma by their clinical course, as described by their names.

Disclosures: None.
[a] Division of Vascular and Interventional Radiology and Vascular Anomalies Center, Children's Hospital Boston and Harvard Medical School, 300 Longwood Avenue, Boston, MA 02115, USA
[b] Department of Radiology, Harvard Medical School, Boston, MA, USA
* Corresponding author.
E-mail address: gulraiz.chaudry@childrens.harvard.edu

Clin Plastic Surg 38 (2011) 21–29
doi:10.1016/j.cps.2010.08.014
0094-1298/11/$ – see front matter

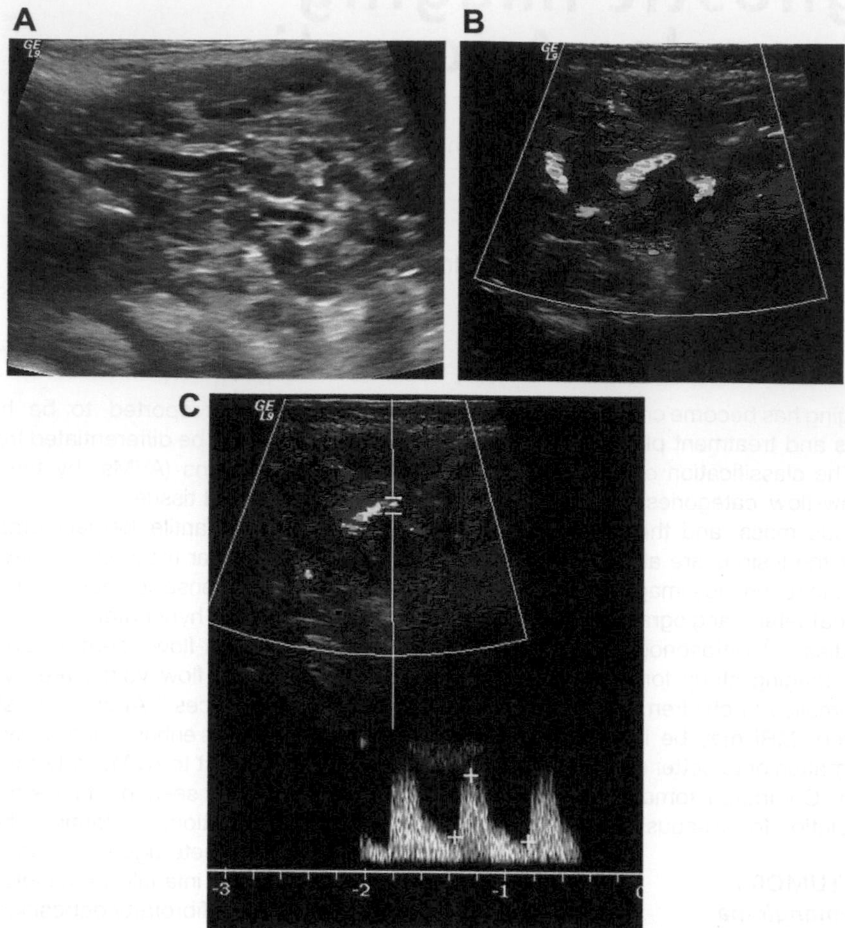

Fig. 1. Ultrasonography in a 7-month-old girl with a parotid infantile hemangioma. (*A*) Two-dimensional image demonstrates a well-defined mass with multiple large internal vessels. (*B*) Color Doppler image shows the marked vascularity of the mass. (*C*) Spectral Doppler trace obtained from an intralesional vessel confirms fast flow.

Unfortunately, these lesions cannot be reliably differentiated from common infantile hemangiomas based on imaging alone. However, some imaging features may be suggestive of a specific lesion. On ultrasonography, the useful differentiating factors are the presence of more visible vessels in congenital hemangiomas in comparison to infantile hemangioma, as well as the presence of intravascular thrombi, calcifications, vascular aneurysms, and arteriovenous shunting (**Fig. 3**).[7,8] RICH and NICH are less likely to be well defined than infantile hemangioma on MRI (**Fig. 4**).[7]

Kaposiform Hemangioendothelioma

Kaposiform hemangioendothelioma (KHE) is a rare vascular neoplasm with locally aggressive characteristics but without metastatic potential. MRI typically shows an ill-defined soft tissue mass that is hypo- or isointense on T1-weighted imaging and hyperintense on T2-weighted imaging. On administration of contrast, there is intense but heterogeneous enhancement (**Fig. 5**). Subcutaneous fat stranding is an important feature that helps differentiate KHE from other benign fast-flow vascular masses. Prominent vascular channels, evidenced by flow voids, are usually present on MRI studies.[9,10]

VASCULAR MALFORMATIONS

Lymphatic Malformation

Lymphatic malformations (LMs) are congenital malformations resulting from abnormal development of the lymphatic channels. The lesions may be classified as macrocystic, microcystic, or combined. On ultrasonography, macrocystic LM appears as a unilocular or mutilocular cystic lesion, usually with thin septations. Doppler imaging often demonstrates vascular channels within the septations.[8] MRI of macrocystic LM

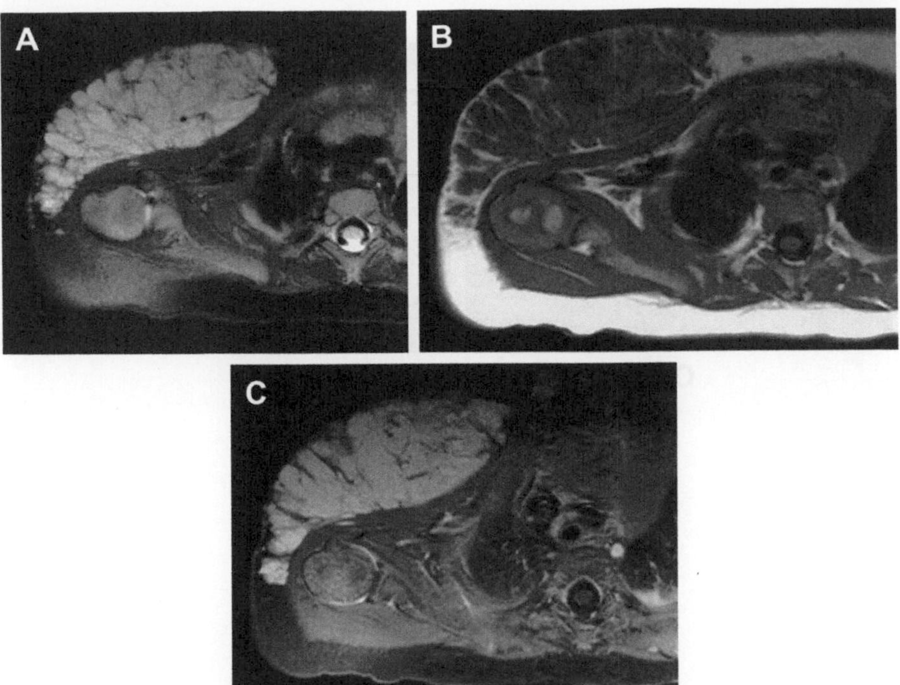

Fig. 2. MRI in a 6-month-old girl with infantile hemangioma of the right anterior chest wall and supraclavicular region. (*A*) T1 axial image shows well-defined low-signal mass with intralesional flow voids. (*B*) T2 axial image. The lesion is uniformly hyperintense on fluid sensitive sequences. (*C*) T1 axial postcontrast image. There is avid homogeneous enhancement of the entire lesion.

shows clearly defined cysts that are hypointense on T1-weighted imaging and hyperintense on T2-weighted imaging. Fluid-fluid levels within the cysts may be present. The septa may enhance, creating a "rings and arcs" appearance (**Fig. 6**). No flow voids or phleboliths are expected within the cysts.[11]

Depending on the size of the cysts, microcystic lesions may appear as ill-defined hyperechoic masses on ultrasonography.[8] Likewise, on MRI, microcystic LMs can appear as solid lesions that are generally hypointense on T1 sequences and hyperintense on T2 sequences. There is minimal enhancement on administration of contrast (**Fig. 7**). Differentiation from soft tissue masses can be difficult.[11] Categorization of LMs as slow-flow lesions and analysis of the extent of the lesions are two important tasks when imaging LMs.[12]

Venous Malformation

Venous malformations (VMs) are congenital slow-flow malformations that are present at birth and typically grow proportionally with the child. VM may take 2 forms: the most common form (cavitary) is a spongy mass of abnormal venous channels containing stagnant blood and the ectatic or dysplastic form presents as multiple irregular varicose veins.[6,8] A combination of the 2 forms can be seen. When VM occurs in an extremity, undergrowth or overgrowth of the affected limb is possible.

Ultrasonography of VM typically shows a well-defined spongelike collection of vessels. Blood can be seen flowing into the cavities, especially after applying and releasing manual compression. Other features include phlebectasia, thickening of subcutaneous tissues, and the presence of phleboliths.[4,8]

MRI studies of VM show multilocular, lobulated, septated masses that are hypo- or isointense to muscle on T1 sequences and hyperintense on T2 sequences. These lesions often infiltrate into adjacent organs, nerves, tendons, muscles, and joints.[6] Slow-flow lesions can be confirmed with gradient-recalled echo imaging, and delayed postcontrast imaging may be used to show central enhancement (**Fig. 8**).[13] Other important characteristics include the presence of phleboliths, best appreciated as focal low-signal areas on gradient-recalled echo

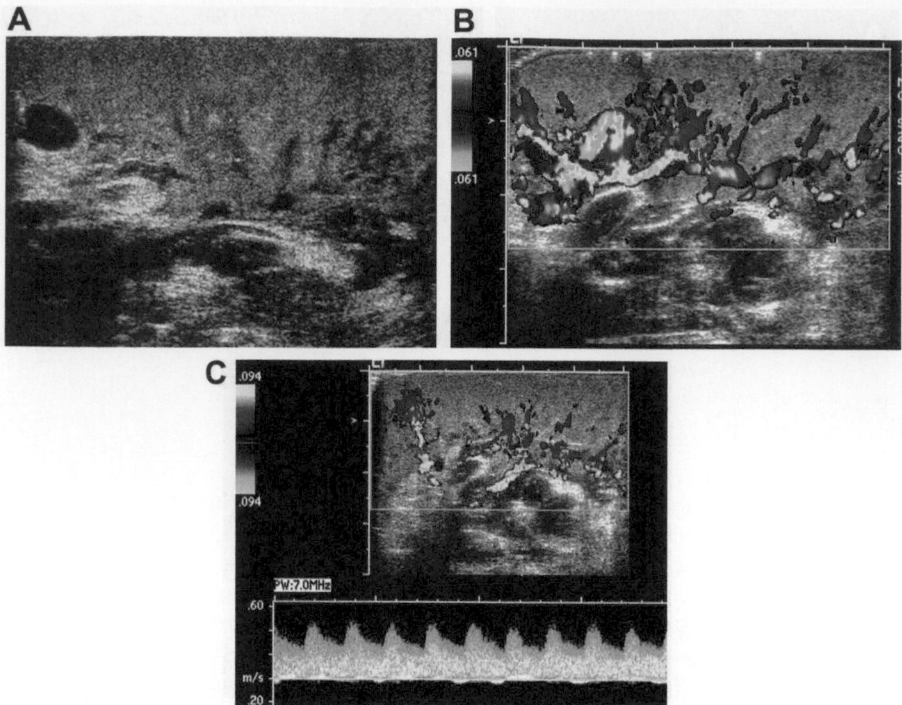

Fig. 3. Ultrasonography of a RICH of the right thigh in a 5-day-old boy. (*A*) Two-dimensional image shows echogenic subcutaneous lesion with prominent vessels and poorly defined borders. (*B*) Color Doppler image. The entire mass is markedly vascular with tortuosity of some intralesional vessels. (*C*) Spectral Doppler trace confirming pulsatile fast flow.

sequences, and the presence of an anomalous venous drainage system.[11] VMs are also more likely than LMs to primarily involve muscle.

Arteriovenous Malformation

AVMs are rare fast-flow lesions that result from dysplastic arterial and venous development, with the absence of a normal intervening capillary bed. Although growth of the lesion is generally proportional to that of the child, AVMs may rapidly enlarge during puberty or after trauma.

On ultrasonography, AVM is a poorly defined hypervascular lesion without a soft tissue mass. Gray-scale imaging is often normal. Multiple tortuous feeding arteries showing increased diastolic flow are best seen with Doppler, power, and spectral imaging. The draining veins are

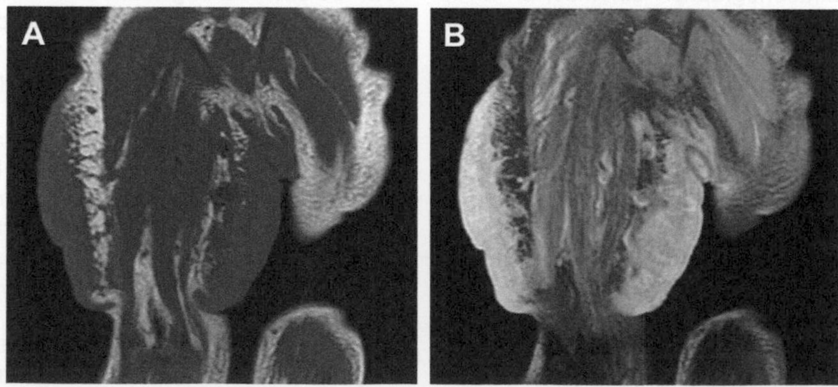

Fig. 4. MRI of a RICH. (*A*) Coronal T1 image. Low-signal subcutaneous lesion is seen with poorly defined borders. (*B*) Coronal T1 postcontrast image. Intense uniform enhancement is seen with stranding of the surrounding fat.

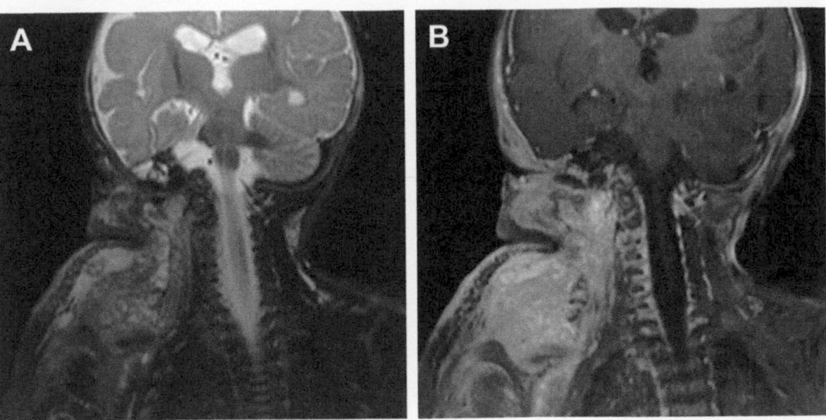

Fig. 5. MRI of a KHE involving the neck, right shoulder, and anterior chest wall in a 4-month-old girl. (*A*) Coronal T2 image. Heterogeneous hyperintensity is seen with involvement of multiple tissue planes. (*B*) Coronal T1 post-contrast image. Avid but heterogeneous enhancement is seen, with evidence of peripheral fat stranding.

enlarged and demonstrate pulsatile high-velocity blood flow.[4,8]

MRI can show the feeding and draining vessels connected by enlarged central channels. Signal voids can be identified on most standard sequences (**Fig. 9**A). Although no soft tissue mass is seen, edema and abnormal enhancement may be present in the surrounding tissues. AVM may result in overlying skin thickening and underlying bony lytic changes.[6,11] Magnetic resonance

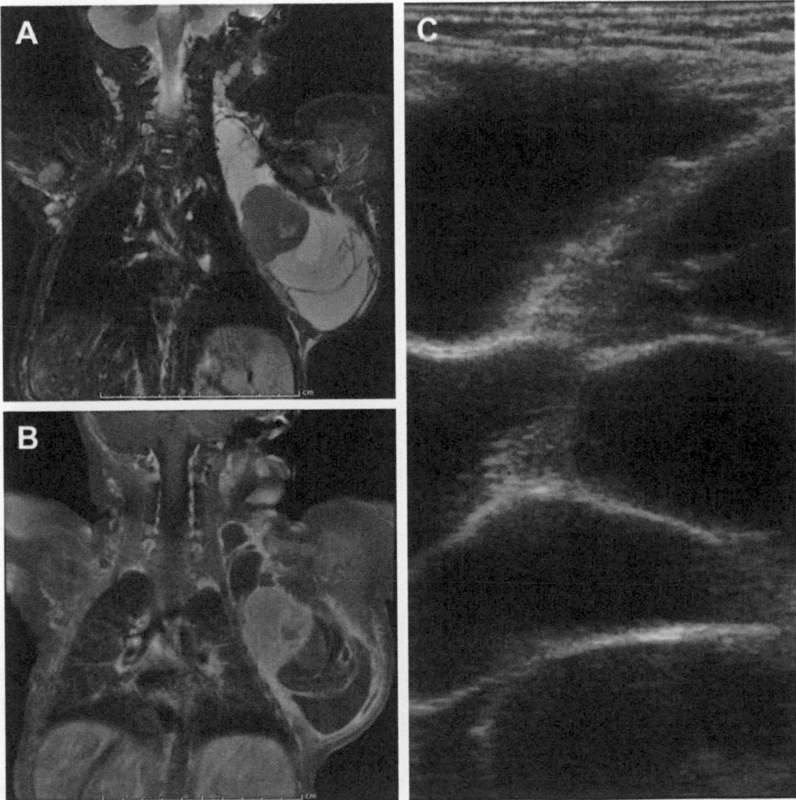

Fig. 6. A 4-month-old girl with a macrocystic LM of the left axilla, lateral chest wall, and neck. (*A*) Coronal T2 MRI. An almost entirely macrocystic lesion is seen. The focal area of low signal corresponds to prior hemorrhage within a macrocyst. (*B*) Coronal T1 postcontrast MRI. Peripheral and septal enhancement is noted. (*C*) Ultrasonography demonstrates the anechoic macrocysts with echogenic intervening septa.

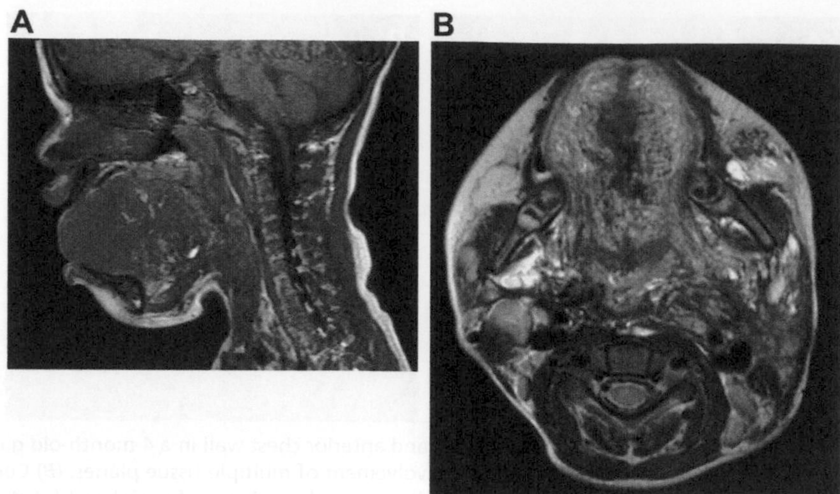

Fig. 7. MRI in a 3-year-old boy with microcystic LM of the tongue and floor of the mouth. (*A*) T1 sagittal image. A grossly enlarged tongue is seen occupying the oral cavity and oropharynx. (*B*) T2 axial image. Heterogeneous high signal is seen throughout the tongue, consistent with microcystic disease.

angiography demonstrates the feeding arterial branches and shows early enhancement of the draining veins.[8]

Catheter angiography of AVM typically shows one or more feeding arteries supplying a nidus formed by entangled vascular loops interconnected by small venules. Several large draining veins are usually seen (see **Fig. 9**B). Although catheter angiography is superior to magnetic resonance angiography in demonstrating the vascular details of AVM, given the invasive nature, it should be reserved as an adjunct to endovascular embolotherapy.[14]

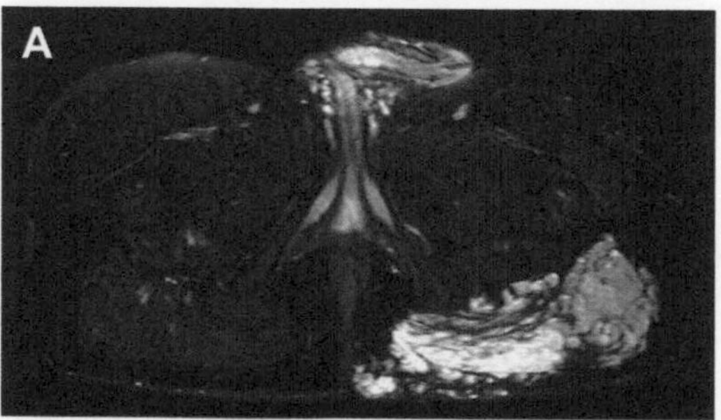

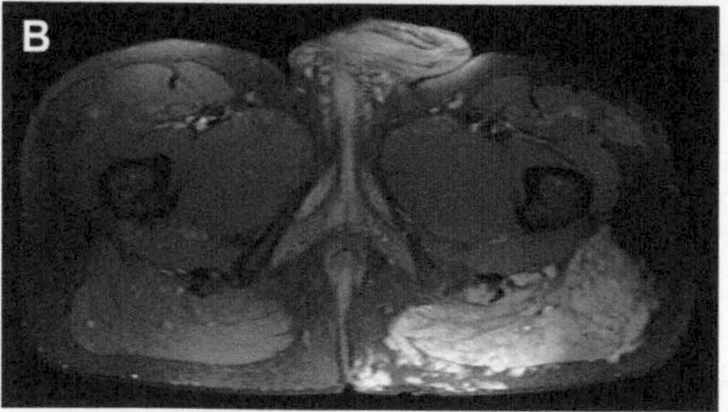

Fig. 8. MRI in a 24-year-old male with a VM of the left buttock, presenting with enlargement and pain on exertion. (*A*) Axial T2 image with fat saturation. Hyperintense lesion with clear lobulated margins is seen in the left gluteus maximus muscle, with subcutaneous extension noted medially. (*B*) Fat-saturated axial T1 postcontrast image showing uniform enhancement of the entire lesion.

COMBINED MALFORMATIONS AND VASCULAR ANOMALY SYNDROMES

Combined Malformations

Combinations of the various types of vascular anomalies are frequently seen. In particular, imaging characteristics of lymphaticovenous malformations have been described.[15,16] These entities display characteristics of both of their individually occurring constituents. In such cases, cross-sectional imaging is useful in excluding fast-flow components and soft tissue masses.

Klippel-Trénaunay Syndrome

Klippel-Trénaunay syndrome (KTS) is characterized by a capillary-lymphaticovenous malformation affecting an extremity with associated overgrowth. Involvement of a lower extremity occurs 95% of the time.[17] Imaging is used for initial diagnosis if the clinical presentation is atypical and it can also be used in the diagnosis and treatment of complications of the disease.

Ultrasonography, CT, and MRI demonstrate soft tissue hypertrophy in KTS and can define the numerous vascular malformations extending throughout the limb (**Fig. 10**). Involvement of vascular lesions in the pelvis and abdomen is

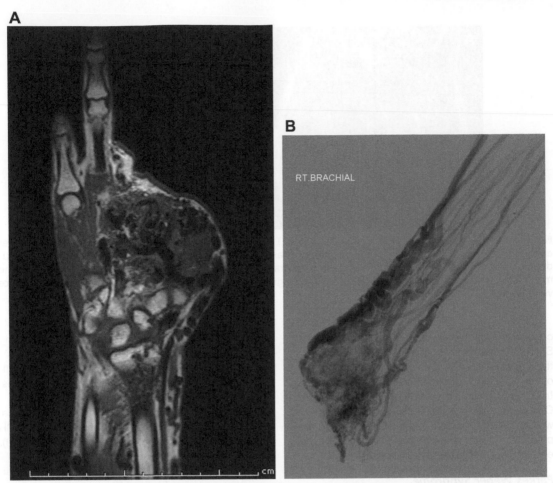

Fig. 9. AVM of the right hand in a 16-year-old boy. (*A*) Coronal T1 MRI showing multiple flow voids without an associated mass. The malformation predominantly involves the thenar muscles, and the second and third rays have been amputated. (*B*) Angiogram with contrast injected into the right brachial artery. The malformation is largely supplied by the enlarged radial artery, with smaller feeding branches from the ulnar artery. There is marked dilatation and tortuosity of the draining veins, with evidence of early filling consistent with arteriovenous shunting.

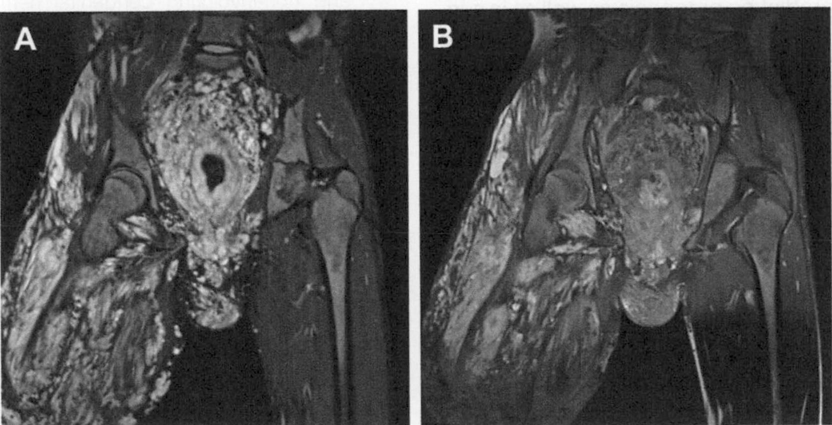

Fig. 10. MRI in a 16-year-old adolescent with KTS, who presented with rectal bleeding. (*A*) Coronal inversion recovery sequence. There is a diffuse high signal within the right thigh, perirectal area, and scrotum. (*B*) Coronal fat-saturated T1 postcontrast image. In the right thigh, there is heterogeneous enhancement of the subcutaneous and intramuscular venous components of the malformation, with minimal enhancement of the perirectal and scrotal LMs.

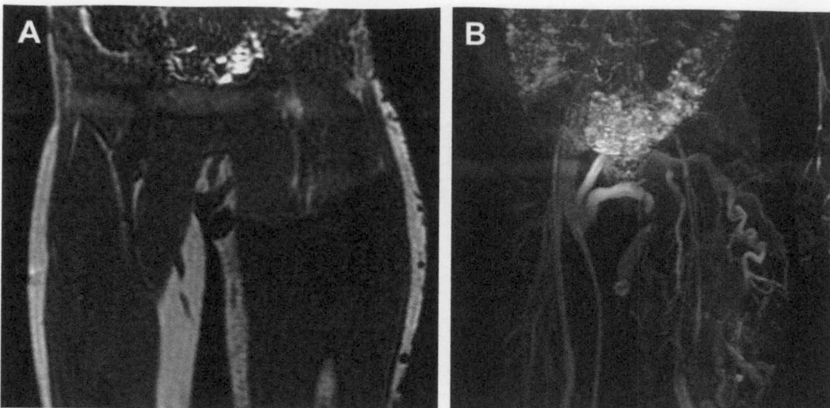

Fig. 11. MRI in a 7-year-old girl with PWS. (*A*) Coronal T1 image showing overgrowth of the affected left lower extremity with multiple subcutaneous flow voids. (*B*) Maximum intensity projection MRA/MRV. Multiple tortuous draining veins are seen on the left. These veins then drain into 2 grossly dilated anomalous veins that cross the midline to empty into the right femoral vein. MRA, magnetic resonance angiography; MRV, magnetic resonance venography.

common. A dilated superficial vein (lateral vein of Servelle) coursing along the subcutaneous fat of the lateral calf and thigh is often identified. Imaging of the vascular abnormalities can direct targeted treatments, such as sclerotherapy and resection. Complications of KTS that are often diagnosed with the aid of medical imaging include thrombophlebitis, deep venous thrombosis, pulmonary embolism, and congestive heart failure.[8,17]

Parkes Weber Syndrome

A combination of arteriovenous fistulae and a cutaneous capillary-lymphatic malformation associated with limb hypertrophy has been termed Parkes Weber syndrome (PWS). This syndrome is often confused with KTS, but the distinction is important in predicting prognosis as well as in suggesting appropriate therapy. The arteriovenous fistulae of PWS are fast-flow lesions that can result in heart failure. These lesions can be identified with ultrasonography, CT, MRI, and catheter angiography (**Fig. 11**). Embolization to reduce shunting may be considered.[18]

REFERENCES

1. Burrows PE, Mulliken JB, Fellows KE, et al. Childhood hemangiomas and vascular malformations: angiographic differentiation. AJR Am J Roentgenol 1983;141(3):483–8.
2. Barnes PD, Burrows PE, Hoffer FA, et al. Hemangiomas and vascular malformations of the head and neck: MR characterization. AJNR Am J Neuroradiol 1994;15(1):193–5.
3. Choi DJ, Alomari AI, Chaudry G, et al. Neurointerventional management of low-flow vascular malformations of the head and neck. Neuroimaging Clin N Am 2009;19(2):199–218.
4. Paltiel HJ, Burrows PE, Kozakewich HP, et al. Soft-tissue vascular anomalies: utility of US for diagnosis. Radiology 2000;214(3):747–54.
5. Meyer JS, Hoffer FA, Barnes PD, et al. Biological classification of soft-tissue vascular anomalies: MR correlation. AJR Am J Roentgenol 1991;157(3): 559–64.
6. Moukaddam H, Pollak J, Haims AH. MRI characteristics and classification of peripheral vascular malformations and tumors. Skeletal Radiol 2009;38(6): 535–47.
7. Gorincour G, Kokta V, Rypens F, et al. Imaging characteristics of two subtypes of congenital hemangiomas: rapidly involuting congenital hemangiomas and non-involuting congenital hemangiomas. Pediatr Radiol 2005;35(12):1178–85.
8. Dubois J, Alison M. Vascular anomalies: what a radiologist needs to know. Pediatr Radiol 2010;40(6): 895–905.
9. Chen YJ, Wang CK, Tien YC, et al. MRI of multifocal kaposiform haemangioendothelioma without Kasabach-Merritt phenomenon. Br J Radiol 2009; 82(975):e51–4.
10. Tamai N, Hashii Y, Osuga K, et al. Kaposiform hemangioendothelioma arising in the deltoid muscle without the Kasabach-Merritt phenomenon. Skeletal Radiol 2010;39(10):1043–6.
11. Stein-Wexler R. MR imaging of soft tissue masses in children. Magn Reson Imaging Clin N Am 2009; 17(3):489–507.
12. Ohgiya Y, Hashimoto T, Gokan T, et al. Dynamic MRI for distinguishing high-flow from low-flow peripheral vascular malformations. AJR Am J Roentgenol 2005; 185(5):1131–7.

13. van Rijswijk CS, van der Linden E, van der Woude HJ, et al. Value of dynamic contrast-enhanced MR imaging in diagnosing and classifying peripheral vascular malformations. AJR Am J Roentgenol 2002;178(5):1181–7.
14. Herborn CU, Goyen M, Lauenstein TC, et al. Comprehensive time-resolved MRI of peripheral vascular malformations. AJR Am J Roentgenol 2003;181(3):729–35.
15. Bisdorff A, Mulliken JB, Carrico J, et al. Intracranial vascular anomalies in patients with periorbital lymphatic and lymphaticovenous malformations. AJNR Am J Neuroradiol 2007;28(2):335–41.
16. Kim EY, Ahn JM, Yoon HK, et al. Intramuscular vascular malformations of an extremity: findings on MR imaging and pathologic correlation. Skeletal Radiol 1999;28(9):515–21.
17. Elsays KM, Menias CO, Dillman JR, et al. Vascular malformations and hemangiomatosis syndromes: spectrum of imaging manifestations. AJR Am J Roentgenol 2008;190(5):1291–9.
18. Ziyeh S, Spreer J, Rossler J, et al. Parkes Weber or Klippel-Trenaunay syndrome? Non-invasive diagnosis with MR projection angiography. Eur Radiol 2004;14(11):2025–9.

Histopathology of Vascular Anomalies

Anita Gupta, MD[a], Harry Kozakewich, MD[b,*]

KEYWORDS

- Hemangioma • Vascular malformation • Vascular tumor
- Pyogenic granuloma • Immunohistochemical stain

Over the past decade, many changes and updates have occurred in the world of vascular anomalies, including their histopathology. A significant step was the adoption of the Mulliken and Glowacki proposal of dividing vascular anomalies into tumors and malformations by the International Society for the Study of Vascular Anomalies in 1996.[1,2] This classification system allowed more meaningful communication between colleagues, helping to eliminate diagnostic and therapeutic errors. Emergence of vascular anomalies centers has facilitated identification of new vascular anomalies and their underlying genetic causes. An appreciation has developed that a combined team approach is optimal in arriving at a correct diagnosis, or at least at an appropriate working diagnosis when uncertainty exists.[2] Furthermore, technical advances such as immunohistochemical stains for GLUT1, an excellent marker for infantile hemangioma,[3–6] and vascular immunostains such as D2-40, PROX1, and vascular endothelial growth factor receptor 3 (VEGFR-3), which distinguish lymphatics from arteries and veins, have been of immense help in daily practice.[7–12]

VASCULAR TUMORS

Infantile Hemangioma

The proliferative phase of cutaneous infantile hemangioma shows a dermal/subcutaneous lesion composed of lobules and sheets of tightly packed, mostly capillary-sized vascular channels (**Fig. 1**A). The endothelial cells are plump and the basement membranes are thin and surrounded by a layer of pericytes (see **Fig. 1**B). The minimal intervascular stroma contains predominantly a few fibroblasts and mononuclear cells, including mast cells. Mitoses are observed. The involutive phase is characterized by diminution in the number of channels, luminal enlargement, flattening of endothelium, waning mitotic activity, apoptotic figures, and thickening of basement membranes (see **Fig. 1**C). The fibrous stroma between channels is increased, mast cells remain, and the arteries and veins in the interlobular stroma appear relatively prominent. In the involuted phase, the fibrofatty background is dominant, the dermis often shows scarring with loss of elastic fibers and absent appendages, and the skin surface is wrinkled. Residual capillaries are sparse, single, or clustered. They are often tiny and "ghost-like" with thick, hyalinized basement membranes, and occluded lumens containing apoptotic debris (see **Fig. 1**D). The large feeding and draining vessels with intimal fibrosis may still be present.[11]

The most useful immunohistochemical marker for diagnosing infantile hemangioma is glucose transporter protein isoform 1 (GLUT1). It is a cytoplasmic endothelial stain expressed in infantile hemangioma at all stages of evolution (see **Fig. 1**E, F).[3–6] Antibodies to CD31 (panendothelial cell marker) and CD34 (vascular endothelial marker) also stain the endothelial cells but are not specific for infantile hemangioma. Smooth muscle actin (SMA) highlights pericytes and vascular smooth muscle. KI-67, a proliferative index marker, may be 20% or greater in the endothelial cells and pericytes in the proliferative phase.

Congenital Hemangiomas

Congenital or fetal hemangiomas[4,5,13–16] differ from infantile hemangiomas in that they are fully

[a] Department of Pathology, Cincinnati Children's Hospital, 3333 Burnet Avenue, Cincinnati, OH 45229, USA
[b] Department of Pathology, Children's Hospital Boston, 300 Longwood Avenue, Boston, MA 02115, USA
* Corresponding author.
E-mail address: kozakewich@hub.tch.harvard.edu

Clin Plastic Surg 38 (2011) 31–44
doi:10.1016/j.cps.2010.08.007
0094-1298/11/$ – see front matter

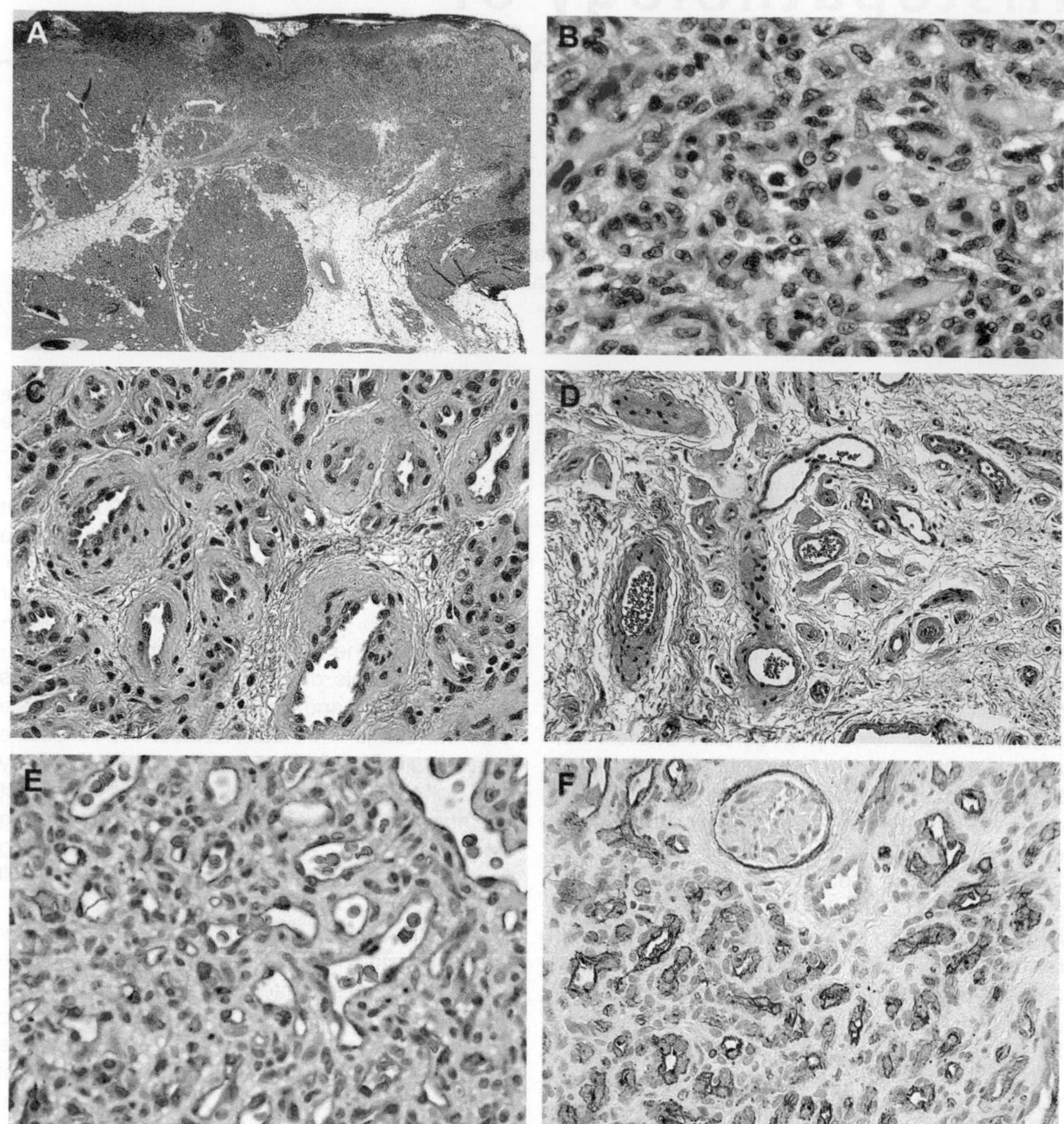

Fig. 1. Infantile hemangioma. (*A*) Proliferative phase composed of lobules and sheets of capillaries within the dermis and subcutis (hematoxylin-eosin, original magnification ×40). (*B*) Proliferative phase shows back-to-back capillaries lined by plump endothelial cells and scattered mitosis (hematoxylin-eosin, original magnification ×600). (*C*) Involuting phase has capillaries with larger lumens, thickening of the capillary basement membranes, less-plump endothelial cells, and separation by fibrous tissue (hematoxylin-eosin, original magnification ×400). (*D*) Involuted phase shows fibrofatty replacement of the lesion and many capillaries with thick basement membranes and small, nearly obliterated lumens (hematoxylin-eosin, original magnification ×400). GLUT1 immunostain highlights the cytoplasm within the lesional capillary endothelial cells in the proliferative (*E*) and involuting phase (*F*). Red cells and perineurium serve as a positive internal control (GLUT1 immunostain, original magnifications ×600 and ×400).

developed at birth with little to no growth postpartum. There are two types of congenital hemangiomas, rapidly involuting congenital hemangiomas (RICH)[14–16] and noninvoluting congenital hemangiomas (NICH).[5]

Rapidly involuting congenital hemangioma

RICH is a circumscribed, raised lesion with a central depression, scar, or ulceration surrounded by a rim of pallor.[14–16] Histology shows dermal and subcutaneous lobules of capillaries, occasionally coalescent, surrounded by abundant fibrous tissue (**Fig. 2**A). The lobular capillaries have moderately plump endothelium and a thin basement membrane surrounded by a layer of pericytes (see **Fig. 2**B). The center of many RICHs shows advanced involution with absence of lobules, abundant fibrous tissue, and residual draining veins, many being large and abnormal

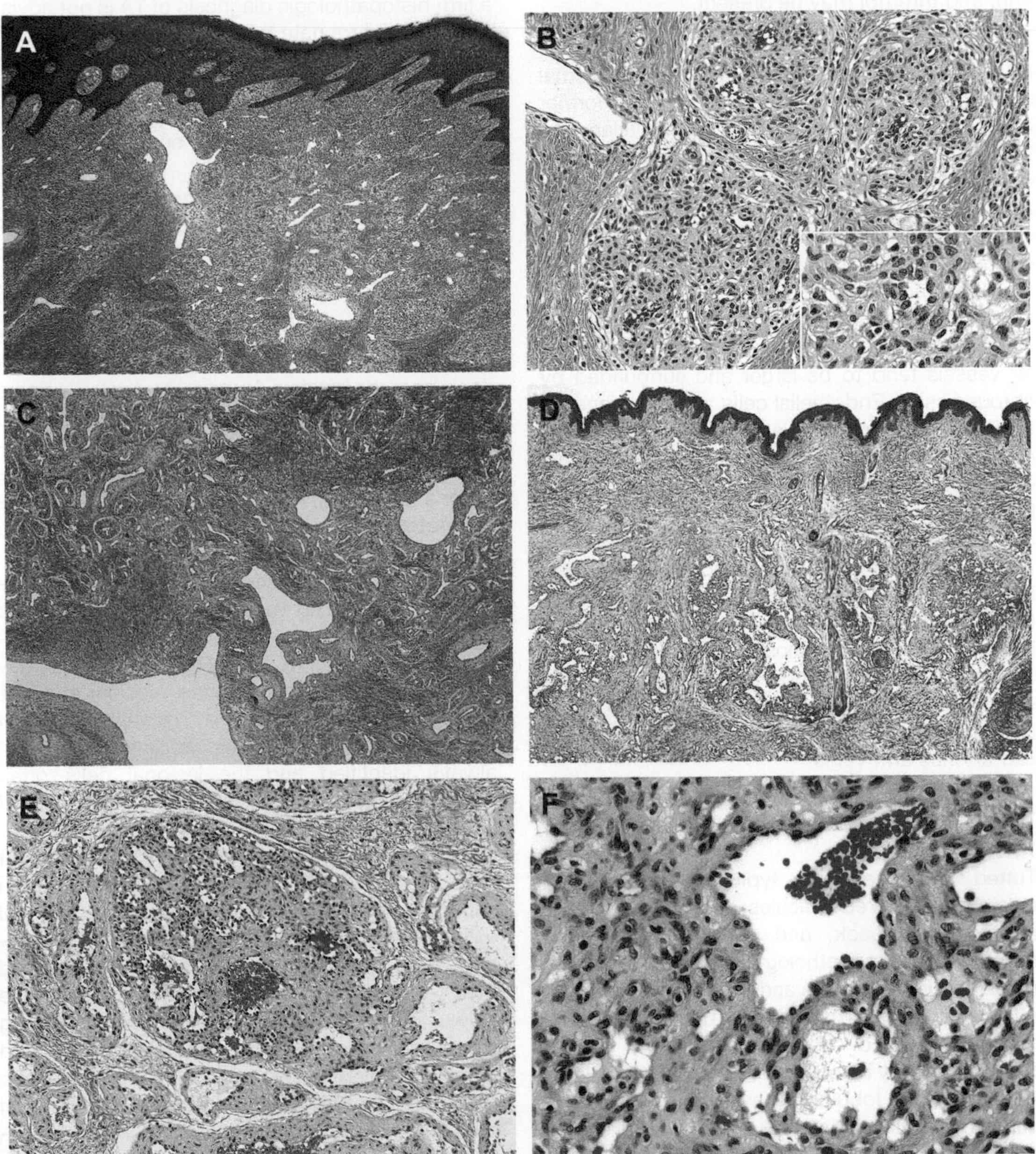

Fig. 2. Congenital hemangioma, rapidly involuting congenital hemangioma (RICH) and noninvoluting congenital hemangioma (NICH) types. (*A*) RICH showing small dermal lobules surrounded by abundant fibrous stroma (hematoxylin-eosin, original magnification ×20). (*B*) Lobules in RICH have capillaries with thin basement membranes, moderately plump endothelial cells (*inset*), and slight separation by fibrous tissue (hematoxylin-eosin, original magnification ×200). (*C*) Many RICHs show loss of lobules and large draining channels in their epicenter (hematoxylin-eosin, original magnification ×40). (*D*) NICH shows variably sized but often large dermal lobules (with larger channels as compared with RICH) (hematoxylin-eosin, original magnification ×20). (*E*) Lobule in NICH with enlarged, thin-walled channels surrounded by fibrous tissue. Note the prominent interlobular arteries and veins (hematoxylin-eosin, original magnification ×10). (*F*) NICH lobular endothelial cells tend to have nuclei that protrude into the lumen (hematoxylin-eosin, original magnification ×200).

with thickened and irregular fibromuscular walls (see **Fig. 2**C). The endothelial cells are immunonegative for GLUT1, although rarely a few cells may be positive. Extramedullary hematopoiesis, arteriovenous shunts, aneurysms, cysts, hemosiderin, and thrombi may be present.

Noninvoluting congenital hemangioma

NICH generally resembles RICH in its external appearance. Minor differences in the former include greater elevation and coarse telangiectases.[5] When NICH is removed at several years of age, histopathology shows lobules that are variable in size and most often large (see **Fig. 2**D) and composed of curved, thin-walled capillaries. The endothelial cells have minimal cytoplasm and small, hyperchromatic nuclei that protrude into the lumen (see **Fig. 2**E, F), and frequently contain cytoplasmic eosinophilic globules. The centrilobular vessels tend to be larger and surrounded by fibrous tissue. Endothelial cells are immunonegative for GLUT1. Interlobular fibrous tissue is abundant and contains prominent arteries and veins, and arteriolobular fistulae may be present. Some lesions have diminished or even few lobules, and are composed primarily of arteries, veins, and fibrous tissue, thereby mimicking a vascular malformation.[5] The histopathologic appearance of NICH removed at an early age, such as 2 years, is similar to RICH without the central zone of advanced involution. NICH, excised in adolescence, tends to have few lobules with the major part of the lesion consisting of prominent interlobular arteries and veins.

Other Vascular Tumors

Tufted angioma

Tufted angioma (TA) typically presents as enlarging pink–red macules and plaques in the upper chest, back, and neck in young children.[17,18] Histopathology shows lobules dispersed in the dermis and subcutaneous tissue, often referred as *cannonball*, because of their frequent rounded shape (**Fig. 3**A). The lobules themselves may be somewhat compartmentalized into miniature lobules. They are composed of capillaries with slightly plump and sometimes spindled endothelial and perithelial cells (see **Fig. 3**B). Focally, the spindled cells are highlighted by the D240 and PROX-1 immunoreaction. Thin-walled draining channels partially surround the lobules.

Some lesions that look like TA clinically have a histopathologic appearance suggestive of, or even indistinguishable from, kaposiform hemangioendothelioma (KHE) with coalescent lobules, microthrombi, hemosiderin deposits, and reactive stroma. Generally, a firm histopathologic diagnosis of TA is not advisable and appropriate therapy will depend on clinical evolution of the lesion. Conversely, selected microscopic fields in KHE may be similar to those seen in TA. Generally, a firm histopathologic diagnosis of TA is not advisable and appropriate therapy will depend on clinical evolution of the lesion. Many observers believe that there is clinical and histopathologic overlap between TA and KHE, with TA being at the less aggressive part of the spectrum.[19,20]

Kaposiform hemangioendotheliomas

KHE are locally aggressive tumors that occur in many locations, particularly skin, subcutis, deep soft tissue, retroperitoneum, mediastinum, and rarely bone.[21–29] Half are congenital and most are present before the age of 2 years. KHEs are grossly, ill-defined vascular stains, plaques, or deep-seated bulging lesions. Vascular tumors larger than 5 cm are often associated with marked thrombocytopenia (Kassabach-Merritt phenomenon). KHEs histopathologically are infiltrative lesions usually involving multiple tissue planes characterized by coalescing and poorly canalized lobules composed of rounded or spindled endothelial cells and pericytes (see **Fig. 3**C, D). The degree of spindling varies among lesions, as do clusters of rounded cells, focally imparting a glomeruloid appearance (see **Fig. 3**E). Nuclei may focally be very small and dense. Nuclear atypia is absent and mitoses are rare. Thrombi or platelet aggregates within the lobular capillaries are almost always identified and the lesional cells often contain hemosiderin. Some KHEs have foci of larger channels containing closely packed erythrocytes, and in some tumors this is a dominant feature (see **Fig. 3**F). Thin-walled channels often surround the lobules (see **Fig. 3**D). The lesional cells are immunoreactive for CD31, and the spindled cells focally for D2-40 (see **Fig. 3**F)[8] and PROX-1. Ki-67 typically shows a low proliferative index. The perilobular stroma shows varying combinations of edema, myxoid change, and fibrosis. Many KHEs have vicinal dilated lymphatic channels (see **Fig. 3** G), and occasionally lesional cells seem to proliferate within them. KHE is negative for HHV-8 by immunostain[29] and reverse transcription–polymerase chain reaction,[22] implying a pathogenesis different from that of Kaposi sarcoma.

Pyogenic granuloma

Pyogenic granuloma (PG), also known as *lobular capillary hemangioma*, is a common acquired lesion of the skin and mucous membranes, most often in the head and neck region. They are

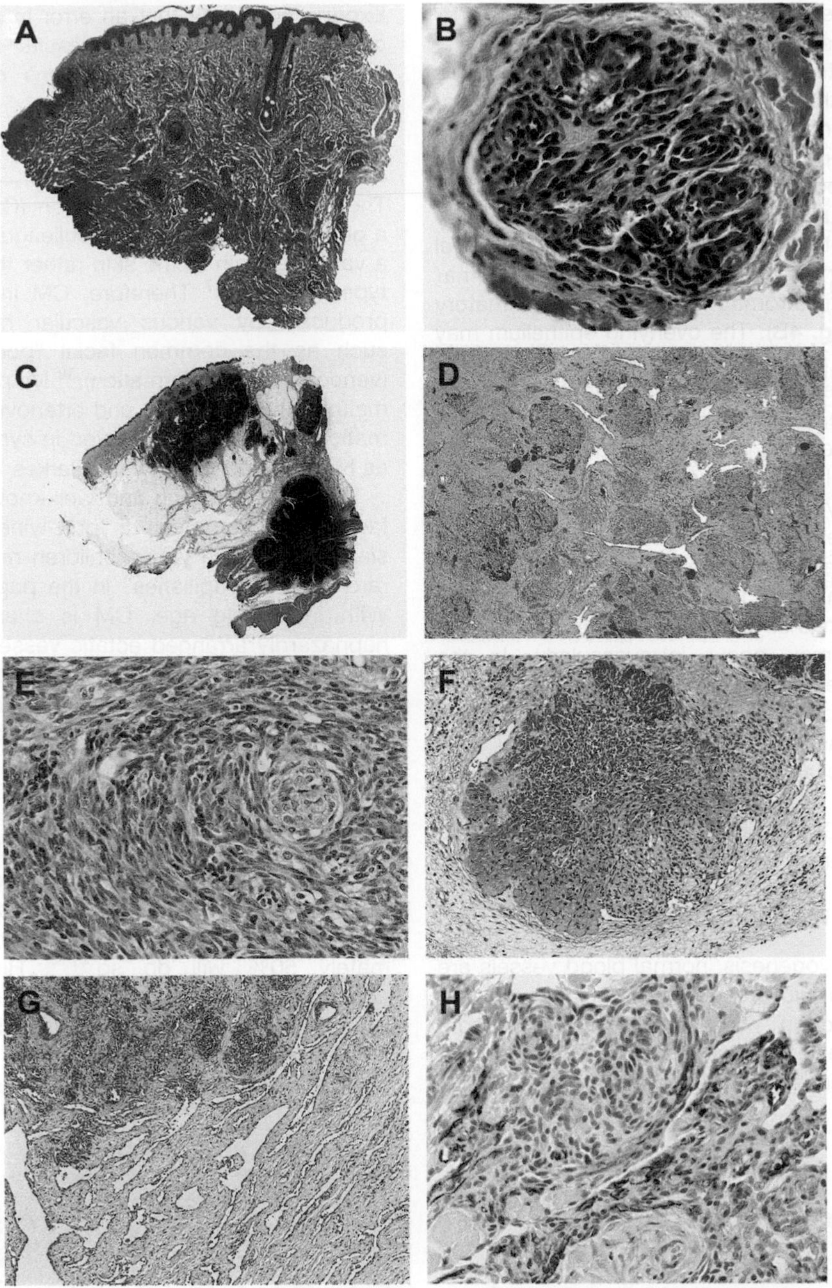

Fig. 3. Tufted angioma (TA) and kaposiform hemangioendothelioma (KHE). (*A*) TA with a few widely dispersed dermal vascular nodules (hematoxylin-eosin, original magnification, ×20). (*B*) TA lobule composed of well-defined capillaries with cuboidal endothelial cells (hematoxylin-eosin, original magnification ×600). (*C*) KHE whole-mount scan shows tightly packed "coalesced" nodules in the dermis, subcutis, and superficial fascia (hematoxylin-eosin stain). (*D*) KHE nodules are surrounded by fibrous tissue and irregular vascular channels (hematoxylin-eosin, original magnification ×20). (*E*) KHE with spindled cells, few channels containing red cells, and a rounded "glomeruloid" cluster (hematoxylin-eosin, original magnification ×400). (*F*) KHE may have capillaries distended with blood, some congealed (hematoxylin-eosin, original magnification ×20). (*G*) KHE with vicinal abnormal and dilated lymphatic channels (hematoxylin-eosin, original magnification ×100). (*H*) KHE endothelial cells are focally immunopositive for D2-40 (*brown*), especially at the periphery of the lobule (D240 immunostain, original magnification ×100).

commonly seen in pregnant women and children[30] and are associated with a history of trauma, hormonal alterations, and medications.[31–33] PGs can arise within a capillary malformation. Congenital solitary and congenital disseminated PGs have also been reported.[34–36]

PG is a polypoid dermal lesion composed of lobules of curved capillaries and venules lined by plump endothelial cells (**Fig. 4**A). The individual capillaries and lobules are separated by edematous to fibrotic stroma with scattered inflammatory cells (see **Fig. 4**B). The overlying epithelium may be atrophic and ulcerated and frequently shows lateral collarettes or indented hyperplastic surface epithelium encasing the lesion (see **Fig. 4**A). A prominent feeding artery is often seen at the base of the lesion. If ulceration ensues, a rind of inflammatory granulation tissue may overlie the lesion. In the late stages, a decreased number of lobules is present and the stroma is more fibrotic. Some lesions are deep-seated and involve the reticular dermis or subcutaneous tissue only, and rarely PG may occur intravascularly. In the absence of epidermal changes, PGs may superficially resemble an infantile hemangioma, but the curved channels, intervascular stroma, and epidermal collarettes in PG are helpful distinguishing features, as is the patient's age. If uncertainty exists, the GLUT1 immunostain will differentiate the two because PGs are negative.

VASCULAR MALFORMATIONS

During embryogenesis, normal blood vessels are derived from two processes: vasculogenesis (the process through which endothelial precursors align themselves to form primitive blood vessels) and angiogenesis (development of new vessels). Experts speculate that an error in both or either one of these processes results in malformed vessels. Vascular malformations occur in less than 1% of the population.

Capillary Malformation

The term *capillary malformation* (CM) is used in a generic sense by clinical colleagues to indicate a vascular stain of the skin rather than a specific type of lesion.[37] Therefore, CM includes stains produced by various vascular malformations, such as the common facial "port-wine" stain (venocapillary malformation),[38] lymphaticovenous malformations, venous and arteriovenous malformations, and those observed in syndromes such as Klippel-Trénaunay[39] and Parkes Weber.

The most common and well-known CM is the facial nevus flammeus or "port-wine" stain. Biopsies of lesions in young children may show only rare dilated "capillaries" in the papillary dermis. With increasing age, CM is characterized by haphazardly arranged ectatic vessels, with small venular morphology in the papillary and occasionally reticular dermis. The channels have flat endothelial cells, thin collagenous walls, and a layer of pericytes (see **Fig. 5**A). Vascular size and the mean vessel area increase with age and correlate with the change in color of the lesion.[40]

A small minority of individuals with a facial CM develop cutaneous thickening, and some also nodularity, and soft tissue and skeletal overgrowth. In Sturge-Weber syndrome, approximately 50% will do so.[41,42] Histopathologic correlates of this phenomenon include enlarged venule-type channels, many with thickened walls composed of collagen, pericytes, and smooth muscle cells surrounded by fibrous tissue (see

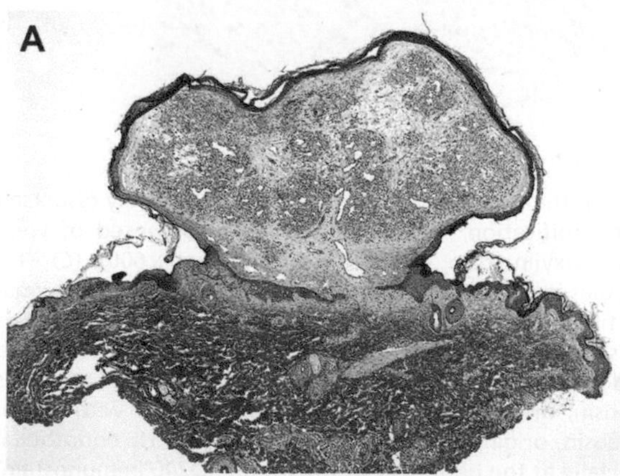

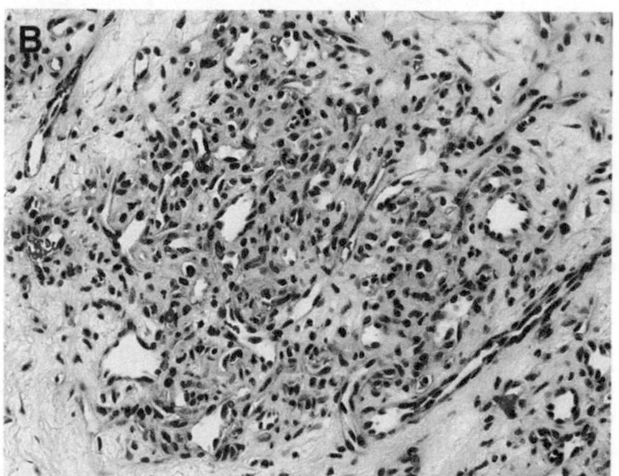

Fig. 4. Pyogenic granuloma. (*A*) Overview shows a polypoid dermal lobular vascular lesion with lateral collarettes (hematoxylin-eosin, original magnification ×20). (*B*) Lobules have thin-walled capillaries lined by flat to round endothelial cells separated by myxoid-to-collagenous stroma, which also surrounds the lobules; occasional scattered inflammatory cells present (hematoxylin-eosin, original magnification ×200).

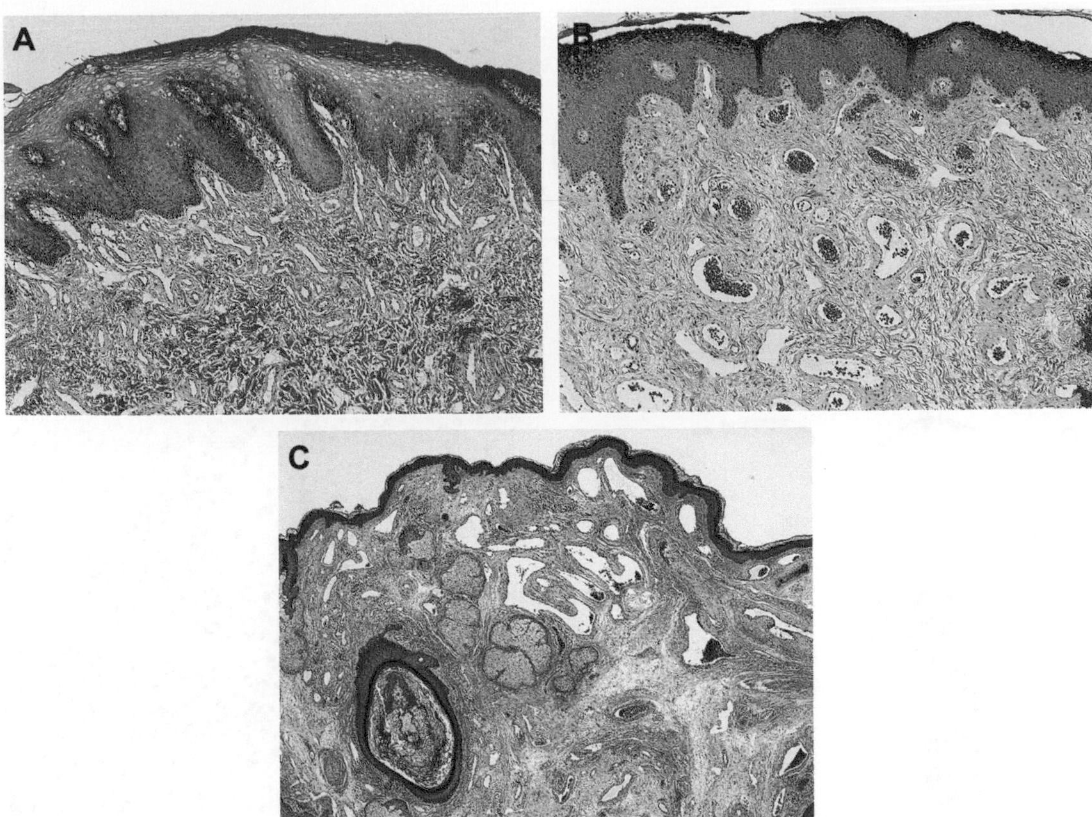

Fig. 5. Capillary malformation (CM). (*A*) Facial CM with lip hypertrophy in a 4-year-old boy showing an excessive number of thin-walled venule-like channels with narrow lumens (hematoxylin-eosin, original magnification ×100). (*B*) Facial CM with lip hypertrophy in a 17-year-old boy has an increased number of enlarged vein-like channels with both thin and thick, mostly fibrous walls. Intervascular fibrous tissue is increased (hematoxylin-eosin, original magnification ×100). (*C*) Facial CM with thickening and nodules in a 35-year-old man with Sturge-Weber syndrome. Nasal skin shows a nodular cluster of large, abnormal vein-like channels. Fibrosis and follicular dilatation and keratin plugging are present (hematoxylin-eosin, original magnification ×40).

Fig. 5B). The channels extend into the deep dermis, subcutis, and skeletal muscle and may form indistinct nodules with abundant fibrous tissue[40] (see **Fig. 5**C). They may also extend into bone. Hyperplasia of the epidermis and dermal appendages occurs, and epidermal and mesenchymal hamartomatous changes have also been reported.[43]

Venous Malformation

Venous malformations (VMs) are still called *cavernous hemangioma*, *venous hemangioma*, and *cavernous angioma* in many medical text books. VMs vary in size, can affect any or all levels of the venous tree, and can involve the dermis, subcutaneous tissue, skeletal muscle,[44] and viscera, including liver and brain.[45]

Histopathologically, VMs are composed of irregular venous-type channels, lined by flat endothelium and surrounded by smooth muscle that is often focally absent or scant relative to channel size (see **Fig. 6**A, B). The channels also vary in size. They may be randomly distributed, in clusters, or back-to-back. The lumens usually contain blood, although some may be empty or contain only sedimented protein or red cells. Luminal thrombi are frequently present, often showing papillary endothelial hyperplasia. Thrombi become organized and incorporated into the wall as fibromyxoid nodules, or form phleboliths. The vascular endothelial cells in VM are highlighted by CD31. SMA highlights the pericytes and smooth muscle within the wall. Ki-67 proliferative index is low. Lymphatic endothelial markers, PROX-1 and D2-40, are negative.

Glomuvenous malformations (GVMs),[46] previously known as *glomangioma*, are single or multiple VMs of a special type. They are characterized by ectatic and malformed veins with smooth

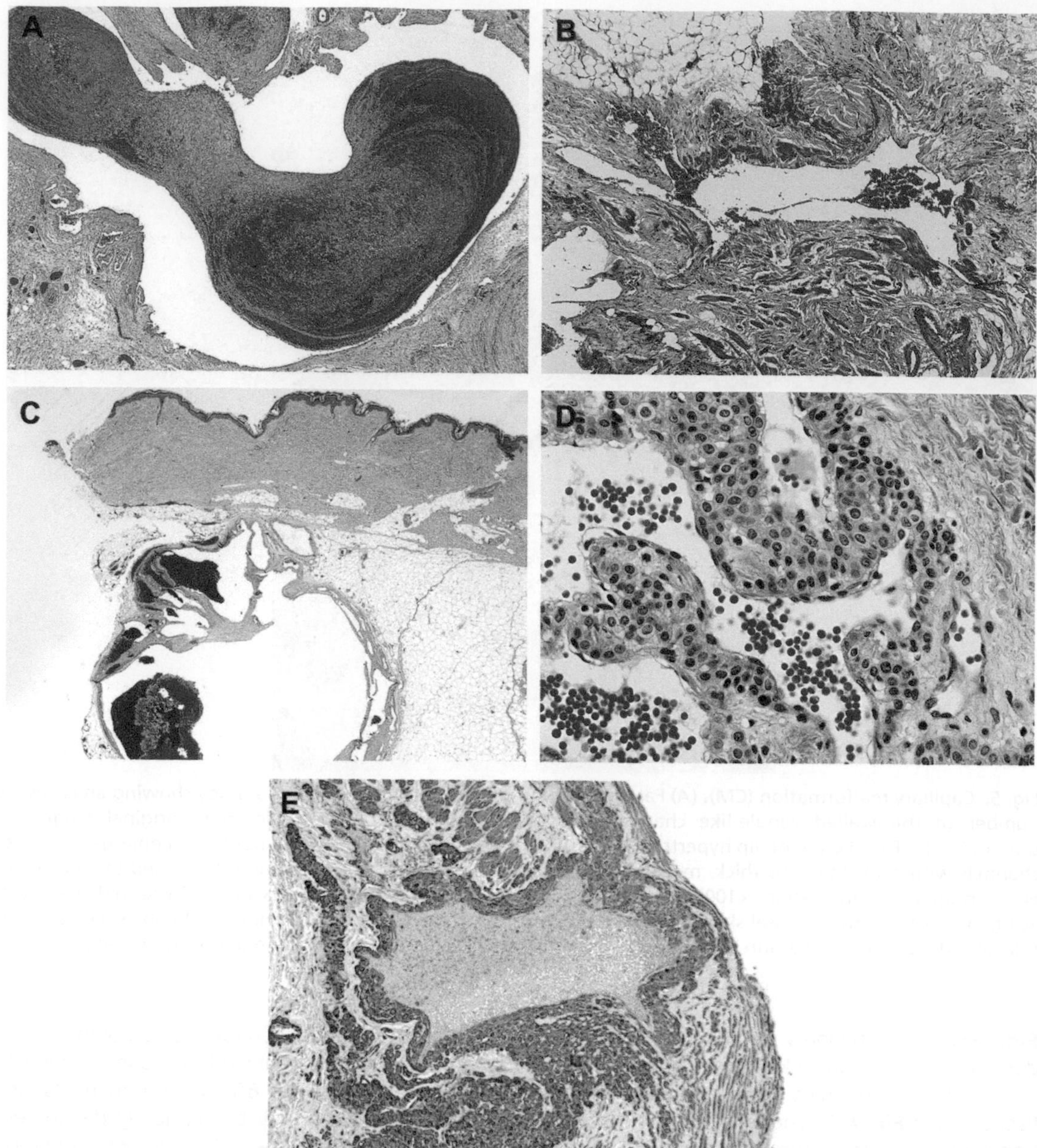

Fig. 6. Venous (VM) and glomuvenous malformation (GVM). (*A*) VM shows malformed venous channels with an organizing thrombus (hematoxylin-eosin, original magnification ×20). (*B*) Venous wall is irregularly muscularized and focally lacks muscle (hematoxylin-eosin, original magnification x100). (*C*) GVM overview of a deep dermal/subcutaneous lesion with organizing thrombi (hematoxylin-eosin, original magnification ×20). (*D*) Vascular channels in GVM have cuboidal glomus cells replacing smooth muscle (hematoxylin-eosin, original magnification ×200). (*E*) Glomus cells are highlighted by smooth muscle actin immunostain (original magnification ×200).

muscle focally, or totally replaced by one or multiple layers of cuboidal "glomus" cells (see **Fig. 6**D), which are immunoreactive for vimentin, SMA (see **Fig. 6**E), and sometimes desmin. Organizing thrombi and phleboliths are common. GVMs occur in the skin, subcutaneous fat, and muscle. Glomus tumors differ from GVMs in that the former almost always occurs in adults as a small well-circumscribed subungual proliferation of clusters and sheets of glomus cells lacking a malformed venous component. Atypical and malignant glomus tumors also occur.[47,48]

Blue rubber bleb nevus syndrome is characterized by soft blue, nodular venous malformations involving the dermis, subcutaneous tissue, and gastrointestinal tract. Cutaneous lesions have large channels with thin walls and little or no smooth muscle. The deeper ones have a layer of smooth muscle, although it may be discontinuous. The smaller gastrointestinal lesions most often involve the submucosa, while larger lesions involve the mucosa, muscular wall, and mesentery.

Other venous anomalies are included under the VM umbrella. Some have characteristic histopathologic features, but many require clinical features for diagnosis. These latter include the so-called hemangioma of bone[28]; cerebral-cavernous malformations (often called *cavernomas*),[49] some of which are associated with cutaneous lesions[50]; and familial cutaneomucosal venous malformations.[51,52]

Lymphatic Malformation

Lymphatic malformations (LMs) reflect the abnormal development of the lymphatic system. Small, localized LMs of the skin and subcutis (previously called *lymphangioma circumscriptum*) are postulated to be duplicated units of the lymphatic system, with no connection to each other or to the normal superficial or deep (intramuscular) lymphatics.[53] Abnormalities of large lymphatic trunks, including the thoracic duct, such as ectasia, lack of valves, or atresia have been shown in extensive or generalized lesions.[54,55] LM is an invariably prominent component in Klippel-Trénaunay syndrome and may occur in other syndromes such as trisomy 21 and Noonan.

LMs used to be called *lymphangioma* or *cystic hygroma*, depending on whether the size of the channels was small or large, respectively. If involvement was extensive or generalized, the term *lymphangiomatosis* was used. LMs vary from small, localized sponge-like lesions to diffuse involvement of a region or organ, to generalized involvement including viscera and bone. They are often classified as microcystic, macrocystic (spaces larger than 1 cm, **Fig. 7**A), or combined.[45] The enlargement of some LMs with time is believed to be caused primarily by distention with fluid. The proliferative index is negligible or low-level.[56]

The cutaneous form of LM, formerly called *lymphangioma circumscriptum*, is seen as hyperkeratotic papules, usually localized to one area.[53] The papillary dermis is expanded by thin-walled lymphatic channels, frequently accompanied by verruciform hyperplasia, ulceration, infection, inflammation, hemorrhage, and thrombosis. The deeper dermis and subcutis are often also involved with the abnormal channels, usually larger with thin muscular walls. Fibrous tissue expands the dermis and subcuticular fibrous septa, and lymphoid collections with or without germinal centers, plasma cells, and polymorphonuclear cells may also be present (see **Fig. 7**B). The subcutaneous fat is increased in amount. The lymphatic channels may be empty or contain a lacy pale or eosinophilic protein, pools of lymphocytes, or occasional macrophages containing red cells or hemosiderin (see **Fig. 7**C). Lumina may also contain blood attributed to prior trauma, the operative procedure, or communication with the venous system. Unilocular or macrocystic LMs usually have thick walls composed of myxoid fibrous tissue containing myofibroblasts and sparse smooth muscle cells. Generalized LM has histopathology similar to solitary LM, but in some lesions the channels are smaller, complex, and permeative; the lymphatic endothelial cells are larger; focal endothelial hyperplasia may be present; and the proliferative index is increased. Gorham-Stout disease, also known as *disappearing bone disease*[28] is almost invariably associated with a microcystic LM with an associated soft tissue component.

Immunoperoxidase markers are valuable in helping to differentiate LMs from other vascular anomalies. *PROX1* (see **Fig. 7**D) and VEGFR-3 are reported to be superior to D2-40 (podoplanin) (see **Fig. 7**E) or lymphatic vessel endothelial receptor 1 (LYVE-1) in staining of the endothelium in LMs, particularly in staining of large channels that usually stain focally or not at all with D2-40 or LYVE-1.[7] Immunoreactivity of the endothelium in LMs for CD31 and factor VIII–related antigen is focal and variable, and for CD34 is usually faint or absent.

Arteriovenous Malformation

Arteriovenous malformations (AVMs), known previously as *arteriovenous hemangioma*, are high-flow lesions involving skin, soft tissue, and viscera, with the head and neck region, including brain, the most common location. Approximately 50% of these lesions are visible at birth.[57] Most of these lesions are sporadic; however, some AVMs are part of inherited syndromes: hereditary hemorrhagic telangiectasia,[58] Parkes Weber syndrome,[59] CM-AVM.[60] An AVM component may be one constituent of the PTEN hamartoma of soft tissue in the PTEN hamartoma tumor syndrome.[61–64]

The histopathology of AVMs of soft tissue shows some variability. Generally, large and tortuous arteries, large and thick-walled veins, thin-walled

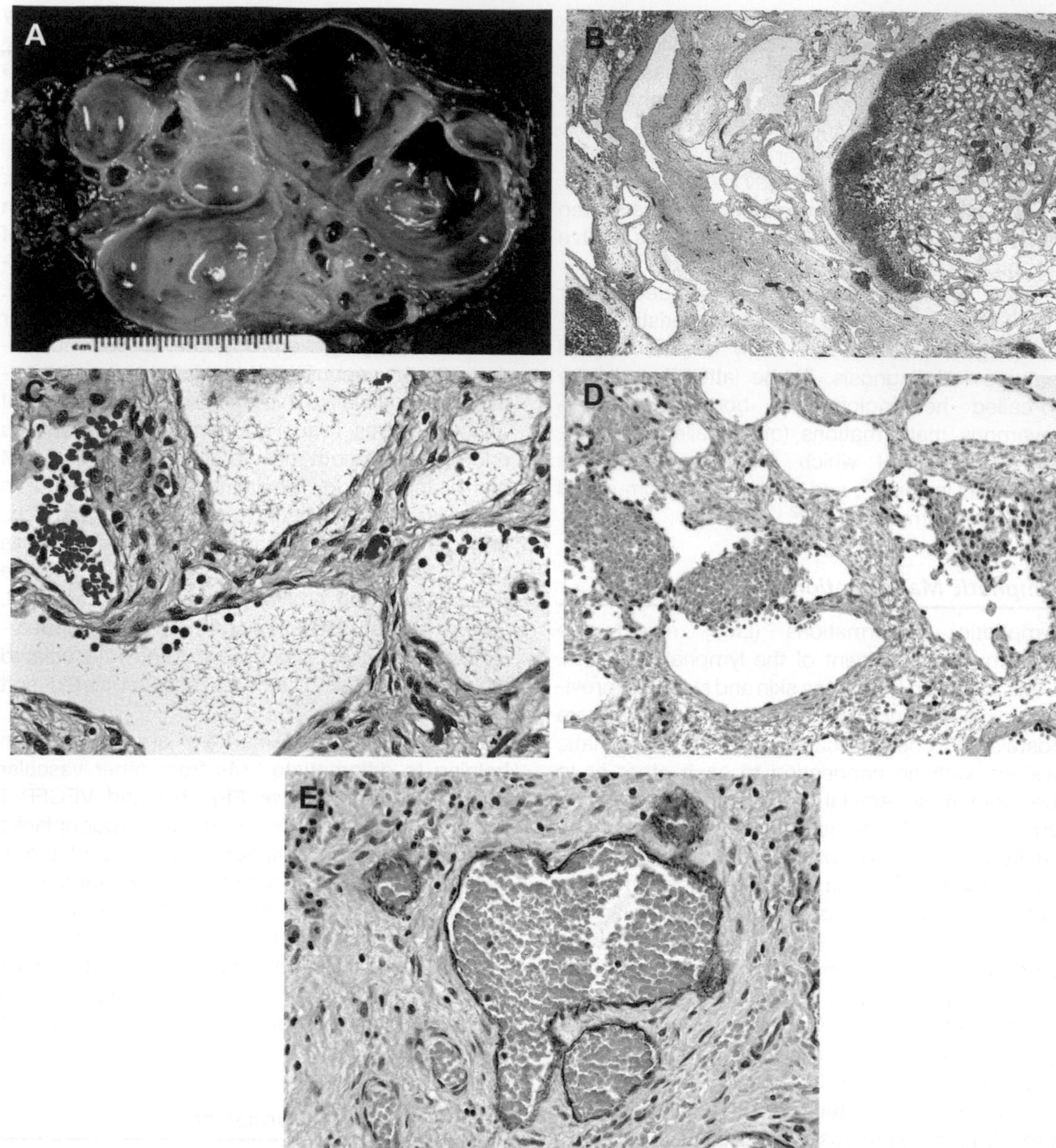

Fig. 7. Lymphatic malformation (LM). (*A*) Macrocystic lymphatic malformation (cyst-like channels are greater or equal to 1 cm. (*B*) Microcystic LM showing vascular channels less than 1 cm (hematoxylin-eosin, original magnification ×2). (*C*) These small thin-walled channels in LM have thin endothelial cells with no apparent muscular wall and lumens contain protein and lymphocytes (hematoxylin-eosin, original magnification ×20). (*D*) lymphatic endothelium is highlighted by PROX-1, brown nuclear stain (PROX-1 immunostain, original magnification ×10) and (*E*) D240, brown cytoplasmic stain (D240 immunostain, original magnification ×20).

structures that are probably abnormal veins, and some number of small vessels (**Fig. 8**A) are present. Some arteries show disruption of the arterial internal elastic lamina, highlighted by the elastic or Verhoeff-van Gieson stain (see **Fig. 8**B), and a transition to indeterminate morphology with channels resembling hypertensive veins, presumably representing sites of shunting. However, these shunts may be small and difficult to show. In the early stage, the veins show hypertrophy of their muscular layer, but later the smooth muscle is replaced by collagen, resulting in thin, fibrotic, inelastic vessels.[65,66] Intimal and adventitial fibrosis in veins is common. A small vessel component of a variable degree is present in most AVMs and is where the proliferative

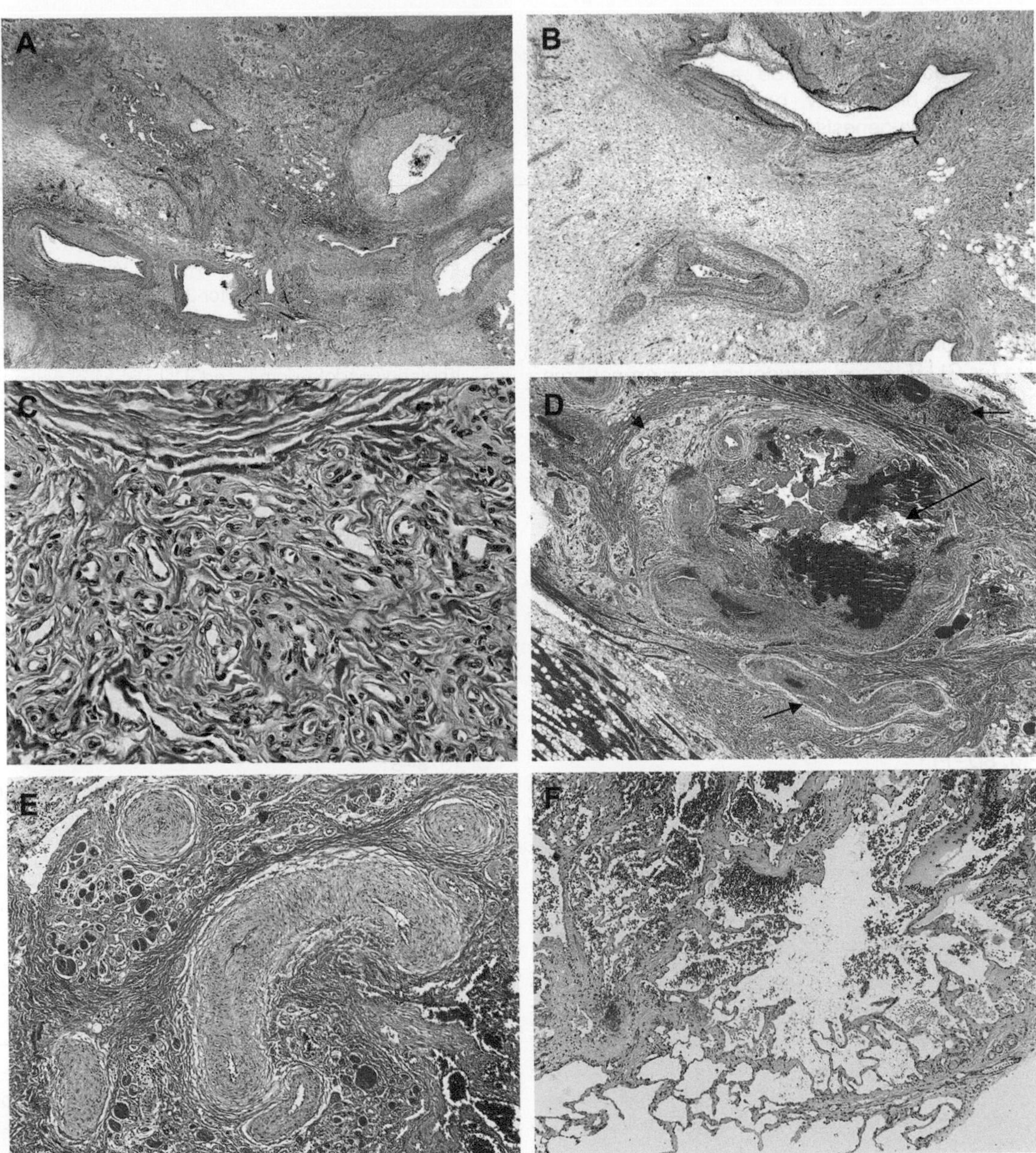

Fig. 8. Arteriovenous malformation (AVM) and PTEN hamartoma of soft tissue (PHOST). (*A*) AVM shows malformed arteries and veins (hematoxylin-eosin, original magnification ×20). (*B*) AVM with Verhoeff-van Gieson stain highlights the disrupted internal elastic lamina in arteries with transition to indeterminate type elastic pattern (*top vessel*; VVG special stain, original magnification ×4). (*C*) Small vessel (proliferative component) in AVM has foci of small channels with plump endothelium and pericytes (hematoxylin-eosin, original magnification ×400). (*D*) Intramuscular PHOST shows a large nodule composed of a large vein (*long arrow*) with a very irregular lumen and focally hypermuscularized wall surrounded by prominent arteries (*shorter arrow*) and dense fibrous tissue containing small myxoid vascular nodules and (*shortest arrow*) and lymphoid clusters (*horizontal arrow*) (hematoxylin-eosin, original magnification ×40). (*E*) PHOST with tortuous arteries showing transmural muscular hyperplasia and small lumens (hematoxylin-eosin, original magnification ×100). (*F*) Some vascular clusters in PHOST are composed of very thin-walled abnormal veins resembling pulmonary alveoli (hematoxylin-eosin, original magnification ×100).

component resides (see **Fig. 8**C). The reason for this proliferation is unknown; however, it has been hypothesized to be a consequence of abounding blood flow, or alternatively may be intrinsic to the genesis of AVM itself. Several overlapping microvascular patterns are present, the most common having dispersed, round, small vessels, measuring approximately 20 to 50 μm in diameter, with thick fibrous walls containing one or more layers of pericytes/smooth muscle cells and sometimes scant elastic fibers. Smaller vessels with pyogenic granuloma-like, infantile hemangioma-like (the endothelial cells are negative for GLUT1), and pseudo-kaposiform patterns may also occur.

One entity that is often misdiagnosed as AVM is PTEN hamartoma of soft tissue.[61–64] These lesions occur most often in children and young adults and are usually intramuscular. Some extend to skin and subcutis, producing an irregular cutaneous capillary stain. The lesions are composed of an overgrowth of fibromyxoid and adipose tissue, tortuous arteries and veins with marked transmural muscular hyperplasia, veins with complex walls and lumens, arteriovenous shunts, lymphoid nodules, and sometimes bone formation and Schwann cell hyperplasia within nerves (see **Fig. 8**D–F).[64]

REFERENCES

1. Mulliken JB, Glowacki J. Hemangiomas and vascular malformations in infants and children: a classification based on endothelial characteristics. Plast Reconstr Surg 1982;69:412–22.
2. Enjolras O, Mulliken JB. Vascular tumors and vascular malformations (new issues). Adv Dermatol 1998;13:375.
3. North PE, Waner M, Mizeracki A, et al. GLUT1: a newly discovered immunohistochemical marker for juvenile hemangiomas. Hum Pathol 2000;3: 11–22.
4. North PE, Waner M, James CA, et al. Congenital non-progressive hemangioma: a distinct clinicopathologic entity unlike infantile hemangioma. Arch Dermatol 2001;137:1607–20.
5. Enjolras O, Mulliken JB, Boon LM, et al. Noninvoluting congenital hemangioma; a rare cutaneous vascular anomaly. Plast Reconstr Surg 2001;107: 1647–54.
6. Takahashi K, Mulliken JB, Kozakewich HP, et al. Cellular markers that distinguish the phases of hemangioma during infancy and childhood. J Clin Invest 1994;93:2357–64.
7. Costa da Cunha Castro E. Galambos C. Prox-1 and VEGFR3 antibodies are superior to D2-40 in identifying endothelial cells of lymphatic malformations: a proposal of a new immunohistochemical panel to differentiate lymphatic from other vascular malformations. Pediatr Dev Pathol 2009;12: 187–94.
8. Debelenko LV, Perez-Atayde AR, Mulliken JB, et al. D2-40 immunohistochemical analysis of pediatric vascular tumors reveals positivity in kaposiform hemangioendothelioma. Mod Pathol 2005;18: 1454–60.
9. Folpe AL, Veikkola T, Valtola R, et al. Vascular endothelial growth factor receptor-3 (VEGFR-3): a marker of vascular tumors with presumed lymphatic differentiation, including Kaposi's sarcoma, kaposiform hemangioendothelioma and Dabska-type hemangioendotheliomas, and a subset of angiosarcomas. Mod Pathol 2000;13:180–5.
10. Galambos C, Nodit L. Identification of lymphatic endothelium in pediatric vascular tumors and malformations. Pediatr Dev Pathol 2005;8:181–9.
11. Glowacki J, Mulliken JB. Mast cells in hemangiomas and vascular malformations. Pediatrics 1982;70:48–51.
12. North PE, Waner M, Buckmiller L, et al. Vascular tumors of infancy and childhood: beyond capillary hemangioma. Cardiovasc Pathol 2006;15:303–17.
13. Boon LM, Fishman SJ, Lund DP, et al. Congenital fibrosarcoma masquerading as a congenital hemangioma: report of two cases. J Pediatr Surg 1995;30: 1378–81.
14. Boon LM, Enjolras O, Mulliken JB. Congenital hemangioma: evidence of accelerated involution. J Pediatr 1996;128:329–35.
15. Mulliken JB, Bischoff J, Kozakewich HPW. Multifocal rapidly involuting congenital hemangioma. A link to chorangioma. Am J Med Genet A 2007;3A:3038–46.
16. Berenguer B, Mulliken JB, Enjolras O, et al. Rapidly involuting congenital hemangioma: clinical and histopathologic features. Pediatr Dev Pathol 2003; 6:495–510.
17. Wilson-Jones E, Orkin M. Tufted angioma (angioblastoma). A benign progressive angioma, not to be confused with Kaposi's sarcoma or low grade angiosarcoma. J Am Acad Dermatol 1989;28:214–25.
18. Padilla RS, Orkin M, Rosai J. Acquired "tufted" angioma (progressive capillary hemangioma). A distinctive entity related to lobular capillary hemangioma. Am J Dermatopathol 1987;9:292–300.
19. Okada E, Tamura A, Ishikawa O, et al. Tufted angiomas (angioblastomas): case report and review of 41 cases in the Japanese literature. Clin Exp Dermatol 2000;25:627–30.
20. Chu CY, Hsaio CH, Chiu HC. Transformation between kaposiform hemangioendothelioma and tufted angioma. Dermatology 2003;206:334–7.
21. Tsang WY, Chan JKC. Kaposi-like infantile hemangioendothelioma: a distinctive vascular neoplasm of the retroperitoneum. Am J Surg Pathol 1991;15 982–9.

22. Zukerberg LR, Nickoloff BJ, Weiss SW. Kaposiform hemangioendothelioma of infancy and childhood. An aggressive neoplasm associated with Kasabach-Merritt syndrome and lymphangiomatosis. Am J Surg Pathol 1993;17:321–8.
23. Sarkar M, Mulliken JB, Kozakewich HP, et al. Thrombocytopenic coagulopathy (Kasabach-Merritt phenomenon) is associated with Kaposiform hemangioendothelioma and not with common infantile hemangioma. Plast Reconstr Surg 1997;100: 1377–86.
24. Enjolras O, Wassef M, Mazoyer E, et al. Infants with Kasabach-Merritt syndrome do not have "true" hemangiomas. J Pediatr 1997;130:631–40.
25. Enjolras O, Mulliken JB, Wassef M, et al. Residual lesions after Kasabach-Merritt phenomenon in 41 patients. J Am Acad Dermatol 2000;42:225–35.
26. Lyons LL, North PE, Mac-Maoune Lai F, et al. Kaposiform hemangioendothelioma: a study of 33 cases emphasizing its pathologic, immunophenotypic, and biologic uniqueness from juvenile hemangioma. Am J Surg Pathol 2004;28:559–68.
27. Gruman A, Liang MG, Mulliken JB, et al. Kaposiform hemangioendothelioma without Kasabach-Merritt phenomenon. J Am Acad Dermatol 2005;52:616–22.
28. Bruder E, Perez-Atayde A, Jundt G, et al. Vascular lesions of bone in children, adolescents, and young adults. Virchows Arch 2009;454:161–79.
29. Cheuk W, Wong KO, Wong CS, et al. Immunostaining for human herpesvirus 8 latent nuclear antigen-1 helps distinguish Kaposi sarcoma from mimickers. Am J Clin Pathol 2004;121:335–42.
30. Patrice SJ, Wiss K, Mulliken JB. Pyogenic granuloma (lobular capillary hemangioma): a clinicopathologic study of 178 cases. Pediatr Dermatol 1991;8: 267–76.
31. Saravana GH. Oral pyogenic granuloma: a review of 137 cases. Br J Oral Maxillofac Surg 2009;47: 318–9.
32. Jafarzadeh H, Sanatkahani M, Mohtasham N. Oral pyogenic granuloma: a review. J Oral Sci 2006;48: 167–75.
33. Pereira CM, de Almeida OP, Correa ME, et al. Oral involvement in chronic graft versus host disease: a prospective study of 19 Brazilian patients. Gen Dent 2007;55:48–51.
34. Browning JC, Eldin KW, Kozakewich HP, et al. Congenital disseminated pyogenic granuloma. Pediatr Dermatol 2009;26:323–7.
35. Walter DL, Parker NP, Kim OS, et al. Lobular capillary hemangioma of the neonatal larynx. Arch Otolaryngol Head Neck Surg 2008;134:272–7.
36. Ogunleye AO, Nwaaorgu OG. Pyogenic granuloma, a cause of a congenital nasal mass: case report. Ann Trop Paediatr 2000;20:137–9.
37. Happle R. What is a capillary malformation? J Am Acad Dermatol 2008;59:1077–9.
38. Finley JL, Noe JM, Arndt K, et al. Port wine stains: morphologic variations and developmental lesions. Arch Dermatol 1984;120:1453–5.
39. Maari C, Frieden IJ. Klippel-Trénaunay syndrome: the importance of "geographic stains" in identifying lymphatic disease and risk of complications. J Am Acad Dermatol 1994;31:391–6.
40. Barsky SH, Rosen S, Geer DE, et al. The nature and evolution of port wine stains: a computer-assisted study. J Invest Dermatol 1980;74:154–7.
41. Greene AK, Tabler SF, Ball KL, et al. Sturge-Weber syndrome: soft-tissue and skeletal overgrowth. J Craniofac Surg 2009;20(Suppl 1):617–21.
42. Mills CM, Lanigan SW, Hughes J, et al. Demographic study of port wine stain patients attending a laser clinic: family history, prevalence of nevus anaemicus with results of prior treatment. Clin Exp Dermatol 1997;22:166–8.
43. Sanchez-Carpintero I, Mihm MC, Mizeracki A, et al. Epithelial and mesenchymal hamartomatous changes in a mature port-wine stain: morphologic evidence for a multiple germ layer field defect. J Am Acad Dermatol 2004;50:608–12.
44. Hein KD, Mulliken JB, Kozakewich HPW, et al. Venous malformations of skeletal muscle. Plast Reconstr Surg 2002;110:1625–35.
45. Mulliken JB, Fishman SJ, Burrows PE. Vascular anomalies. Curr Probl Surg 2000;37:517–84.
46. Boon LM, Mulliken JB, Enjolras O, et al. Glomuvenous malformation (glomangioma) and venous malformation; distinct clinicopathologic and genetic entities. Arch Dermatol 2004;140:971–6.
47. Folpe AL, Fanburg-Smith JC, Miettinen M, et al. Atypical and malignant glomus tumors: analysis of 52 cases, with a proposal for the reclassification of glomus tumors. Am J Surg Pathol 2001;25: 1–12.
48. Weiss SW, Goldblum JR, editors. Enzinger and Weiss's soft tissue tumors. Philadelphia: Mosby, Elsevier; 2008.
49. Del Curling O, Kelly DL, Elster AD, et al. An analysis of the natural history of cavernous angiomas. J Neurosurg 1991;75:702–8.
50. Sirventi A, Enjolras O, Wassef M, et al. Frequency and genotypes of cutaneous vascular malformations in a consecutive series of 417 patients with familial cerebral cavernous malformations. J Eur Acad Dermatol Venereol 2009;9:1066–72.
51. Vikkula M, Boon LM, Enjolras O, et al. Vascular dysmorphogenesis caused by an activating mutation in the receptor tyrosine kinase TIE2. Cell 1996;87: 1181–90.
52. Wouters V, Limaye N, Uebelhoer A, et al. Hereditary cutaneomucosal venous malformations are caused by *TIE2* mutations with widely variable hyperphosphorylating effects. Eur J Hum Genet 2010; 18:414–20.

53. Whimster IW. The pathology of lymphangioma circumscriptum. Br J Dermatol 1976;94:473–86.
54. Kinmonth JB. The lymphatics. London: Edward Arnold; 1982.
55. Fishman SJ, Burrows PE, Hendren WH. Life-threatening anomalies of the thoracic duct: anatomic delineation dictates management. J Pediatr Surg 2001;36:1269–72.
56. Meijer-Jorna LB, van der Loos CM, de Boer OJ, et al. Microvascular proliferation in congenital vascular malformations of skin and soft tissue. J Clin Pathol 2007;60:798–803.
57. Garzon MC, Huang JT, Enjolras I, et al. Vascular malformations. Part 1. J Am Acad Dermatol 2007; 56:353–70.
58. Khalid SK, Garcia-Tsao G. Hepatic vascular malformations in hereditary hemorrhagic telangiectasia. Semin Liver Dis 2008;28:247–58.
59. Revencu N, Boon LM, Mulliken JB, et al. Parkes Weber syndrome, vein of Galen aneurysmal malformation, and other fast-flow vascular anomalies are caused by RASA1 mutations. Hum Mutat 2008;29: 959–65.
60. Eerola I, Boon LM, Mulliken JB, et al. Capillary malformation-arteriovenous malformation-arteriovenous malformation, a new clinical and genetic disorder caused by RASA1 mutations. Am J Hum Genet 2003;73:1204–9.
61. Fargnoli MC, Orlow SJ, Semel-Concepcion J, et al. Clinicopathologic findings in the Bannayan-Riley-Ruvalcaba syndrome. Arch Dermatol 1996;132: 1214–8.
62. Tan WH, Baris HN, Burrows PE, et al. The spectrum of vascular anomalies in patients with PTEN mutations: implications for diagnosis and treatment. J Med Genet 2007;44:594–602.
63. Zhou XP, Marsh DJ, Hampel H, et al. Germline and germline mosaic PTEN mutations associated with a Proteus-like syndrome of hemihypertrophy, lower limb asymmetry, arteriovenous malformations and lipomatosis. Hum Mol Genet 2000;22:765–8.
64. Howard EL, Tennant LB, Upton J, et al. PTEN-associated vascular anomaly [abstract]. Mod Pathol 2005;18:309.
65. Leu HJ. Zur Morphologie der arteriovenosen Anastomosen bei kongenitalen Angiodysplasien [in German]. Morphol Med 1982;2:99.
66. Mulliken JB, Dethlefson SM. A preliminary morphologic study of an arteriovenous malformation and adjacent vasculature. In: Belov ST, Loose DA, Weber J, editors. Periodica angiologica. Hamburg (Germany): Einhorn-Presse Verlag; 1989. p. 16–50.

Management of Hemangiomas and Other Vascular Tumors

Arin K. Greene, MD, MMSc

KEYWORDS

- Hemangioma • Kaposiform hemangioendothelioma
- Pyogenic granuloma • Vascular anomaly • Vascular tumor

Vascular tumors of childhood are typically benign. The 4 most common types are infantile hemangioma (IH), congenital hemangioma (CH), kaposiform hemangioendothelioma (KHE), and pyogenic granuloma (PG). Vascular tumors *must* be differentiated from vascular malformations. Although tumors and malformations may appear as raised, blue, red, or purple lesions, their management differs significantly.

INFANTILE HEMANGIOMA

Clinical Features

IH is a benign tumor of the endothelium, and the most common tumor of infancy.[1,2] IH affects approximately 4% to 5% of Caucasian infants and is rare in dark-skinned individuals.[3–5] It is more frequent in premature children (23% of infants <1200 g) and females (3:1 to 5:1).[6,7] IH typically is single (80%) and involves the head and neck (60%), trunk (25%), or extremity (15%).[2] The median age of appearance is 2 weeks, although 30% to 50% of lesions are noted at birth as a telangiectatic stain or ecchymotic area.[8] IH grows faster than the rate of the child during the first 9 months of age (proliferating phase); 80% of its size is achieved by 3.2 ($\pm$1.7) months.[9] When IH involves the superficial dermis it appears red. A lesion beneath the skin may not be appreciated until 3 to 4 months of age when it has grown large enough to cause a visible deformity; the overlying skin may appear bluish. By 9 to 12 months of age the growth of IH plateaus to approximate that of the infant.[9] After 12 months of age the tumor begins to shrink (involuting phase); the color fades and the lesion flattens (**Fig. 1**). Involution stops in most children by 5 years of age (involuted phase).[10] After involution, one-half of children have an abnormality: residual telangiectasias, anetoderma from loss of elastic fibers, scarring, fibrofatty residuum, redundant skin, or destroyed anatomic structures.

Diagnosis

Ninety percent of IH are diagnosed by history and physical examination (**Fig. 2**). Deeper lesions may be more difficult to appreciate because they are noted later than superficial tumors, and may not have significant overlying skin changes. Diagnosis of subcutaneous IH is facilitated using a hand-held Doppler device showing fast flow. When history and physical examination are equivocal, ultrasonography is the first-line confirmatory study to differentiate IH from other lesions. IH appears as a soft-tissue mass with fast flow, decreased arterial resistance, and increased venous drainage.[11] Magnetic resonance imaging (MRI) can differentiate vascular anomalies, although young children require sedation.[12] During the proliferating phase, IH is isointense on T1 images, hyperintense on T2 sequences, and enhances with contrast. IH appears as a mass with dilated feeding and draining vessels; signal voids represent fast flow and shunting.[13] Involuting IH has increased lobularity and adipose tissue; the number of vessels and flow is reduced.[12]

Disclosures: none.

Department of Plastic and Oral Surgery, Vascular Anomalies Center, Children's Hospital Boston, Harvard Medical School, 300 Longwood Avenue, Boston, MA 02115, USA
E-mail address: arin.greene@childrens.harvard.edu

Clin Plastic Surg 38 (2011) 45–63
doi:10.1016/j.cps.2010.08.001
0094-1298/11/$ – see front matter

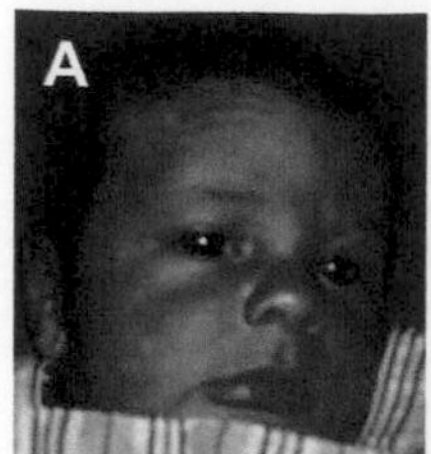

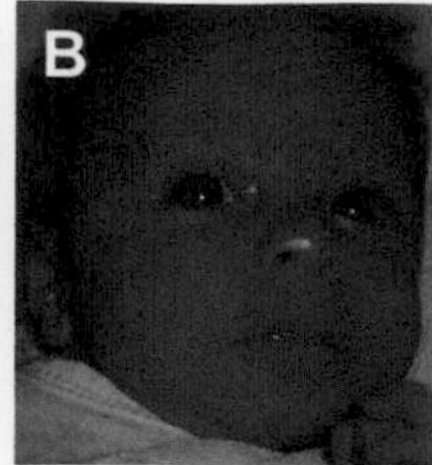

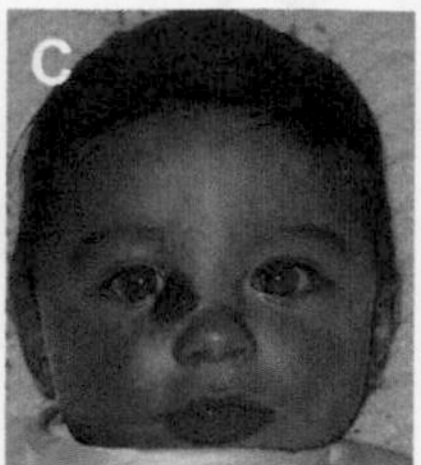

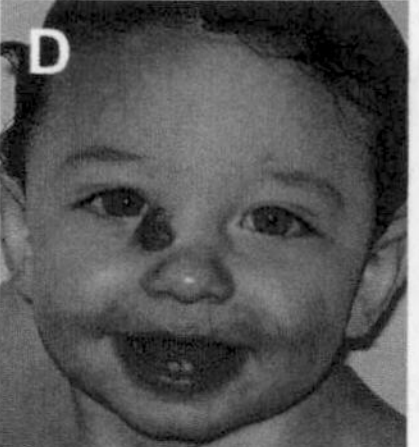

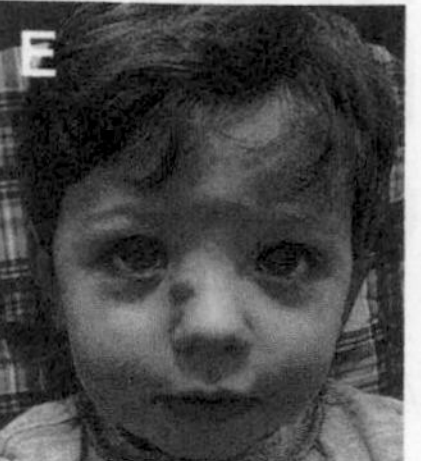

Fig. 1. Proliferation and involution of infantile hemangioma. (*A*) Age 2 weeks. (*B*) Age 5 weeks. (*C*) Age 6 months. (*D*) Age 12 months. (*E*) Age 18 months.

Rarely, biopsy is indicated if malignancy is suspected or if the diagnosis remains unclear following imaging studies. Tumors or fast-flow lesions that may be confused with IH include arteriovenous malformation, CHs, cutaneous leukemia (chloroma), hemangioendotheliomas, infantile fibrosarcoma, infantile myofibromatosis, lymphoma, metastatic neuroblastoma, PTEN-associated vascular anomaly, and PG.[14–18] In the liver, the differential diagnosis of hemangioma includes arteriovenous malformation, hepatoblastoma, or metastatic neuroblastoma. Because an erythrocyte-type glucose transporter (GLUT1) is specifically expressed in IH, immunostaining for GLUT1 can differentiate IH from other tumors and malformations.[19]

Clinical Considerations

Head and neck hemangiomas

Ten percent of proliferating IH cause significant deformity or complications, usually when located on the head or neck.[20] Ulcerated lesions may destroy the eyelid, ear, nose, or lip. IH of the scalp or eyebrow can injure hair follicles, resulting in alopecia. Obstruction of the external auditory canal can cause otitis externa, but sensorineural hearing loss does not occur if the contralateral canal is patent. Periorbital hemangioma can block the visual axis or distort the cornea causing deprivation or astigmatic amblyopia, respectively. IH involving the upper eyelid is more likely to be problematic than a lesion involving the lower eyelid. Infants with periorbital IH are referred to an ophthalmologist; the noninvolved eye may be patched for a minimum of 2 hours per day to stimulate use of the affected eye. Subglottic hemangioma, associated with large cervicofacial lesions, may obstruct the airway; patients are referred to an otolaryngologist for evaluation. Although the patency of the airway is usually maintained with oral corticosteroid, laser treatment or tracheostomy may be necessary.[21,22]

Multiple hemangiomas

Although 20% of infants have more than one IH, occasionally a child will have 5 or more small (<5 mm), dome-like lesions termed disseminated hemangiomatosis.[8] These children are at increased risk for IH of internal organs, although the risk is low. The liver is most commonly affected; the brain, gut, or lung are rarely involved. Ultrasonography should be considered to rule out hepatic IH. However, because intervention is not necessary for an incidentally found liver lesion, families may not elect to pursue imaging. In addition, infants with problematic hepatic IH are usually symptomatic early in infancy, before they are referred for evaluation of the cutaneous lesions. If symptomatic

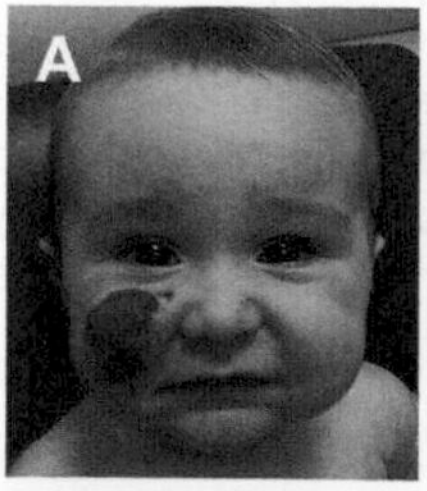

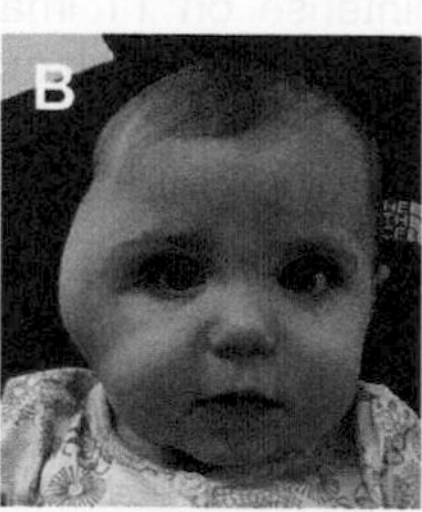

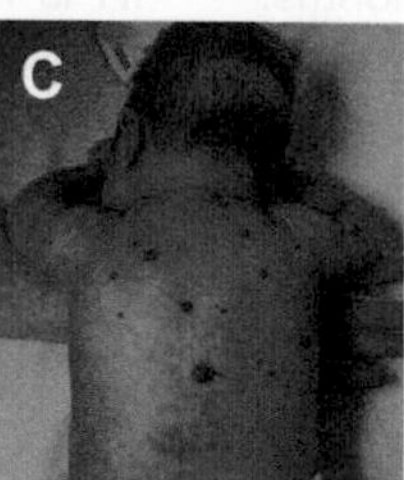

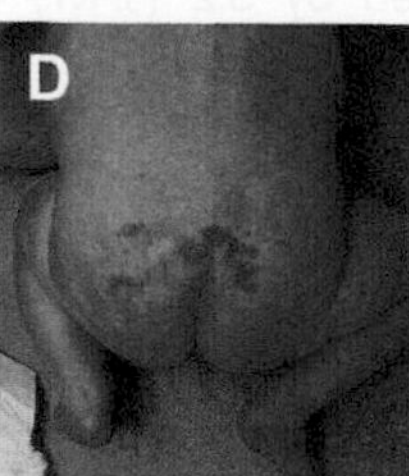

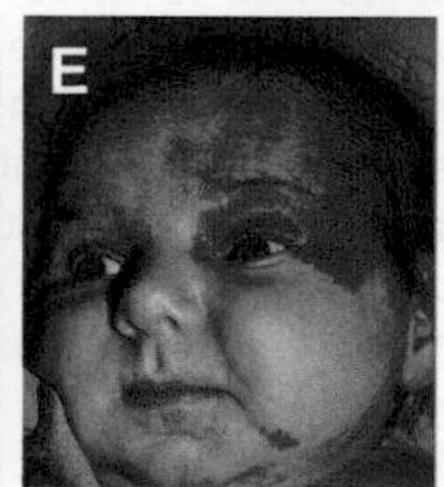

Fig. 2. Clinical features of infantile hemangioma (IH). (*A*) A 5-month-old male with a superficial tumor of the cheek. (*B*) A 12-month-old female with a deep IH of the cheek and temporal area without overlying skin changes. (*C*) A 2-month-old infant with hemangiomatosis, including hepatic hemangioma. (*D*) A 2-month-old female with midline lumbosacral IH and underlying lipomyelomeningocele. (*E*) An infant female with PHACE association (*P*osterior fossa brain malformation, *H*emangioma, *A*rterial cerebrovascular anomalies, *C*oarctation of the aorta and cardiac defects, *E*ye/*E*ndocrine abnormalities) and cerebrovascular anomalies.

brain, gut, or lung lesions are suspected, MRI is considered.

Hepatic hemangiomas

The liver is the most common extracutaneous site for IH, which may be focal, multifocal, or diffuse.[23] Although hepatic IH usually are nonproblematic and discovered incidentally, large tumors can cause heart failure, hepatomegaly, anemia, or hypothyroidism. Ninety percent of fast-flow hepatic lesions are hemangioma; arteriovenous malformation, hepatoblastoma, and metastatic neuroblastoma are less common and do not demonstrate significant shunting on imaging.[24] Focal hepatic IH usually is asymptomatic and not associated with cutaneous lesions; it is discovered incidentally on prenatal or antenatal ultrasonography. A focal liver hemangioma may not be IH but rather rapidly involuting congenital hemangioma (RICH), because it undergoes rapid postnatal involution and does not stain for GLUT1.[23] Multifocal hepatic IH may be associated with cutaneous lesions and is immunopositive for GLUT1. Although usually asymptomatic, multifocal lesions can cause high-output cardiac failure because of shunting which is managed by corticosteroids with or without embolization.[23] Diffuse hepatic IH can cause massive hepatomegaly, respiratory compromise, or abdominal compartment syndrome. Infants also are at risk for hypothyroidism and irreversible brain injury because the tumor expresses a deiodinase that inactivates thyroid hormone.[25] Patients require thyroid-stimulating hormone monitoring and, if abnormal, intravenous thyroid replacement until the IH has involuted.

Reticular hemangioma

Reticular hemangioma is an uncommon variant of IH that most commonly affects the lower extremity and perineum; the involved limb is often undergrown.[26] The macular lesion stains for GLUT1 and females (83%) usually are affected. Unlike typical IH, reticular tumors are: (1) infiltrative and not lobular; (2) involve fascia, muscle, or bone; and (3) are more likely to ulcerate and cause cardiac overload.[26] Reticular hemangioma also may be associated with hepatic hemangioma as well as ventral-caudal anomalies (omphalocele, rectovaginal fistula, vaginal/uterine duplication, solitary/duplex kidney, imperforate anus, tethered cord).[26] After involution small veins often remain, which may be treated by sclerotherapy.

Lumbosacral hemangioma

Large, superficial, plaque-like, or reticular IH rarely may be associated with underlying spinal, urogenital, or anorectal malformations when it is located in the lumbosacral midline (tethered cord, imperforate anus, abnormal genitalia, renal anomalies, lipomyelomeningocele).[27–31] Ultrasonography is obtained to rule out associated anomalies in infants younger than 4 months. MRI is indicated in older infants or when ultrasonography is equivocal.

PHACE association

PHACE association affects 2.3% of all patients with IH, and consists of a plaque-like IH in a "segmental" or trigeminal dermatomal distribution of the face with at least one of the following anomalies: *P*osterior fossa brain malformation, *H*emangioma, *A*rterial cerebrovascular anomalies, *C*oarctation of the aorta and cardiac defects, *E*ye/*E*ndocrine abnormalities.[32] When ventral developmental defects (*S*ternal clefting or *S*upraumbilical raphe) are present the condition is termed PHACES association.[32] Ninety percent of infants are female and cerebrovascular anomalies are the most common associated finding (72%).[33] Less than one-third of children have more than one extracutaneous feature. Because 8% of children with PHACE have a stroke in infancy and 42% have a structural brain anomaly, patients with suspected PHACE association should have an MRI to evaluate the brain and cerebrovasculature.[34] If an anomaly is present, neurologic consultation is obtained. Aspirin therapy may be considered to reduce the risk of stroke if a cerebrovascular malformation is noted.[33] Patients also should be referred for ophthalmologic, endocrine, and cardiac evaluation to rule out associated anomalies.[34]

Nonoperative Management

Observation

Most IH are managed by observation because 90% are small, localized, and do not involve aesthetically or functionally important areas (**Fig. 3**).[8] Infants are followed closely, on a monthly basis, during the proliferative phase if a lesion has the potential to cause obstruction, destruction, or ulceration requiring intervention. Once the IH has stabilized in growth, patients are followed annually during the involuting phase if intervention may be necessary in childhood for excess skin, residual fibrofatty tissue, or to reconstruct damaged structures.

Wound care

During the proliferative phase at least 16% of hemangiomas ulcerate at a median age of 4 months; labial, neck, and anogenital tumors are most likely to ulcerate.[35] Superficial IH is prone to skin breakdown because the integument is damaged by the tumor. In addition, arteriovenous

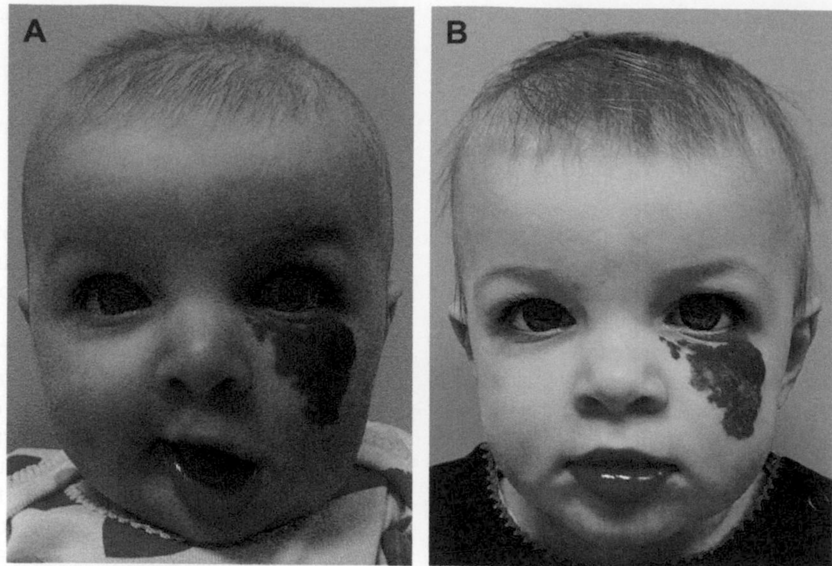

Fig. 3. Observation of IH. (*A*) A 3-month-old female with a superficial tumor not threatening vital structures. (*B*) The IH is involuting at 12 months of age.

shunting reduces capillary oxygen delivery and thus the skin is ischemic. Consequently, desiccation or minor injury can cause a wound to form; tumors located in trauma-prone areas are most likely to ulcerate. To reduce the risk of ulceration, the IH is kept moist during the proliferative phase with hydrated petroleum to minimize desiccation as well as to protect against accidental shearing of the skin. IH in the anogenital area may be further protected by using a petroleum gauze barrier to prevent friction from the diaper.

If ulceration develops, the wound is washed gently with soap and water at least twice daily. Small, superficial areas are managed by topical antibiotic ointment and occasionally with a petroleum gauze barrier (**Fig. 4**). Large, deep wounds require damp-to-dry dressing changes. To minimize discomfort, a small amount of topical lidocaine may be applied no more than 4 times daily to avoid toxicity. EMLA (eutectic mixture of local anesthetics) contains prilocaine and should not be used in infants younger than 3 months because of the risk of methemoglobinemia.

If bleeding occurs it is minor, and is treated by applying direct pressure. Almost all ulcerations heal with local wound care and the elimination of extrinsic factors that may have contributed to the ulceration. If the ulceration fails to heal with

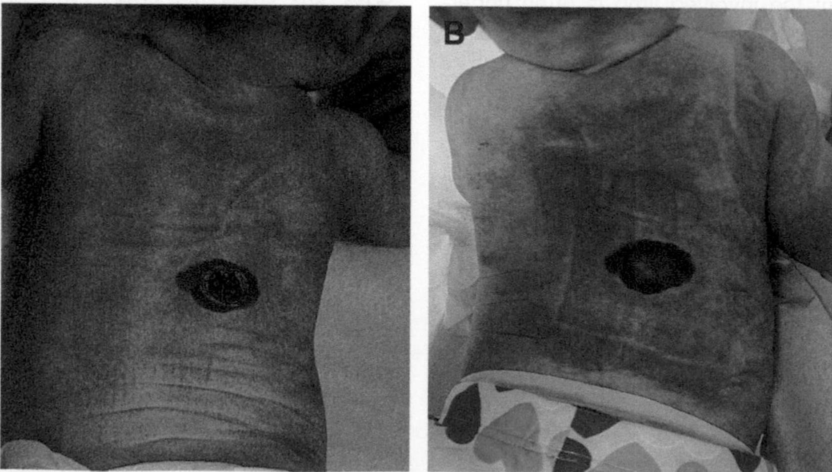

Fig. 4. Management of ulcerated IH. (*A*) A 4-month-old female with an ulcerated tumor of the posterior trunk. (*B*) The ulceration has healed 3 weeks following local wound care.

conservative measures and continues to be problematic, intralesional or oral corticosteroid may be necessary to provide a more favorable intrinsic environment for wound healing. By stabilizing the growth of the IH, pharmacotherapy reduces the tumor burden of the skin, arteriovenous shunting, and ischemia.

Topical corticosteroid

Topical corticosteroid has minimal efficacy, especially against IH involving the deep dermis and subcutis. Ultrapotent agents (clobetasol propionate 0.05% twice a day) may be effective for small, superficial IH, particularly in the periorbital area. However, their efficacy is inferior to intralesional corticosteroid. Although lightening may occur, if an underlying mass is present it will not be affected.[36–38] Adverse effects include hypopigmentation, skin atrophy, and possible adrenal suppression.[39]

Intralesional corticosteroid

Small, well-localized IH that obstruct the visual axis or nasal airway, or those at risk for damaging aesthetically sensitive structures (ie, eyelid, lip, nose) are best managed by intralesional corticosteroid. Corticosteroid accelerates involution of IH because it is antiangiogenic; it inhibits macrophage function and its production of vascular endothelial growth factor and basic fibroblast growth factor.[40] Corticosteroid also inhibits phospholipase A2, the enzyme that releases arachidonic acid, the precursor to the proangiogenic prostaglandins.[40]

Corticosteroid injection (triamcinolone 3 mg/kg) stabilizes the growth of the lesion in at least 95% of patients, and 75% of tumors decrease in size (**Fig. 5**).[41] The corticosteroid lasts 4 to 6 weeks and thus young children may require additional injections during the proliferative phase. Intralesional corticosteroid may cause subcutaneous fat atrophy. Blindness has been reported following injection of periorbital hemangioma, possibly due to embolic occlusion of the retinal artery.[42,43] Adrenal suppression may occur with large volume injections, although adverse sequelae have not been reported.[44]

Systemic corticosteroid

Problematic IH that is too large to treat with intralesional corticosteroid is managed by daily oral prednisolone (Orapred). The patient is started on 3 mg/kg/d for 1 month, which then is tapered by 0.5 mL every 2 to 4 weeks until it is discontinued between 9 and 10 months of age when the tumor is no longer proliferating. One dose is given in the morning to facilitate compliance and minimize adrenal suppression. Live attenuated vaccines are not administered during treatment. The dose should be weaned slowly to prevent rebound growth and should not be stopped abruptly to avoid adrenal crisis.

Recently, propranolol has been described for the treatment of IH, but its efficacy and safety compared with corticosteroid has not been studied.[45,46] Although preliminary data appear promising, bradycardia, hypotension, and hypoglycemia have been reported in infants receiving propranolol for IH.[47,48] Corticosteroid, in contrast, has been used to treat IH for more than 40 years and has proven to be very safe and effective.[49–53] Overall, 84% of patients treated with different doses of corticosteroid have (1) stabilization of growth or (2) accelerated regression.[51] Almost all patients, however, respond to 3 mg/kg (**Fig. 6**).[51]

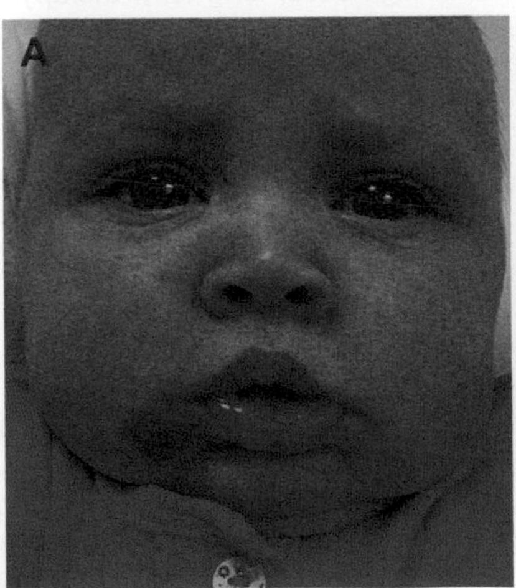

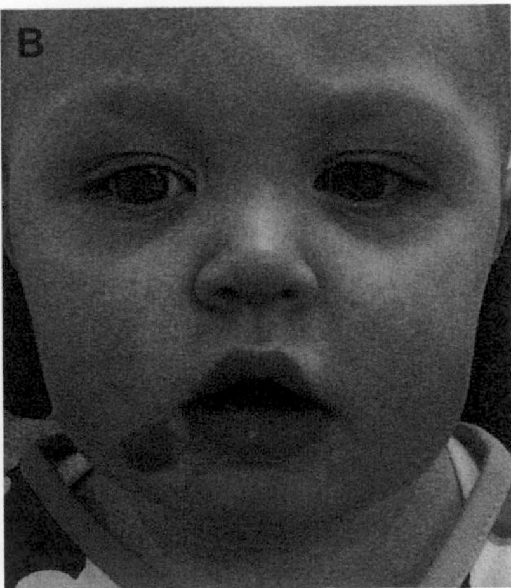

Fig. 5. Management of IH with intralesional corticosteroid. (*A*) A 2.5-month-old female with a localized, rapidly enlarging tumor treated with triamcinolone injection. (*B*) Accelerated involution at 11 months of age.

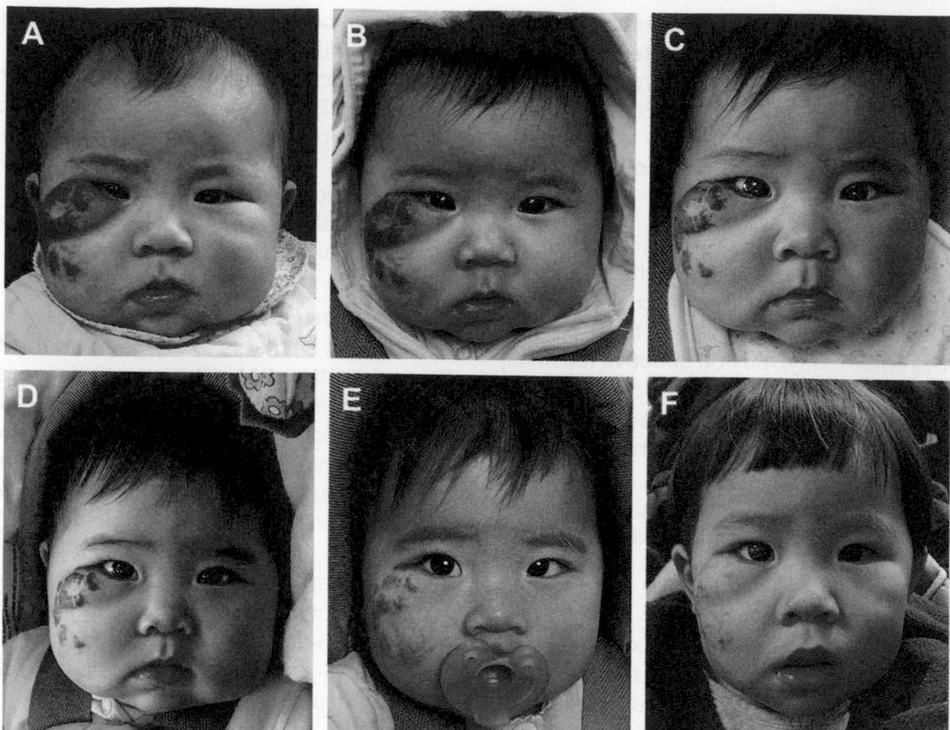

Fig. 6. Treatment of problematic IH with oral corticosteroid. (*A*) A 4-month-old female with an enlarging tumor causing a significant deformity and threatening vision. (*B*) Age 5 months, 1 month after starting daily oral prednisolone 3 mg/kg. Note opening of palpebral fissure and reduced size of IH (*C*) Age 8 months, IH continues to involute after 4 months on corticosteroid taper. (*D*) Age 10 months, weaning off prednisolone. (*E*) Age 12 months, off corticosteroid. (*F*) Age 24 months with minimal residual deformity as the IH continues to involute.

Treatment response usually is evident within 1 week of therapy by signs of involution: decreased growth rate, fading color, and softening of the lesion. The location of the hemangioma does not affect response rate.[54] For the rare lesion that fails to stabilize with corticosteroid, the dose may be increased up to 5 mg/kg.[55] Alternatively, the child may be switched to vincristine.[56–59] Interferon is not advocated in children younger than 12 months because it may cause spastic diplegia.[60–62]

Short-term side effects of corticosteroid treatment for IH are reversible after cessation of therapy, and may include cushingoid face, personality change, or gastric irritation; cutaneous fungal growth and myopathy are rare.[50] Approximately one-third of infants exhibit decreased gain in height, but they return to their pretreatment growth curve by 24 months of age.[50,63] This risk falls to 12% for patients treated after 3 months of age for less than 6 months.[50] Although some infants may become hypertensive, the clinical significance of this is unclear and no side effects have been reported.[50,64] No increased risk of infection has been shown in patients receiving corticosteroid for infantile hemangioma.[50,51,64] In fact, corticosteroid often is given to accelerate healing of infected, ulcerated tumors.

Long-term complications of corticosteroid (ie, adverse neurodevelopment, aseptic necrosis of the femoral head, diabetes, osteoporosis, adrenal insufficiency, cataracts, glaucoma) are associated with high-dose, long-term therapy[65,66] and have not been observed in patients treated with corticosteroid for IH.[50–53,63,64,67] Unlike patients with hypercortisolism or those taking chronic corticosteroid for inflammatory disorders, children with infantile hemangioma are only treated for several months. In addition, the dose of the drug is rapidly weaned as (1) the infant gains weight and (2) the physician lowers the dose every few weeks.

Embolic therapy

Large IH, most commonly multifocal hepatic lesions, may cause high-output congestive heart failure. Embolization may be indicated for the initial control of heart failure while the therapeutic effects of systemic corticosteroid are pending. Cardiac failure often recurs even after initial improvement, and drug therapy should be continued after embolization until the child is approximately 9 to 10 months of age, when natural involution begins.

Laser therapy

Pulsed-dye laser treatment for proliferating IH is contraindicated. The laser penetrates only 0.75 to 1.2 mm into the dermis and thus only affects the superficial portion of the tumor. Although lightening may occur, the mass is not affected and accelerated involution does not occur.[68,69] Instead, patients have an increased risk of skin atrophy and hypopigmentation.[69] The thermal injury delivered by the laser to the ischemic dermis increases the risk of ulceration and thus pain, bleeding, and scarring.[70] The pulsed-dye laser is indicated, however, during the involuted phase to treat residual telangiectasias. Unlike the pulse-dye laser, a carbon dioxide laser may be useful for the treatment of a proliferating subglottic IH.[21]

Operative Management

Indications

Ninety percent of IH proliferate and involute without sequelae; no intervention is required.[20] During the proliferative phase, however, 10% ulcerate, bleed, or destroy/obstruct important structures. First-line therapy for a problematic proliferating IH usually is corticosteroid; operative treatment in infancy generally is not recommended. The tumor is highly vascular during this period and the patient is at risk for blood loss, iatrogenic injury, and an inferior aesthetic outcome, as compared with excising residual tissue after the tumor has regressed.[54,71–73] Anesthetic morbidity also is 3 to 8 times greater in infants than in children older than 1 year.[74–77] Although operative treatment of hemangioma during the proliferating phase is uncommon, patients may require intervention in childhood because approximately 50% of IH leave residual fibrofatty tissue, redundant skin, or damaged structures after involution.[8]

Timing

Proliferative phase (infancy) Although operative intervention for IH generally is not advocated in infancy, occasionally the benefits of resection outweigh the risks. Factors that lower the threshold for excision of a problematic proliferating IH include (1) failure or contraindication to corticosteroid, (2) well localized in an anatomically safe area, (3) complicated reconstruction is not required, and (4) resection will be necessary in the future and the scar will be the same (**Figs. 7** and **8**).[8] For example, a localized, ulcerated scalp IH may be better managed by excision because the risk of iatrogenic injury is low, the laxity of the scalp in infancy facilitates resection, and the patient will require a procedure in early childhood to correct alopecia. By contrast, a large, problematic lesion located in a sensitive area of the face should be managed by corticosteroid because the extent of resection, risk of iatrogenic injury, and scar length is greater, in comparison to allowing the IH to become smaller and less vascular before resection in childhood.

Involuting phase (early childhood) Although operative management of IH generally is avoided during the proliferative phase, resection during involution is much safer because the lesion is less vascular and smaller. Because the extent of the excision and reconstruction is reduced, the aesthetic outcome is superior. Approximately 50% of IH leave behind fibrofatty tissue or damaged skin after the tumor regresses, causing a deformity.[8] Less often, children require reconstruction of damaged structures (ie, nose, ear, lip).

Staged or total excision should be considered during this period, rather than waiting for complete involution if (1) it is clear that the patient will require resection (ie, postulceration scarring, destroyed structures, expanded skin, significant fibrofatty residuum), (2) the length of the scar would be similar if the procedure was postponed to the involuted phase, or (3) the scar is in a favorable location (**Figs. 9** and **10**). The advantage of operative intervention during this period as compared with late childhood is that reconstruction is performed before the child's development of memory or awareness of body differences. Consequently, low self-esteem and psychosocial morbidity may be prevented. If it is obvious that a patient requires excision of residual fibrofatty tissue, scarred/excess skin, or reconstruction of damaged structures, it is preferable to intervene before 3.5 years of age when long-term memory and personal identity begin to develop.[78–80] At this time, the IH has had at least 2 years to regress, the patient does not have a memory of the procedure, and the deformity is corrected early to prevent psychosocial morbidity. Some parents, however, may elect to wait until the child is older and able to make the decision to proceed with operative intervention, especially if the deformity is minor.

Involuted phase (late childhood) Waiting until the IH has fully involuted before resection ensures that the least amount of fibrofatty residuum and excess skin is resected, giving the smallest possible scar. Allowing full involution to occur, however, must be weighed against the psychosocial morbidity of maintaining a deformity until late childhood. Allowing full involution is advocated for lesions when it is

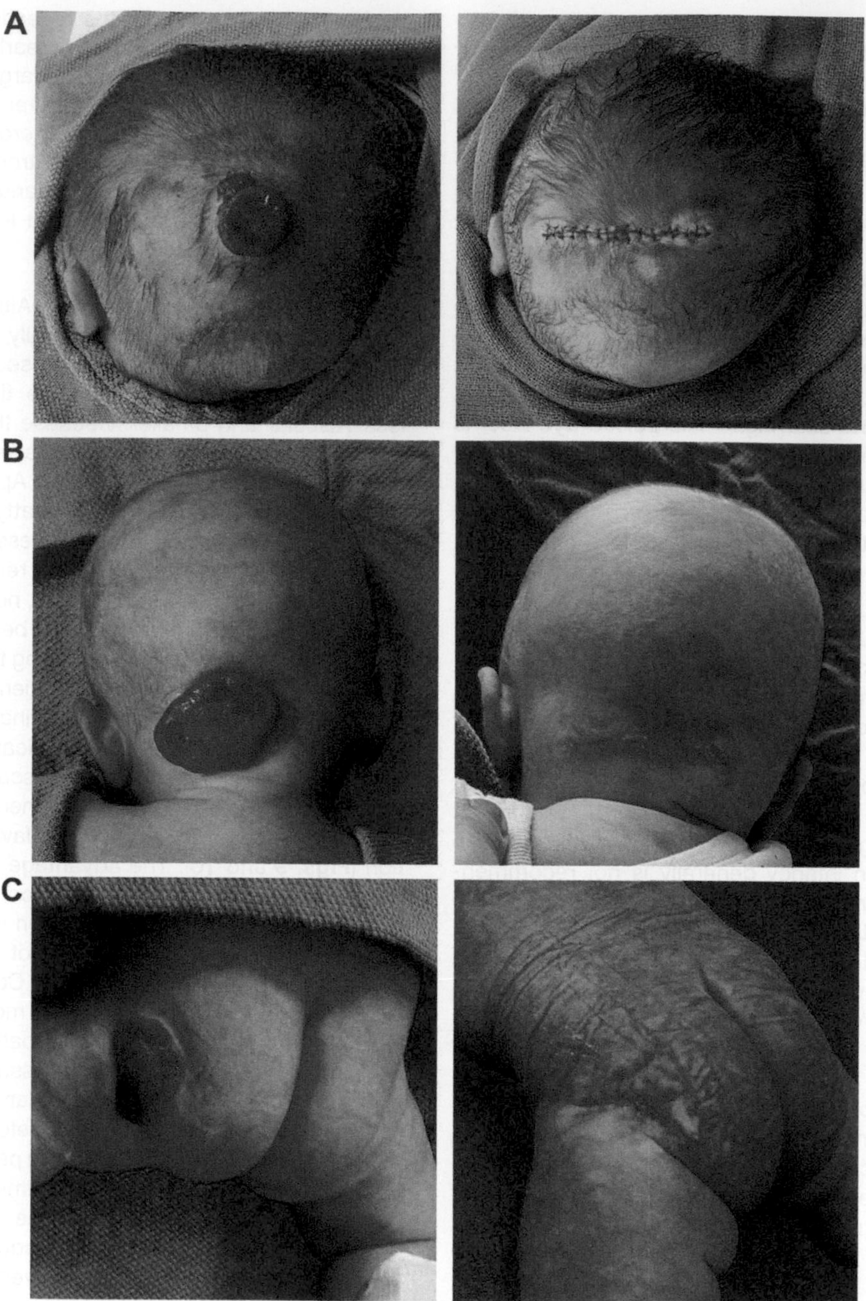

Fig. 7. Operative management of proliferating IH with lenticular excision and linear closure. (*A*) A 4-month-old male with an ulcerated scalp IH that would ultimately require resection for residual fibrofatty tissue and alopecia. Note the length of the scar is approximately 3 times the diameter of the circular tumor. (*B*) A 5-month-old female with an ulcerated neck IH. (*C*) A 3-month-old female with an ulcerated IH of the left buttock.

unclear if a surgical scar would leave a worse deformity than the appearance of the residual hemangioma.

Operative Principles and Techniques

Before excising a proliferating IH, the area should be infiltrated with an epinephrine-containing local anesthetic to minimize blood loss and iatrogenic injury; a tourniquet may be used when resecting an extremity lesion. Because the tumor acts as a tissue expander, usually there is adequate skin to allow primary, linear closure of the wound. Circular lesions located in visible areas, particularly the face, are best treated by circular excision

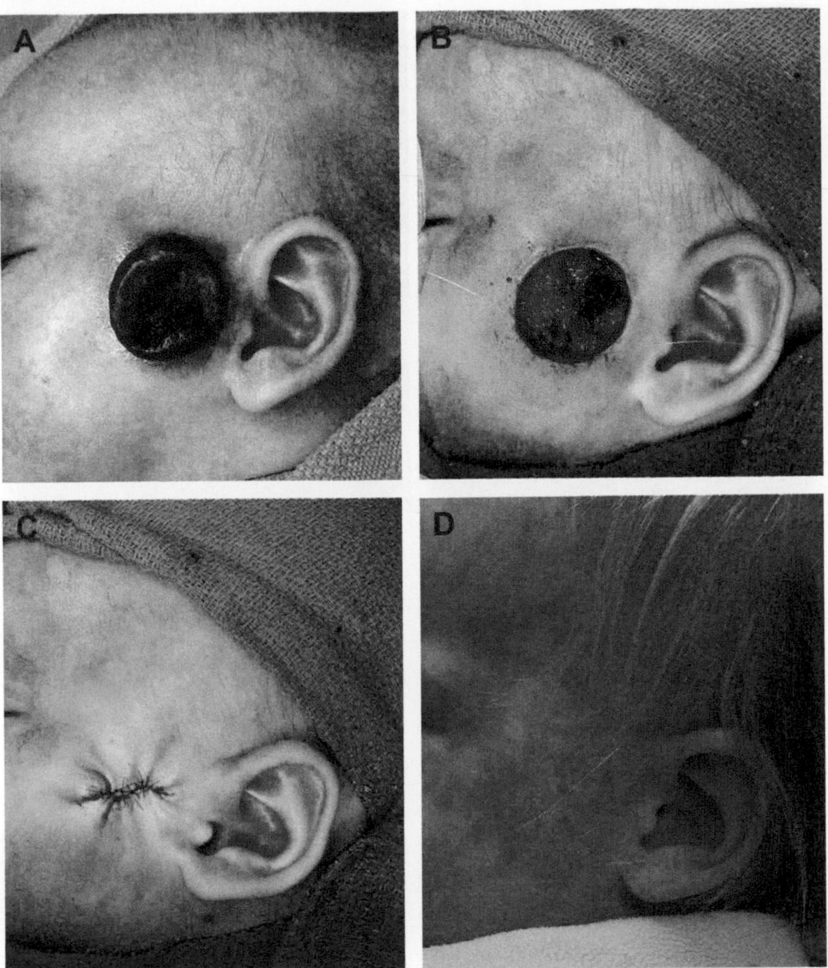

Fig. 8. (*A–D*) Operative management of proliferating IH with circular excision and purse-string closure. A 6-month-old female with a localized, ulcerated IH of the cheek not involving sensitive structures. Resection would ultimately be required for residual fibrofatty residuum and damaged skin. Circular excision and purse-string closure was chosen to limit scar length to the original diameter of the lesion.

and purse-string closure.[81] This technique takes advantage of the skin laxity produced by the hemangioma and minimizes the length of the scar as well as distortion of surrounding structures. A lenticular excision of a circular hemangioma results in a scar as long as 3 times the diameter of the lesion, whereas a 2-stage circular resection followed by lenticular excision 6 to 12 months later leaves a scar approximately the same length as the diameter of the original hemangioma.[81] For larger lesions, multiple circular excisions and purse-string closures can minimize the length of the scar. Approximately one-half of families do not elect for a second stage to convert the circular scar into a line. The circular scar can be difficult to appreciate; it may appear similar to an acne or chicken-pox scar. The disadvantage of circular excision and purse-string closure is that a second stage may be required, and the skin around the edges of the circular scar may not flatten for several weeks. In the scalp, lenticular excision and linear closure is preferred to circular excision/purse-string closure because (1) the length of the scar in the scalp is not critical because it is covered by hair, (2) the procedure has one stage, (3) the scalp lacks skin redundancy necessary for purse-string closure, and (4) the circular scar may leave an area of alopecia necessitating another stage (see **Fig. 7**).

CONGENITAL HEMANGIOMA

Clinical Features

CH is fully grown at birth and does not illustrate postnatal growth.[82–84] CH has a different appearance to IH; it is red-violaceous with coarse

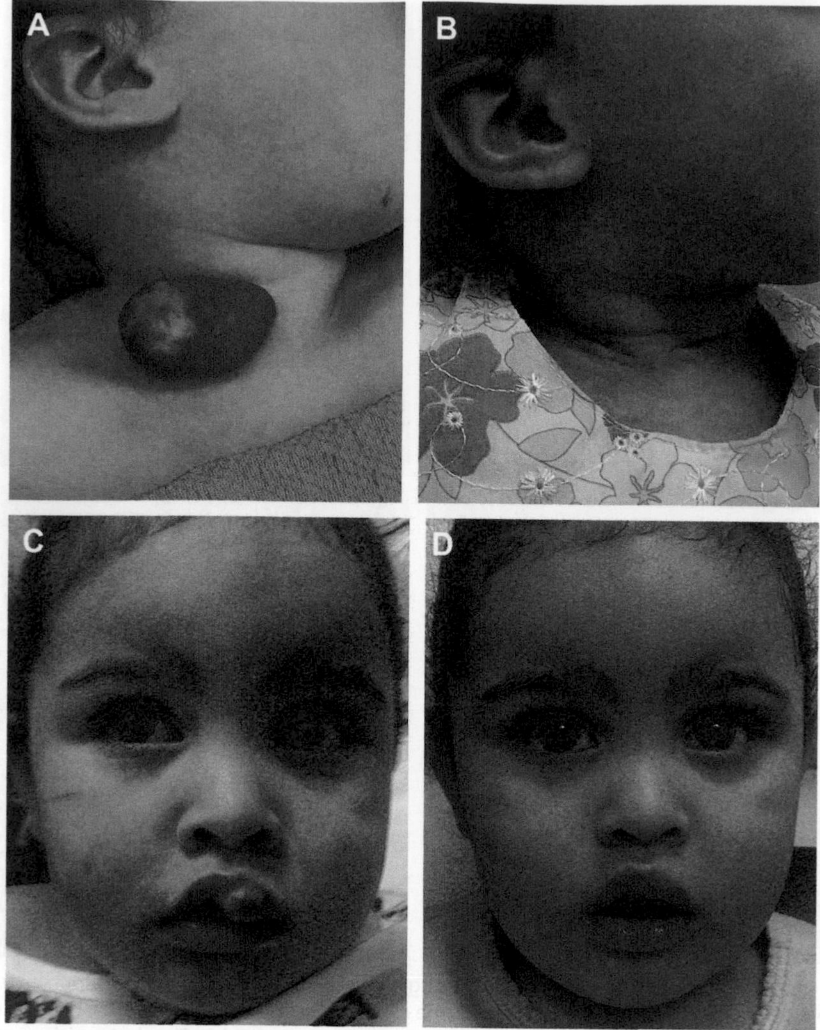

Fig. 9. Operative management of an involuting IH. (*A*) A 2.5 year-old female with an IH complicated by fibrofatty residuum and a large scar secondary to ulceration in infancy. (*B*) A one-stage lenticular excision was chosen because the length-to-width ratio favored linear closure, and the scar is concealed in a relaxed skin tension line. (*C*) A 2.5-year-old female with a residual fibrofatty IH of the upper lip. (*D*) The lesion was removed using a transverse mucosal incision.

telangiectasias, central pallor, and a peripheral pale halo. Unlike IH, CH is more common in the extremities, has an equal sex distribution, and is solitary, with an average diameter of 5 cm.[82–84] Two types of CH exist: rapidly involuting congenital hemangioma (RICH) and noninvoluting congenital hemangioma (NICH). RICH involutes immediately after birth and 50% of lesions have completed regression by 7 months of age; the remaining tumors are fully involuted by 14 months (**Fig. 11**).[82,84] RICH affects the head or neck (42%), limbs (52%), or trunk (6%).[82,84] After involution, RICH does not leave behind a significant adipose component, unlike IH.[84] NICH, in contrast, does not undergo involution and rarely ulcerates (**Fig. 12**).[83] NICH involves the head or neck (43%), limbs (38%), or trunk (19%).[83]

Management

Rapidly involuting congenital hemangioma

RICH does not require operative management in infancy because it undergoes accelerated postnatal regression; tumors are observed. Occasionally, RICH is complicated by congestive heart failure, which is controlled by corticosteroid or embolization as the lesion involutes. After regression RICH may cause a residual deformity, usually atrophic skin and subcutaneous tissue (**Fig. 13**).

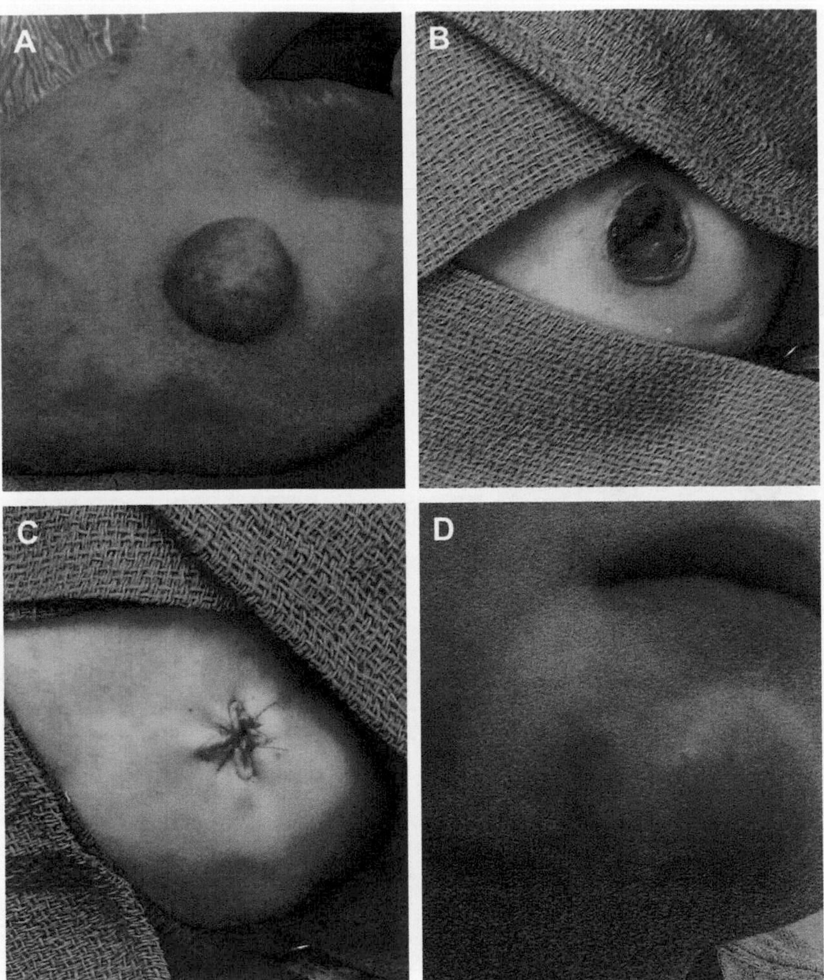

Fig. 10. (*A–D*) Operative management of an involuting IH with circular excision and purse-string closure. A 2.5-year-old male with a residual fibrofatty IH of the chin. Circular excision and purse-string closure was chosen to limit the length of the scar to the diameter of the original lesion.

Reconstruction of damaged skin or atrophic subcutaneous tissue can begin as early as 3.5 years of age, before memory and self-esteem begin to form. Alternatively, some families may elect to wait until the child wishes to have the area improved later in childhood or during adolescence. Operative intervention for RICH must not create a more obvious deformity than the lesion. Because RICH may leave behind atrophic tissue, reconstruction with autologous grafts (fat, dermis) or acellular dermis may be indicated. Residual telangiectasias can be lightened with a pulsed-dye laser.

Noninvoluting congenital hemangioma

NICH is rarely problematic in infancy and is observed. Because NICH is benign, asymptomatic tumors do not require excision. However, the threshold for resection of a problematic NICH is lower than that for IH because NICH does not involute or respond to pharmacotherapy. Symptomatic lesions in infancy are managed with either embolization or resection. Most NICH, however, are nonproblematic and do not cause a significant deformity.

Resection may be indicated to improve the appearance of the affected area, as long as the surgical scar is less noticeable than the lesion. Parents may elect to have a visible lesion excised in early childhood before the onset of memory, or wait until the child makes his or her decision to remove the lesion when they are older. Patients with a NICH may not elect for resection if the intervention would leave a more noticeable deformity than

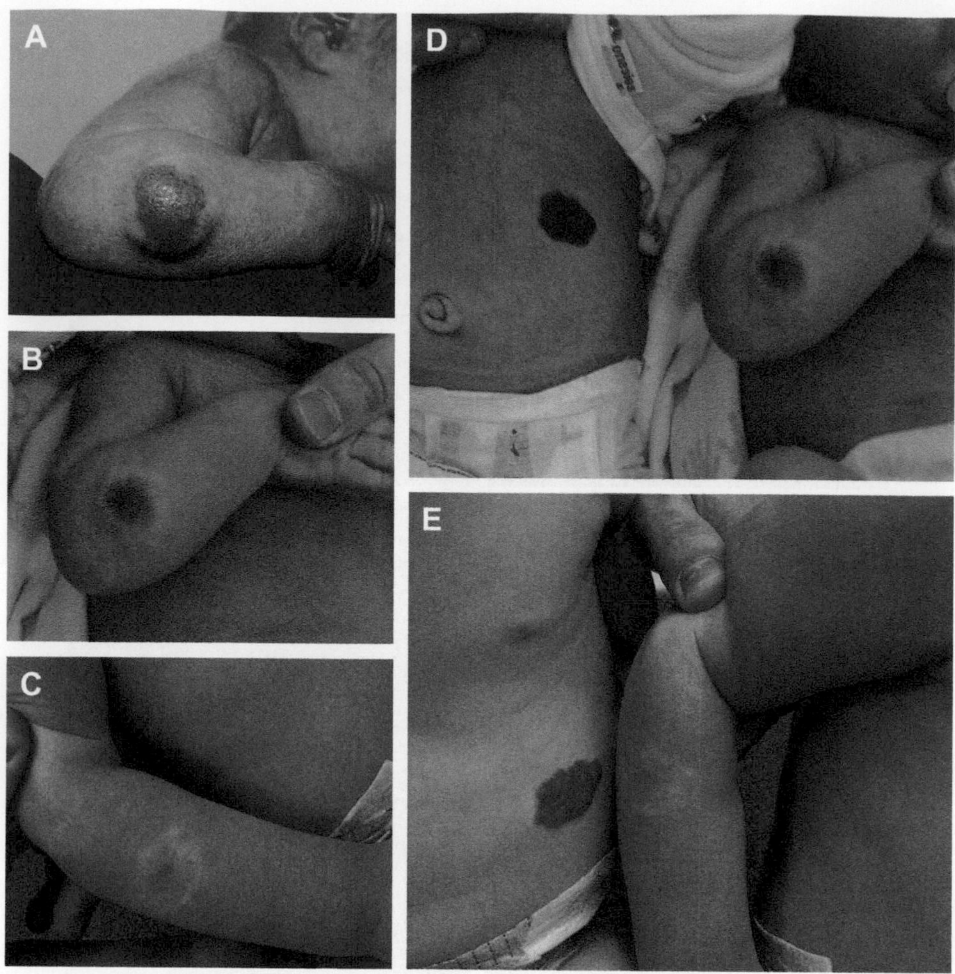

Fig. 11. Rapidly involuting congenital hemangioma (RICH). (*A–C*) A newborn male with RICH of the upper extremity (*A*); rapid regression at 6 weeks of age (*B*); complete involution at 12 months of age (*C*). (*D, E*) Comparison of RICH with twin sister's infantile hemangioma of the trunk at 6 weeks of age (*D*) and at 12 months of age (*E*); the RICH has completely involuted, unlike the infantile hemangioma.

the tumor. Pulsed-dye laser therapy may improve the appearance of the NICH by eliminating telangiectasias.

KAPOSIFORM HEMANGIOENDOTHELIOMA

Clinical Features

Kaposiform hemangioendothelioma (KHE) is a rare vascular neoplasm that is locally aggressive, but does not metastasize.[85–88] Although one-half of lesions are present at birth, KHE may develop during infancy (58%), between age 1 and 10 years (32%), or after 11 years of age (10%).[89] In contrast to IH, KHE has an equal sex distribution, is solitary, and affects the head/neck (40%), trunk (30%), or extremity (30%).[89,90] The tumor is often greater than 5 cm in diameter, and thus larger than the typical IH.[87,91]

KHE causes a visible deformity as well as pain. In addition, 50% of patients have Kasabach-Merritt phenomenon (KMP) (thrombocytopenia <25,000/mm^3, petechiae, bleeding).[86–88,91] Fibrinogen is low and fibrin-split products (D-dimers) are elevated. KHE enlarges in early childhood and then partially regresses after 2 years of age; it usually persists long term, causing chronic pain and stiffness.[92] KHE has overlapping clinical and histopathological features with another tumor, tufted angioma, suggesting they are on the same neoplastic spectrum. KMP also may complicate tufted angioma, which has a similar anatomic distribution as KHE but is more erythematous and plaque-like.[14,88]

Although KHE is considered a pediatric tumor, adult onset has been described.[93,94] In adults, the mean age at diagnosis is 42.9 years (range

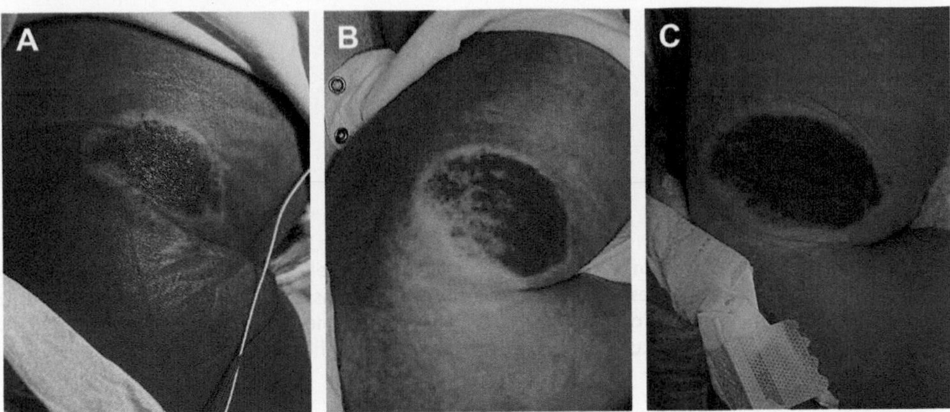

Fig. 12. Noninvoluting congenital hemangioma (NICH). (*A*) A newborn with congenital hemangioma present at birth. Note purple color, telangiectasias, and peripheral halo. (*B*) Age 3 months with minimal changes since birth. (*C*) Age 9 months; no signs of involution.

22–64 years) and males are usually affected (80%).[94] Although the anatomic distribution is similar to children with KHE, lesions are smaller; two-thirds are less than 2 cm (average 4.5 cm; range 0.6–15 cm).[94] The small size of these tumors may explain why adult-onset KHE does not cause KMP; lesions less than 8 cm are less likely to cause a platelet abnormality.[91,95]

Diagnosis

KHE is diagnosed by history and physical examination. Unlike IH, it is usually present at birth as a flat, reddish-purple, edematous lesion that does not exhibit rapid postnatal growth; it is also associated with KMP. MRI is indicated for diagnostic confirmation and to evaluate the extent of the tumor. MRI shows poorly defined margins, small vessels, and invasion of adjacent tissues.[12,87,94] In addition, lymphatic involvement causes T2 hyperintensity in subcutaneous tissue as well as postgadolinium enhancement on T1-weighted images. Hemosiderin can cause signal voids in the absence of fast flow.[12,87,94]

Histologically, KHE shows infiltrating sheets or nodules of endothelial cells lining capillaries.[86,93,94] Hemosiderin-filled slit-like vascular spaces with red blood cell fragments, as well as dilated lymphatics, are present.[86,93] Tufted angioma may be distinguished from KHE by small tufts of capillaries (“cannonballs”) in the middle to lower third of the dermis.[14]

Nonoperative Management

Treatment of KHE depends on the size of the lesion and presence of KMP. A localized tumor can be resected, depending on its location. However, because most lesions are large and involve multiple tissues, complete extirpation usually is not possible. Patients with KMP require systemic treatment to prevent life-threatening

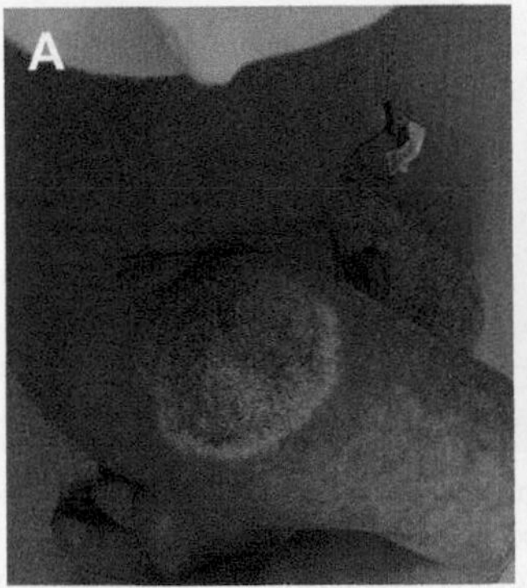

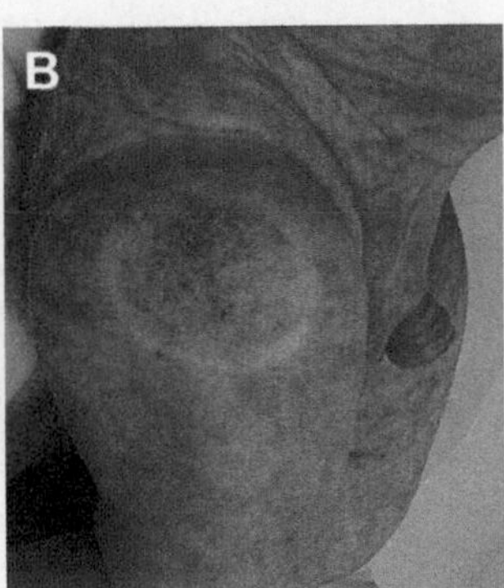

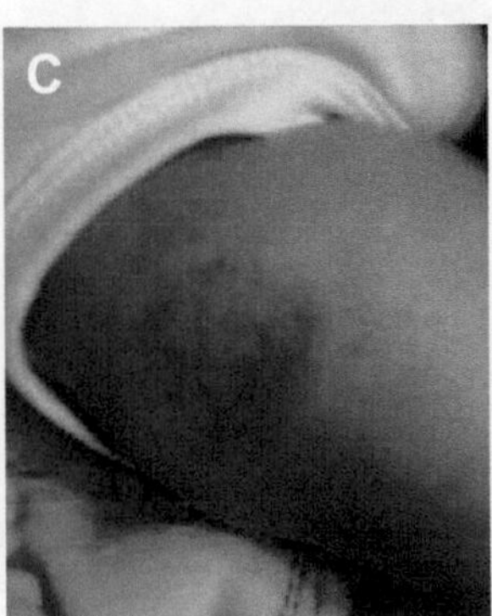

Fig. 13. Residual deformity after regression of a RICH. (*A*) A 2-week-old infant with a RICH present at birth. (*B*) Lesion is involuting at 8 weeks of age. (*C*) Atrophic skin and subcutaneous tissue remain after the tumor has completed regression at age 8 months.

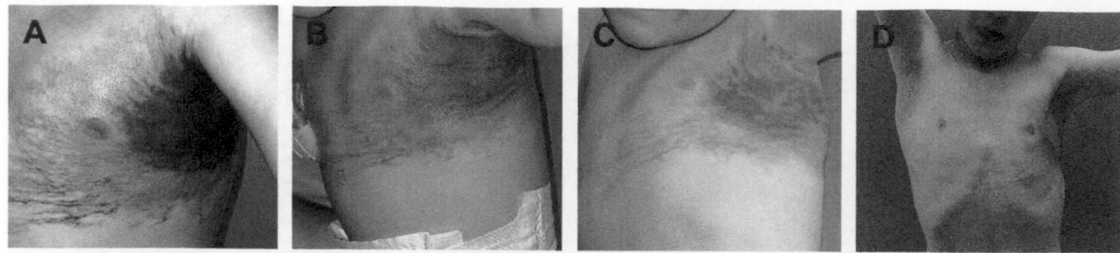

Fig. 14. Pharmacologic management of kaposiform hemangioendothelioma (KHE). (*A*) A 20-month-old male with diffuse KHE involving the left chest and axilla complicated by Kassabach-Merritt phenomenon. (*B*) At 27 months of age the tumor shows regression after treatment with vincristine. (*C*) At age 5 years the lesion continues to slowly regress. (*D*) Residual axillary contracture secondary to tumor fibrosis at 9 years of age.

complications (**Fig. 14**). Large, asymptomatic tumors also are managed with pharmacotherapy to minimize fibrosis and subsequent long-term pain and stiffness. KHE responds best to vincristine (90%), which is first-line therapy.[57] Vincristine is administered 0.05 to 0.065 mg/kg intravenously, weekly for 6 months. KHE does not respond as well to second-line drugs, interferon (50%), or corticosteroid (10%).[57,91] Thrombocytopenia does not improve after platelet transfusion because the platelets are trapped in the lesion, worsening the swelling. Platelet transfusion should

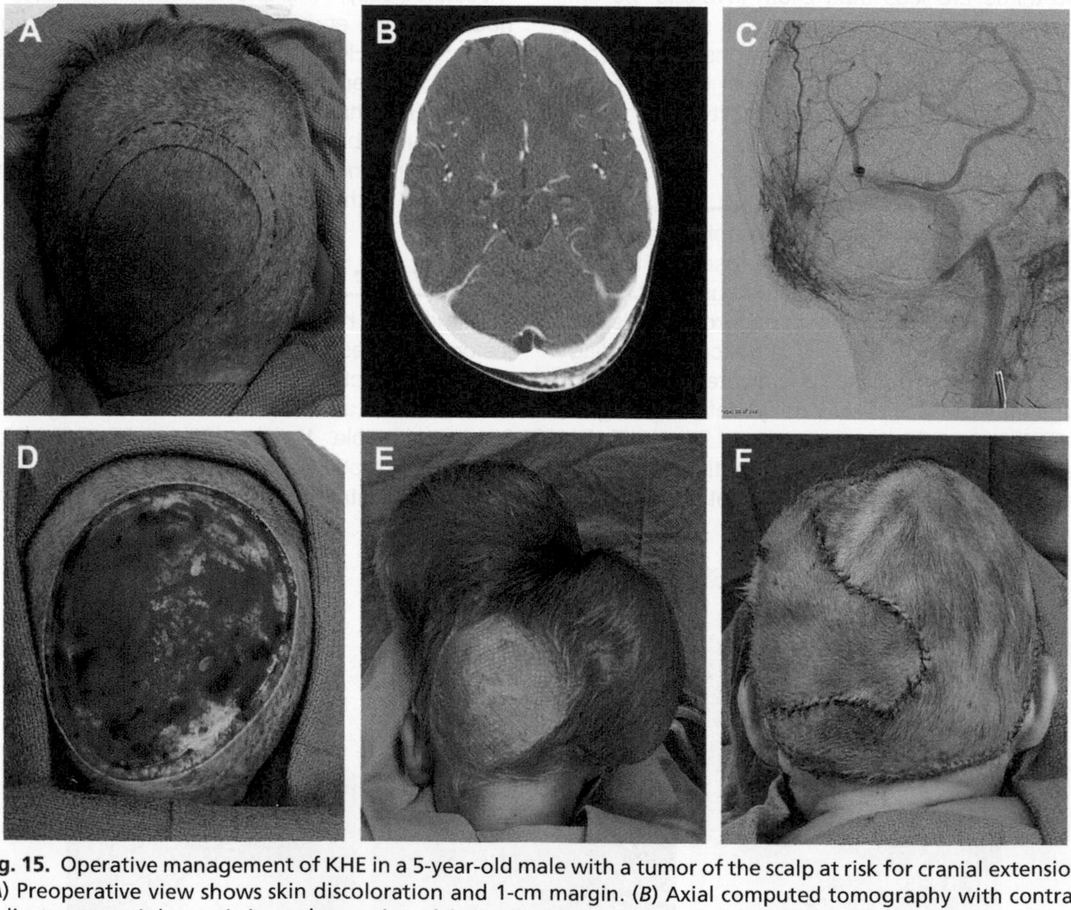

Fig. 15. Operative management of KHE in a 5-year-old male with a tumor of the scalp at risk for cranial extension. (*A*) Preoperative view shows skin discoloration and 1-cm margin. (*B*) Axial computed tomography with contrast indicates tumor is located above the cranium. (*C*) Preoperative angiography shows hypervascular tumor blush. (*D*) Intraoperative view following tumor resection. (*E*) Completed tissue expansion and healed split-thickness skin graft over the extirpation site. (*F*) Restoration of hair-bearing scalp after replacement of the skin graft with expanded flaps.

be avoided unless there is active bleeding or a surgical procedure is indicated. Heparin is not given because it can stimulate growth of the tumor, aggravate platelet trapping, and worsen bleeding. By 2 years of age, the tumor often undergoes partial involution and the platelet count normalizes.

Operative Management

Most patients with KHE have diffuse tumors involving multiple tissue planes and important structures, and thus are difficult to resect; they are best managed with chemotherapy until they "burn-out" in early childhood. Operative management may be possible for small lesions that more commonly present in older children and adults. Removal of larger areas also may be indicated for symptomatic patients with relatively localized tumors or who have failed chemotherapy (**Fig. 15**). During childhood, reconstruction for secondary deformities caused by the tumor (ie, contractures) may be necessary. Resection is not required for lesions that are not causing functional problems because KHE is benign. The risks of the resection and the resulting deformity should be weighed against the appearance of the tumor.

PYOGENIC GRANULOMA

Clinical Features

PG has been called lobular capillary hemangioma.[96] PG is a solitary red papule that grows rapidly, forming a stalk. PG is small, with an average diameter of 6.5 mm (range 2–20 mm); 75.0% of lesions are less than 1 cm in diameter.[97] The male:female ratio is 2:1. PG is commonly complicated by bleeding (64.2%) and ulceration (36.3%). The mean age of onset is 6.7 years; only 12.4% develop during the first year of life. The presentation is inversely correlated with age: younger than 5 years (42.1%), 5 to 10 years (30.4%), 10 to 15 years (23.0%), and 15 to 20 years (4.5%).[97] PG primarily involves the skin (88.2%), but can involve mucous membranes as well (11.8%). It is distributed on the head or neck (62%), trunk (19%), upper extremity (13%), or lower extremity (5%). Within the head and neck, affected sites include cheek (28.8%), oral cavity (13.5%), scalp (10.8%), forehead (9.9%), eyelid

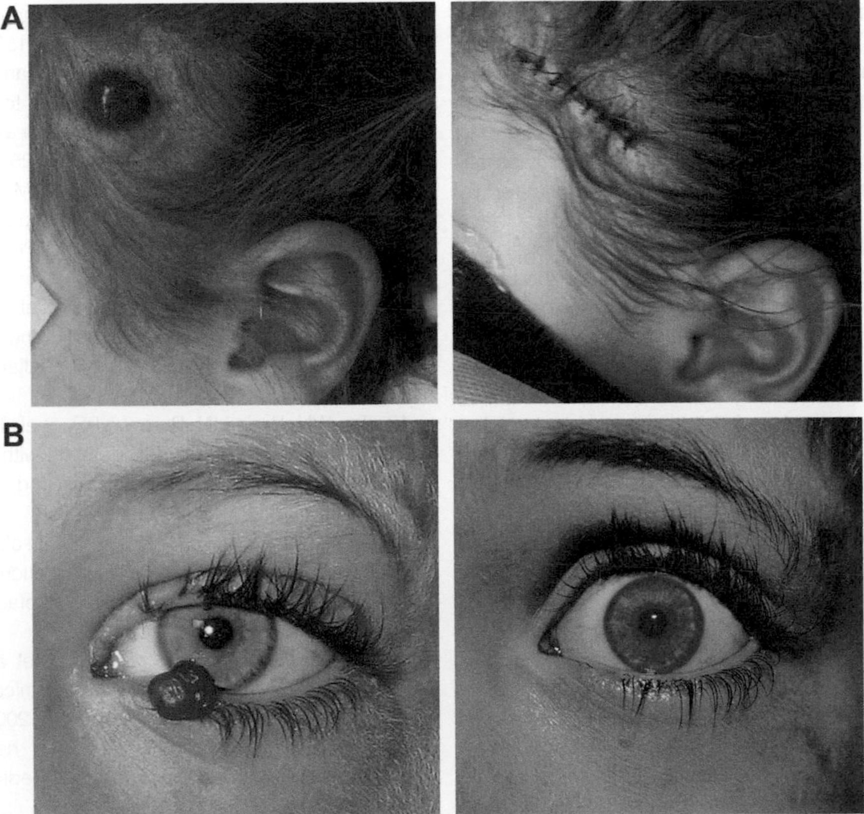

Fig. 16. Operative management of pyogenic granuloma. (*A*) A 5-year-old female with a 3-month history of an enlarging, bleeding lesion of the temporal scalp. (*B*) A 5-year-old male with a 2-month history of a bleeding lower eyelid lesion.

(9.0%), or lips (9.0%).[97] Twenty-five percent of patients have a history of trauma or an underlying cutaneous condition (ie, capillary malformation).

Diagnosis

PG rarely appears within the first month of life, unlike IH, CH, or KHE. Instead it commonly develops in the head and neck of young children. PG is smaller than IH, CH, or KHE, with an average size of 6.5 mm. In addition, unlike IH, CH, or KHE, the lesion is often pedunculated and complicated by frequent bleeding.

PG has normal numbers of mast cells, in contrast to a proliferating IH.[97] It appears as an exophytic mass attached to a narrow stalk on low power. The superficial lesion typically shows immature capillaries with interspersed fibroblastic tissue, resembling granulation tissue in an edematous matrix. The deeper portion of the lesion has proliferating capillaries arranged in a lobular pattern extending into the deep dermis, with a dense, fibrous stroma.[96,97]

Management

PG usually is complicated by ulceration and bleeding; it also causes a visible deformity because it is commonly located on the face. Consequently, most patients with PG require operative intervention. PG should be treated after diagnosis to prevent ulceration and bleeding complications. PG may become temporarily smaller after bleeding and crusting, which is followed by regrowth. Numerous treatment methods have been described for PG: curettage, shave excision, laser therapy, or excision.[97,98] Because the lesion can involve the reticular dermis, it may be out of the reach of the pulsed-dye laser, cautery, or shave excision. Consequently these modalities have a recurrence rate of 43.5%, and definitive management requires full-thickness skin excision (**Fig. 16**).[97]

REFERENCES

1. Mulliken JB, Glowacki J. Hemangiomas and vascular malformations in infants and children: a classification based on endothelial characteristics. Plast Reconstr Surg 1982;69:412–22.
2. Finn MC, Glowacki J, Mulliken JB. Congenital vascular lesions: clinical application of a new classification. J Pediatr Surg 1983;18:894–900.
3. Holmdahl K. Cutaneous hemangiomas in premature and mature infants. Acta Paediatr Scand 1955;44: 370–9.
4. Jacobs AH, Walton RG. The incidence of birthmarks in the neonate. J Pediatr 1976;58:218–22.
5. Kilcline C, Frieden IJ. Infantile hemangiomas: how common are they? A systematic review of the medical literature. Pediatr Dermatol 2008;25: 168–73.
6. Amir J, Metzker A, Krikler R, et al. Strawberry hemangioma in preterm infants. Pediatr Dermatol 1986;3:331–2.
7. Drolet BA, Swanson EA, Frieden IJ. Infantile hemangiomas: an emerging health issue linked to an increased rate of low birth weight infants. J Pediatr 2008;153:712–5.
8. Mulliken JB, Fishman SJ, Burrows PE. Vascular anomalies. Curr Probl Surg 2000;37:517–84.
9. Chang LC, Haggstrom AN, Drolet BA, et al. Growth characteristics of infantile hemangiomas: implications for management. Pediatrics 2008;122:360–7.
10. Bowers RE, Graham EA, Tomlinson KM. The natural history of the strawberry nevus. Arch Dermatol 1960; 82:667–80.
11. Paltiel H, Burrows PE, Kozakewich HPW, et al. Soft-tissue vascular anomalies: utility of US for diagnosis. Radiology 2000;214:747–54.
12. Burrows PE, Laor T, Paltiel H, et al. Diagnostic imaging in the evaluation of vascular birthmarks. Dermatol Clin 1998;16:455–88.
13. Meyer JS, Joffer FA, Barnes PD, et al. Biological classification of soft-tissue vascular anomalies: MR correlation. Am J Roentgenol 1991;157:559–64.
14. Jones EW, Orkin M. Tufted angioma (angioblastoma): a benign progressive angioma, not to be confused with Kaposi's sarcoma or low grade angiosarcoma. J Am Acad Dermatol 1989;20:214–25.
15. Chung KC, Weiss SW, Kuzon WM Jr. Multifocal congenital hemangiopericytomas associated with Kasabach-Merritt syndrome. Br J Plast Surg 1995; 48:240–2.
16. Boon LM, Fishman SJ, Lund DP, et al. Congenital fibrosarcoma masquerading as congenital hemangioma: report of two cases. J Pediatr Surg 1995; 30:1378–81.
17. Tan WH, Baris HN, Burrows PE, et al. The spectrum of vascular anomalies in patients with PTEN mutations: implications for diagnosis and management. J Med Genet 2007;44:594–602.
18. Merrell SC, Rahbar R, Alomari AI, et al. Infantile myofibroma or lymphatic malformation: differential diagnosis of neonatal cystic cervicofacial lesions. J Craniofac Surg 2010;21:422–6.
19. North PE, Waner M, Mizeracki A, et al. GLUT1. A newly discovered immunohistochemical marker for juvenile hemangiomas. Hum Pathol 2000;31:11–22.
20. Enjolras O, Gelbert F. Superficial hemangiomas: associations and management. Pediatr Dermatol 1997;14:173–9.
21. Sie KC, McGill T, Healy GB. Subglottic hemangioma: ten years experience with carbon dioxide laser. Ann Otol Rhinol Laryngol 1994;103:167–72.

22. Rahbar R, Nicollas R, Roger G, et al. The biology and management of subglottic hemangioma: past, present, future. Laryngoscope 2004;114:1880–91.
23. Christison-Lagay ER, Burrows PE, Alomari A, et al. Hepatic hemangiomas: subtype classification and development of a clinical practice algorithm and registry. J Pediatr Surg 2007;42:62–7.
24. Boon LM, Burrows PE, Paltiel HJ, et al. Hepatic vascular anomalies in infancy: a twenty-seven-year experience. J Pediatr 1996;129:346–54.
25. Huang SA, Tu HM, Harney JW, et al. Severe hypothyroidism caused by type 3 iodothyronine deiodinase in infantile hemangiomas. N Engl J Med 2000;343:185–9.
26. Mulliken JB, Marler JJ, Burrows PE, et al. Reticular infantile hemangioma of the limb can be associated with ventral-caudal anomalies, refractory ulceration, and cardiac overload. Pediatr Dermatol 2007;24: 356–62.
27. Goldberg NS, Hebert AA, Esterly NB. Sacral hemangiomas and multiple congenital anomalies. Arch Dermatol 1986;122:684–7.
28. Albright AL, Gartner JC, Wiener ES. Lumbar cutaneous hemangiomas as indicators of tethered spinal cords. Pediatrics 1989;83:977–80.
29. Bouchard S, Yazbeck S, Lallier M. Perineal hemangioma, anorectal malformation, and genital anomaly: a new association? J Pediatr Surg 1999;34:1133–5.
30. Girard C, Bigorre M, Guillot B, et al. PELVIS syndrome. Arch Dermatol 2006;142:884–8.
31. Stockman A, Boralevi F, Taieb A, et al. SACRAL syndrome: spinal dysraphism, anogenital, cutaneous, renal and urological anomalies, associated with an angioma of lumbosacral localization. Dermatology 2007;214:40–5.
32. Freiden IJ, Reese V, Cohen D. PHACE syndrome. The association of posterior fossa brain malformations, hemangiomas, arterial anomalies, coarctation of the aorta and cardiac defects and eye abnormalities. Arch Dermatol 1996;132:307–11.
33. Metry DW, Haggstrom AN, Drolet BA, et al. A prospective study of PHACE syndrome in infantile hemangiomas: demographic features, clinical findings, and complications. Am J Med Genet 2006; 140A:975–86.
34. Metry DW, Garzon MC, Drolet BA, et al. PHACE syndrome: current knowledge, future directions. Pediatr Dermatol 2009;26:381–98.
35. Chamlin SL, Haggstrom AN, Drolet BA, et al. Multicenter prospective study of ulcerated hemangiomas. J Pediatr 2007;151:684–9.
36. Elsas FJ, Lewis AR. Topical treatment of periocular capillary hemangioma. Strabismus 1994;31:153–6.
37. Cruz OA, Zarnegar SR, Myers SE. Treatment of periocular capillary hemangioma with topical clobetasol propionate. Ophthalmology 1995;102:2012–5.
38. Garzon MC, Lucky AW, Hawrot A, et al. Ultrapotent topical corticosteroid treatment of hemangiomas of infancy. J Am Acad Dermatol 2005;52:281–6.
39. Gilbertson EO, Spellman MC, Piacquadio DJ, et al. Super potent topical corticosteroid use associated with adrenal suppression: clinical considerations. J Am Acad Dermatol 1998;38:318–21.
40. Crum R, Szabo S, Folkman J. A new class of steroids inhibits angiogenesis in the presence of heparin or a heparin fragment. Science 1985;230:1375–8.
41. Sloan GM, Renisch JF, Nichter LS, et al. Intralesional corticosteroid therapy for infantile hemangiomas. Plast Reconstr Surg 1989;83:459–67.
42. Ruttum MS, Abrams GW, Harris GJ, et al. Bilateral retinal embolization associated with intralesional steroid injection for capillary hemangioma of infancy. J Pediatr Ophthalmol Strabismus 1993;30:4–7.
43. Egbert JE, Schwartz GS, Walsh AW. Diagnosis and treatment of an ophthalmic artery occlusion during an intralesional injection of corticosteroid into an eyelid capillary hemangioma. Am J Ophthalmol 1996;121:638–42.
44. Goyal R, Watts P, Lane CM, et al. Adrenal suppression and failure to thrive after steroid injections for periocular hemangioma. Ophthalmology 2004;111:389–95.
45. Leaute-Labreze C, Dumas de la Roque E, Hubiche T, et al. Propranolol for severe hemangiomas of infancy. N Engl J Med 2008;358:2649–51.
46. Sans V, Dumas de la Roque E, Berge J, et al. Propranolol for severe infantile hemangiomas: follow-up report. Pediatrics 2009;124:423–31.
47. Lawley LP, Siegfried E, Todd JL. Propranolol treatment for hemangioma of infancy: risks and recommendations. Pediatr Dermatol 2009;26:610–4.
48. Frieden IL, Drolet BA. Propranolol for infantile hemangiomas: promise, peril, pathogenesis. Pediatr Dermatol 2009;26:642–4.
49. Zarem HA, Edgerton MT. Induced resolution of cavernous hemangiomas following prednisolone therapy. Plast Reconstr Surg 1967;39:76–83.
50. Boon LM, MacDonald DM, Mulliken JB. Complications of systemic corticosteroid therapy for problematic hemangiomas. Plast Reconstr Surg 1999;104: 1616–23.
51. Bennett ML, Fleischer AB, Chamlin SL, et al. Oral corticosteroid use is effective for cutaneous hemangiomas. Arch Dermatol 2001;137:1208–13.
52. Greene AK. Corticosteroid treatment for problematic infantile hemangioma: evidence does not support an increased risk for cerebral palsy. Pediatrics 2008; 126:1251–2.
53. Greene AK. Systemic corticosteroid is effective and safe treatment for problematic infantile hemangioma. Pediatr Dermatol 2010;27:322–3.
54. Greene AK, Rogers G, Mulliken JB. Management of parotid hemangioma in 100 children. Plast Reconstr Surg 2004;113:53–60.

55. Sadan N, Wolach B. Treatment of hemangiomas of infants with high doses of prednisone. J Pediatr 1996;128:141–6.
56. Moore J, Lee M, Garzon M, et al. Effective therapy of a vascular tumor of infancy with vincristine. J Pediatr Surg 2001;36:1273–6.
57. Haisley-Royster C, Enjolras O, Frieden IJ, et al. Kasabach-Merritt phenomenon: a retrospective study of treatment with vincristine. J Pediatr Hematol Oncol 2002;24:459–62.
58. Fawcett SL, Grant I, Hall PN, et al. Vincristine as a treatment for a large haemangioma threatening vital functions. Br J Plast Surg 2004;57:168–71.
59. Enjolras O, Breviere GM, Roger G, et al. Vincristine treatment for function- and life-threatening infantile hemangioma. Arch Pediatr 2004;11:99–107.
60. Barlow CF, Priebe C, Mulliken JB, et al. Spastic diplegia as a complication of interferon-alfa-2a treatment of hemangiomas of infancy. J Pediatr 1998; 132:527–30.
61. Dubois J, Hershon L, Carmant L, et al. Toxicity profile of interferon-alfa-2b in children: a prospective evaluation. J Pediatr 1999;135:782–5.
62. Michaud AP, Bauman NM, Burke DK, et al. Spastic diplegia and other motor disturbances in infants receiving interferon-alpha. Laryngoscope 2004; 114:1231–6.
63. Lomenick JP, Backeljauw PF, Lucky AW. Growth, bone mineral accretion, and adrenal function in glucocorticoid-treated infants with hemangiomas—a retrospective study. Pediatr Dermatol 2006;23: 169–74.
64. George ME, Sharma V, Jacobson J, et al. Adverse effects of systemic glucocorticosteroid therapy in infants with hemangiomas. Arch Dermatol 2004; 140:963–9.
65. Seale JP, Compton MR. Side-effects of corticosteroid agents. Med J Aust 1986;144:139–42.
66. Fardet L, Abdulrhaman K, Cabane J, et al. Corticosteroid-induced adverse events in adults. Drug Saf 2007;30:861–81.
67. Lomenick JP, Reifschneider KL, Lucky AW, et al. Prevalence of adrenal insufficiency following systemic gluocorticoid therapy in infants with hemangiomas. Arch Dermatol 2009;145:262–6.
68. Scheepers JH, Quaba AA. Does the pulsed tunable dye laser have a role in the management of infantile hemangiomas: observations based on 3 years experience. Plast Reconstr Surg 1995;95:305–12.
69. Batta K, Goodyear HM, Moss C, et al. Randomized controlled study of early pulsed dye laser treatment of uncomplicated childhood haemangiomas: results of a 1-year analysis. Lancet 2002;360:521–7.
70. Witman PM, Wagner AM, Scherer K, et al. Complications following pulsed dye laser treatment of superficial hemangiomas. Lasers Surg Med 2006;38: 116–23.
71. Scarcella JV, Dykes ER, Anderson R. Hemangiomas of the parotid gland. Plast Reconstr Surg 1965;36:38–47.
72. Williams HB. Hemangiomas of the parotid gland in children. Plast Reconstr Surg 1975;56:29–34.
73. Little KE, Cywes S, Davies MR, et al. Complicated giant hemangioma: excision using cardiopulmonary bypass and deep hypothermia. J Pediatr Surg 1976; 11:533–6.
74. Tiret L, Nivoche Y, Hatton F, et al. Complications related to anesthesia in infants and children. Br J Anaesth 1988;61:263–9.
75. Cohen MM, Cameron CB, Duncan PG. Pediatric anesthesia morbidity and mortality in the perioperative period. Anesth Analg 1990;70:160–7.
76. Tay CL, Tan GM, Ng SA. Critical incidents in paediatric anaesthesia: an audit of 1000 anaesthetics in Singapore. Paediatr Anaesth 2001;11:711–8.
77. Murat I, Constant I, Maudhuy H. Perioperative anaesthetic morbidity in children: database of 24165 anaesthetics over a 30-month period. Paediatr Anaesth 2004;14:158–66.
78. Charlesworth R. The toddler: affective development. In: Charlesworth R, editor. Understanding child development. 6th edition. Clifton Park (NY): Delmar Learning; 1994. p. 304.
79. Santrock JW. The self and identity. In: Santrock JW, editor. Child development. 7th edition. Columbus (OH): McGraw-Hill; 1996. p. 378–85.
80. Neisser U. Memory development: new questions and old. Dev Rev 2004;24:154.
81. Mulliken JB, Rogers GF, Marler JJ. Circular excision of hemangioma and purse-string closure: the smallest possible scar. Plast Reconstr Surg 2002;109:1544–54.
82. Boon LM, Enjolras O, Mulliken JB. Congenital hemangioma: evidence of accelerated involution. J Pediatr 1996;128:329–35.
83. Enjolras O, Mulliken JB, Boon LM, et al. Noninvoluting congenital hemangioma: a rare cutaneous vascular anomaly. Plast Reconstr Surg 2001;107:1647–54.
84. Berenguer B, Mulliken JB, Enjolras O, et al. Rapidly involuting congenital hemangioma: clinical and histopathologic features. Pediatr Dev Pathol 2003; 6:495–510.
85. Kasabach HH, Merritt KK. Capillary hemangioma with extensive purpura: report of a case. Am J Dis Child 1940;59:1063–70.
86. Zukerberg LR, Nikoloff BJ, Weiss SW. Kaposiform hemangioendothelioma of infancy and childhood: an aggressive neoplasm associated with Kasabach-Merritt syndrome and lymphangiomatosis. Am J Surg Pathol 1993;17:321–8.
87. Sarkar M, Mulliken JB, Kozakewich HP, et al. Thrombocytopenic coagulopathy (Kasabach-Merritt phenomenon) is associated with kaposiform hemangioendothelioma and not with common infantile hemangioma. Plast Reconstr Surg 1997;100: 1377–86.

88. Enjolras O, Wassef M, Mazoyer E, et al. Infants with Kasabach-Merritt syndrome do not have "true" hemangiomas. J Pediatr 1997;130:631–40.
89. Lyons LL, North PE, Mac-Moune Lai F, et al. Kaposiform hemangioendothelioma: a study of 33 cases emphasizing its pathologic, immunophenotypic, and biologic uniqueness from juvenile hemangioma. Am J Surg Pathol 2004;28:559–68.
90. Debelenko LV, Perez-Atayde AR, Mulliken JB, et al. D2-40 immunohistochemical analysis of pediatric vascular tumors reveals positivity in kaposiform hemangioendothelioma. Mod Pathol 2005;18: 1454–60.
91. Mulliken JB, Anupindi S, Ezekowitz RA, et al. Case 13-2004: a newborn girl with a large cutaneous lesion, thrombocytopenia, and anemia. N Engl J Med 2004;350:1764–75.
92. Enjolras O, Mulliken JB, Wassef M, et al. Residual lesions after Kasabach-Merritt phenomenon in 41 patients. J Am Acad Dermatol 2000;42:225–35.
93. Mentzel T, Mazzoleni G, Dei Tos AP, et al. Kaposiform hemangioendothelioma in adults. Clinicopathologic and immunohistochemical analysis of three cases. Am J Clin Pathol 1997;108:450–5.
94. Karnes JC, Lee BT, Phung T, et al. Adult-onset kaposiform hemangioendothelioma in a post-traumatic site. Ann Plast Surg 2009;62:456–8.
95. Gruman A, Liang MG, Mulliken JB, et al. Kaposiform hemangioendothelioma without Kasabach-Merritt phenomenon. J Am Acad Dermatol 2005;52:616–22.
96. Mills SE, Cooper PH, Fechner RE. Lobular capillary hemangioma: the underlying lesion of pyogenic granuloma. Am J Surg Pathol 1980;4:470–9.
97. Patrice SJ, Wiss K, Mulliken JB. Pyogenic granuloma (lobular capillary hemangioma): a clinicopathologic study of 178 cases. Pediatr Dermatol 1991;8: 267–76.
98. Kirschner RE, Low DW. Treatment of pyogenic granuloma by shave excision and laser photocoagulation. Plast Reconstr Surg 1999;104:1346–9.

Management of Capillary Malformations

Sheilagh M. Maguiness, MD*, Marilyn G. Liang, MD

KEYWORDS

- Vascular malformation • Capillary malformation
- Port wine stain • Nevus simplex • Nevus flammeus
- Pulsed dye laser • Sturge-Weber syndrome

Capillary malformations (CMs) are the most common vascular malformations. They are comprised of the small vessels of the capillary network in skin and mucous membranes. In the vast majority of affected individuals, CMs are isolated and not associated with any underlying abnormalities. Depending on size and location, however, they may cause significant morbidity due to stigmatization or disfigurement and, rarely, herald the presence of an underlying syndrome.

FADING CAPILLARY STAIN (NEVUS SIMPLEX)

The fading capillary stain, also known as salmon patch or stork bite, is the most common vascular stain, present in up to 40% of infants. It consists of dilated capillaries within the papillary dermis. Some postulate that they are due to lack of autonomic regulation of local vessels in the affected skin. In general, fading capillary stains on the face diminish over time and those on the nape of neck tend to persist. Fading capillary stains are distinct from CMs and other vascular malformations. They are often observed on the glabella, eyelids, nose, and philtrum and even more frequently seen on the posterior neck. The lumbosacral spine can also be affected and some clinicians think that in this location it can rarely be associated with occult spinal dysraphism.[1,2] Many infants have stains on multiple sites. Unlike true CMs, fading capillary stains on the face do not occur in a dermatomal distribution and are not associated with the Sturge-Weber syndrome (SWS). Large and persistent stains on the face, however, are sometimes seen in association with other underlying diseases or syndromes, such as the Beckwith-Wiedemann syndrome and macrocephaly-CM syndrome (M-CM).[3,4]

Usually, no treatment is required. In persistent stains on cosmetically sensitive locations (ie, facial), however, treatment with the pulsed dye laser (PDL) is effective and can be considered. In infants and children with persistent stains, a detailed history and physical examination to rule out associated abnormalities, such as macrocephaly, hypotonia, or other clinical features seen in M-CM and Beckwith-Wiedemann syndrome, could help facilitate the diagnosis of one of these conditions. In patients with lumbosacral stains, particularly those with the reportedly characteristic butterfly shape, it may be appropriate to consider imaging studies, such as duplex ultrasound or MRI, to rule out underlying occult spinal dysraphism.[1,5] This is controversial, however, and prospective studies are needed to determine the true association, which is probably low.

CAPILLARY MALFORMATIONS

CM is equated with port wine stain, which is what it is still most commonly referred to in the literature. CM is also known as nevus flammeus. CM is common and occurs in approximately 0.3% of all newborns. Histolopathologically, initially CM is

Disclosure: Dr Marilyn G. Liang for Pierre-Fabre Dermatology.
Department of Dermatology, Harvard Medical School, Children's Hospital Boston, 300 Longwood Avenue, Boston, MA 02115, USA
* Corresponding author.
E-mail address: maguinesss@derm.ucsf.edu

Clin Plastic Surg 38 (2011) 65–73
doi:10.1016/j.cps.2010.08.010

composed of normal capillaries in the superficial dermis with no evidence of cellular proliferation. Telangiectasias and vascular ectasias become more evident over time. CMs are true vascular malformations and as such are present at birth and persist throughout life. They can occur anywhere on the body. Growth is proportionate with that of the affected child. On the face, they usually present in a dermatomal distribution and respect the midline. In some cases, however, there is involvement of neighboring dermatomes. CMs are initially bright pink, red, or violaceous in color. They often seem to lighten significantly over the first few months of life, probably due to a drop in circulating blood hemoglobin concentration. This physiologic lightening is not indicative of spontaneous resolution.[6] Most CMs become darker, thicker, and more nodular over time, particularly within facial lesions. Local complications of CM include the development of pyogenic granulomas[7] and eczematous dermatitis[8] occurring within the stain. The differential diagnosis of CM includes a host of other vascular lesions, both tumors and malformations, including fading capillary stain, early infantile hemangioma, telangiectatic or nonproliferative infantile hemangioma, vascular stain associated with arteriovenous malformation (AVM), and other vascular malformations, including lymphatic and/or combined malformations (ie, capillary-lymphatic-venous malformation [CLVM]). Early in infancy it can sometimes be difficult to distinguish between CM and infantile hemangiomas located on the face. Clues to the diagnosis include the distribution (dermatomal in CM versus regional or segmental in infantile hemangiomas)[9] or the presence of small, brightly erythematous islands of proliferation characteristic of infantile hemangioma (**Fig. 1**). To differentiate between CM and underlying AVM, Doppler assessment of flow can be helpful along with auscultation for a bruit and palpation for the thrill of an AVM.

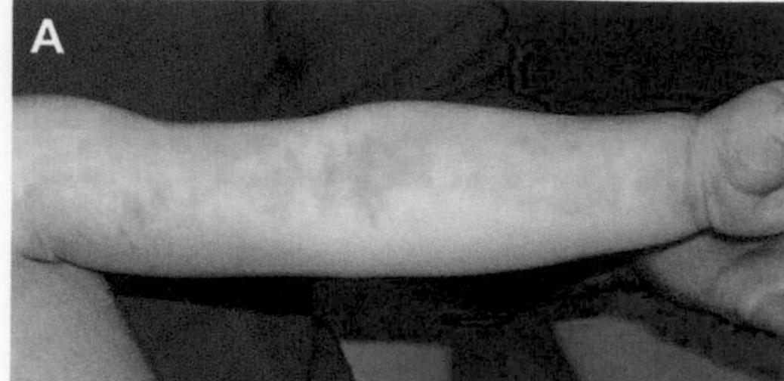

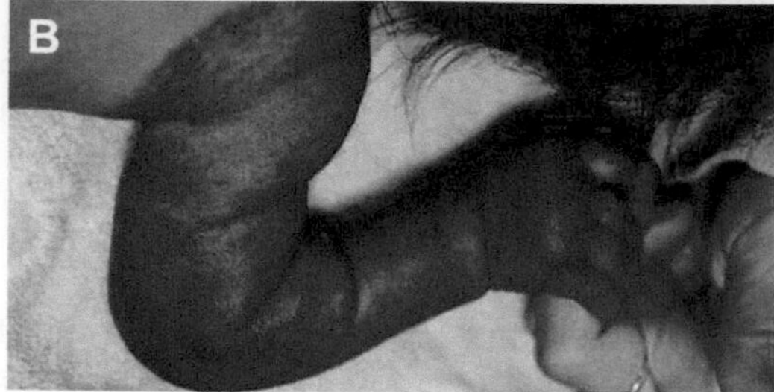

Fig. 1. CM (*A*) and regional infantile hemangioma (*B*). Note the distinct, brightly erythematous islands of proliferation present in the infantile hemangioma but not within the CM.

Associated Syndromes

Inherent in the management of infants and children with CM is the initial evaluation and continued monitoring for associated syndromes. Although rare, CM can present as manifestations of several distinct syndromes. In the past, many different vascular malformations were confused with CM; however, since the advent of the International Society for the Study of Vascular Anomalies (ISSVA) and the development of a specific and updated classification framework for vascular lesions,[10] vascular malformations can now be more precisely identified and separated into their respective vessels of origin. Syndromes that exhibit true CM include SWS (which is the most common), M-CM, capillary malformation-arteriovenous malformation syndrome (CM-AVM), cutis marmorata telangiectatica congenita (CMTC), and overgrowth syndromes, such as Klippel-Trénaunay syndrome (KT). Several of these entities, including KT and CM-AVM, are described in subsequent articles.

Sturge-Weber syndrome, OMIM 185300

SWS refers to the triad of a facial CM in the V1 distribution, ipsilateral leptomeningeal vascular malformation, and choroidal vascular malformation of the eye, which can lead to ipsilateral glaucoma and buphthalmos. The cause is unknown; cases are sporadic with no clear evidence of genetic predisposition.

Approximately 6% to 10% of patients with a CM in the V1 distribution have SWS.[11] Bilateral involvement and involvement of the other trigeminal dermatomes may also occur and increase the risk of central nervous system (CNS) involvement.[12] There does not seem to be any direct relationship between the size of the CM and the severity of the brain involvement in affected patients.[13] Common neurologic manifestations include contralateral seizures, hemiparesis or hemiplegia, migraine headaches, and intellectual impairment. Seizures occur in 75% of patients; these are usually generalized tonic-clonic type and onset is usually before age 1.[14] Developmental delay occurs in approximately half of affected children and prolonged or uncontrolled seizures can worsen CNS outcomes (ie, poor intellectual development, behavioral abnormalities, and learning disabilities). Aggressive seizure management is often warranted.[14]

The incidence of glaucoma in association with V1 CM has been reported as between 7% and 52%.[11,12,15] Like CNS involvement, the incidence of glaucoma is much higher when V1 and V2 dermatomes are involved.[12,15] The presence of a CM in the V2 distribution has not been associated with the development of glaucoma. Regular ophthalmologic examinations (every 6 to 12 months) should be performed in all affected patients, because glaucoma can develop early. Early detection of raised intraocular pressure is important in preventing progressive disease. Long-term follow-up is also necessary because glaucoma can arise as a late complication. When glaucoma is present early on, associated bupthalmos (bull's eye/large eye secondary to enlarged cornea) can also occur. Diffuse vascular malformation of the choroid ipsilateral to the CM is another characteristic feature of SWS that may be found in up to 71% of SWS cases.[12] Myopia, coloboma, cataract, and iris heterochromia have also been seen in association with SWS.[12]

Children with facial CM in the V1 or multiple dermatomal distributions should be evaluated for possible SWS. A complete fundoscopic eye examination and evaluation of intraocular pressure should be performed at regular intervals. In those patients with known eye complications, early-onset seizures, or other symptoms, neuroimaging to identify leptomeningeal (pial) vascular malformations should be performed. MRI with gadolinium contrast is the most sensitive study for diagnosis and evaluation of SWS. In addition to the ipsalateral vascular malformations, cerebral cortex atrophy or characteristic calcifications can also often observed in affected patients.

The management of SWS depends on the clinical manifestations. Seizures require aggressive anticonvulsant therapy and regular follow-up with neurology.[14] In very severe, refractory cases, surgical intervention, such as localized resection of the involved brain tissue or hemispherectomy, may be warranted.[16] In some cases, early neurosurgical intervention may improve outcomes.[16]

Laser treatment of the CM can begin early (ie, when seizures are controlled by anticonvulsants). Patients often require many treatments and even repeated laser ablation (discussed later) years later because CMs are known to undergo redarkening.[17] Many patients with SWS have associated soft tissue and bony overgrowth of the affected areas. Gum hypertrophy, a common finding in patients with V2 involvement and overgrowth of the maxilla, is exacerbated by antiepileptic medications but can be amenable to surgical resection.[18] The lip and surrounding soft tissue hypertrophy are the most common sites requiring surgical intervention.[18] Overgrowth of the maxilla creates an occlusion deformity and crossbite requiring regular orthodontic evaluation and follow-up. Patients with SWS benefit from a multidisciplinary approach with the expertise of neurologists, ophthalmologists, pediatricians, neurosurgeons, dermatologists, plastic surgeons, maxillofacial surgeons, otolaryngologists, and neuroradiologists. The Sturge-Weber Foundation is an active support group for patients and families (http://www.sturge-weber.org/).

Macrocephaly–capillary malformation, OMIM 602501

M-CM was previously known as macrocephaly-CMTC (M-CMTC). Recently more appropriately named,[3,4] M-CM is a rare, sporadic syndrome characterized by either CM or persistent nevus simplex with macrocephaly, hypotonia, and developmental delay. The vascular stain of M-CM is characteristically ill defined or blotchy and is not be confused with true CMTC because it lacks the fixed livedoid pattern, atrophy, or ulceration, which can occur with CMTC. In M-CM, the vascular stain is usually located on the face; the philtrum and glabella are often involved. Other associated features include hydrocephalus, seizures, developmental delay, connective tissue defects (soft skin and joint hypermobility), toe syndactyly, frontal bossing, and, rarely, hemihypertrophy.[3]

Capillary malformation–arteriovenous malformation, OMIM 608354

CM-AVM is an autosomal dominant condition recently found to be due to underlying mutations in the RASA1 gene (RASA1 is an inhibitor of the Ras-Map kinase pathway).[19,20] The disorder is characterized by small, multifocal CMs in association with underlying AVMs/arteriovenous fistulas and occasionally Parkes Weber syndome.[21] Affected patients demonstrate atypical-appearing CM, manifesting as randomly distributed, multifocal, pink to dull red annular papules/plaques with a surrounding halo of vasoconstriction. The lesions often demonstrate high flow or a bruit on doppler examination. In patients with multifocal CM, a Doppler examination is helpful to determine if there is an underlying AVM. Genetic counseling may be indicated.

Cutis marmorata telangiectatica congenita

CMTC is an unusual, distinctive vascular malformation usually noted at birth. The cause is unknown and there is no known genetic basis. Infants present with a fixed coarse, violaceous, livedoid (or net-like) pattern of vasculature, which is unresponsive to local warming. Most commonly, these malformations occur in a regional distribution and respect the midline. Usually, the extremitites are involved (**Fig. 2**). The affected limb may demonstrate hyper- or hypoplasia. Limb asymmetry is the most common associated finding (33%–68%), but lesions can also present with cutaneous atrophy or ulceration.

Neurologic complications, syndactyly, arterial stenosis, and ophthalmologic anomalies have also been reported, although less frequently.[22,23] Histopathologically, CMTC consists of dilated capillaries and venules along with occasional atrophy and ulceration.[24] The livedoid stains tend to improve in appearance over time. Follow-up with orthopedics is important when limb length discrepency is a concern.

Klippel Trenaunay, OMIM 149000

Traditionally, KT has been characterized as the triad of CM, visible venous varicosities, and bony and/or soft tissue overgrowth. It has become accepted, however, that the vascular malformation associated with true KT is actually a complex, combined vascular malformation (CLVM) associated with bony and soft tissue overgrowth of the affected limb. In most patients with KT, the CLVM presents as a well-demarcated, geographic violaceous plaque,[25] often with visible nodules (lymphatic blebs), which become thicker over time.

Reticulate or blotchy CM on the extremities can also be associated with overgrowth and venous varicosities but are less likely to demonstrate extensive underlying lymphatic malformation. These patients with diffuse or blotchy CM of an extremity and stable overgrowth have a significantly better overall prognosis than those with true KT (**Fig. 3**). In KT, progressive worsening of the venous stasis and/or lymphedema is inevitable, and ulceration, coagulopathy, thrombosis, pulmonary emboli, and pulmonary artery hypertension have all been associated.[26,27]

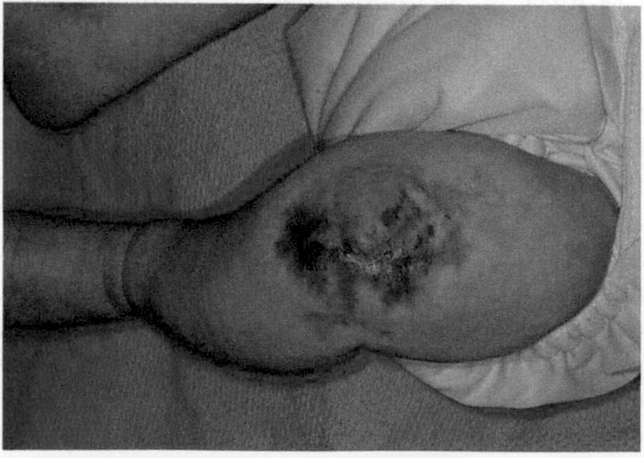

Fig. 2. CMTC of the lower extremity. Note the fixed, livedoid vascular pattern and scarring from previous ulceration.

MANAGEMENT OF CAPILLARY MALFORMATIONS

In children with CM, the decision about if, when, and how to treat usually depends on the size and location of the stain. CMs in extrafacial locations do not necessarily require treatment (ie, laser ablation). In addition, CMs that are not on visually prominent areas may never become an aesthetic concern to the patient and thus treatment may not be necessary. The mainstay and gold standard therapy for facial or aesthetically sensitive CM is still the flashlamp PDL at 595-nm wavelength, although other lasers are being used more frequently.

The risks and benefits of any treatment must be fully discussed with the patient and family. Parents should be advised regarding the natural history of CM and given realistic expectations regarding specific therapies. In infants and young children, or in older patients with extensive CM, a brief, general anesthetic during the procedure may be required.

In the case of facial CM, most pediatric dermatologists recommend early intervention with PDL in attempt to lighten the stain before school age,[28,29] but there is currently no prospective evidence that early laser treatment reduces complications, such as overgrowth of the underlying bone or soft tissue or darkening/thickening of the CM with time.[30] There is a known psychosocial benefit to early intervention, however, because the stigma associated with facial CM can lead to teasing, stress, and lowered self-esteem.[31]

Pulsed Dye Laser

The flashlamp PDL is the mainstay of therapy for CM. PDL was developed for the selective ablation of vascular lesions and has greatly advanced the ability to successfully treat aesthetically compromising CM. Most PDL units have a wavelength of 595 nm. Settings of 0.45- to 1.5-ms pulse duration, 6- to 10-J/cm^2 fluences, and 7- to 10-mm spot size and ideally a coolant system (dynamic cooling device) are used in the majority of lesions. The PDL has now been used for more than 15 years in children and young infants and is a safe and

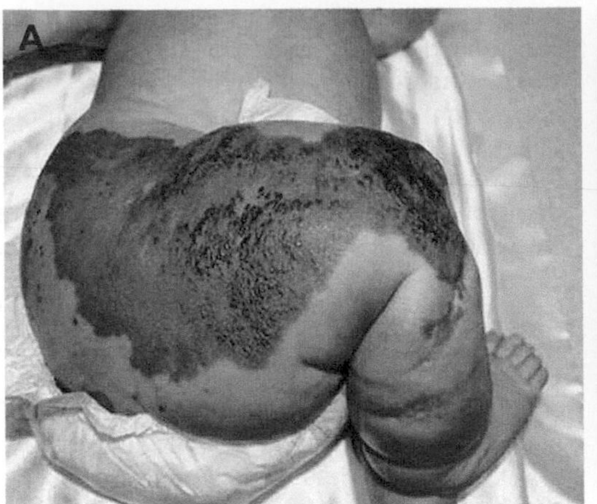

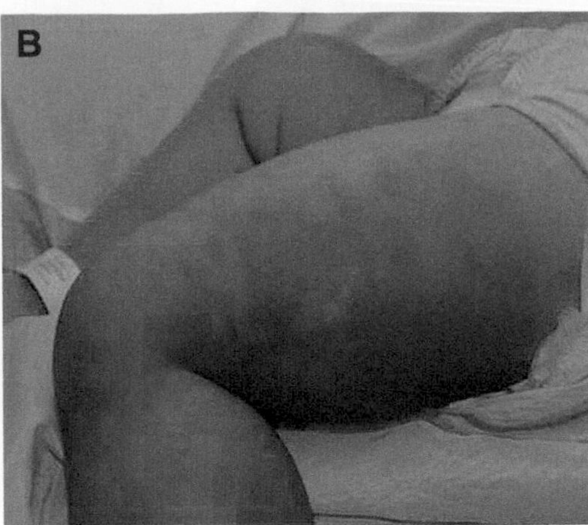

Fig. 3. An example of KT with characteristic geographic CLVM and massive hypertrophy of the limb (*A*). Note the distinction between the patient with CM and slight overgrowth of the leg (*B*).

effective treatment modality with a low risk of scarring and good rate of clinical response.[32–35] In general, multiple treatments (4–8) are needed for maximum clinical response (**Fig. 4**). Complications are infrequent but include pigmentary alteration, scarring, and rarely, infection. Although uncommon, there are several case reports documenting infection as a complication of PDL therapy for CM. These include local reactivation of herpes simplex infection,[36] bacterial superinfection, molluscum contagiosum,[37] and the development of extensive flat warts.[38]

To minimize potential complications, patients and parents should be advised to use sunblock and avoid direct sun exposure post treatment, which may help minimize dyspigmentation. Liberal use of barrier emollients, such as petrolatum or Aquaphor, can help protect the treated skin from abrasion and bacterial infection. In those patients with known herpes simplex infection, oral acyclovir can be used as prophylaxis during and for several days post treatment to prevent an outbreak or more disemminated infection in the treated areas.

Laser ablation with the PDL is reportedly effective in approximately 20% of cases, where almost complete lightening is achieved. In most patients, however, PDL treatments result in lightening of the stain, but not total response, with 50% of patients achieving approximately 70% improvement.[39] Approximately 20% to 30% of CMs do not respond well to PDL therapy. It is important to disclose these facts to parents before embarking on treatment so that expectations are realistic.

Response to treatment often depends on the size and location of the CM. Large CMs associated

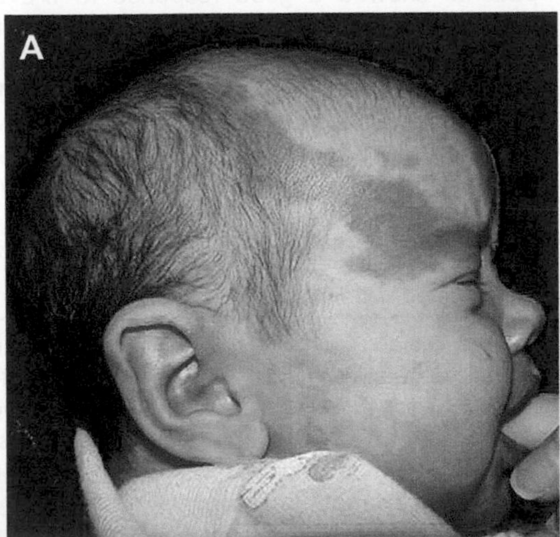

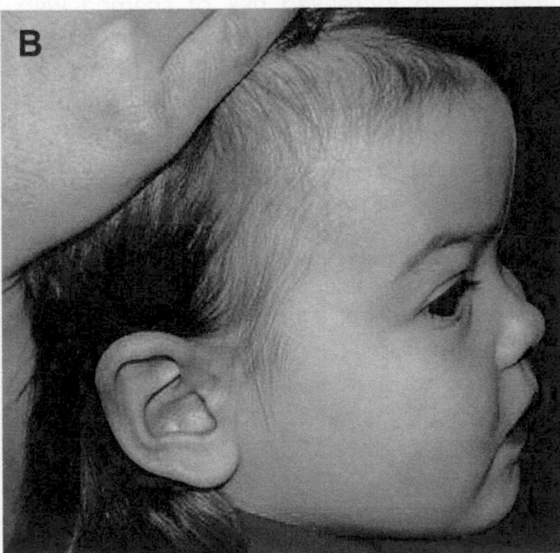

Fig. 4. CM of the face before (*A*) and after (*B*) 10 PDL treatments.

with soft tissue overgrowth and those located in the V2 distribution tend to respond less well to laser therapy. The reason for this is unknown but most likely related to vessel size, depth, and skin type of the patient.

In treatment-resistant CM, many other laser modalities have been used and studied in an attempt to decrease thickness, color, and nodularity of the lesions. These include the long-pulsed neodymium:yttrium-aluminum-garnet (Nd:YAG) laser, the combined PDL and Nd:YAG laser, and the alexandrite laser. Other novel therapies have recently been studied and show some initial promise in treatment-resistant CM, including intense pulsed light (IPL), photodynamic therapy (PDT), and application of topical antiangiogenic factors (imiquimod and rapamycin) in conjunction with laser ablation. These are discussed later.

Long-pulsed Nd:YAG

The long-pulsed-Nd:YAG is a 1064-nm laser that penetrates more deeply than the PDL. In treatment-resistant CM, the deeper, larger vessels are not ablated by the PDL, which only penetrates to approximately 1 mm in depth. Therefore, nodularity and dark color can persist despite repeated treatment, which is why many other laser modalities have been used to try to lighten CMs even further. There are some studies documenting the efficacy of long-pulsed Nd:YAG in this setting,[40] specifically for use of treatment-resistant hypertrophic CM of the lip.[41] Although the majority of treated patients in one pilot study showed similar efficacy to PDL, one patient suffered hypertrophic scarring after the Nd:YAG was used at a fixed dosage.[40] Subsequent patients in this study were treated at their individual minimum purpuric doses and did not suffer scarring.[40] Due to depth of penetration and increased risk of scarring with long-pulsed Nd:YAG over PDL, the long-pulsed Nd:YAG should be reserved for use in treatment-resistant cases only, as a second-line therapy for dermatologists or plastic surgeons with experience in this area.

Combined PDL and Nd:YAG Laser Systems

New combined modality laser systems, such as the Cynergy MultiPlex (Cynosure, Westford, MA, USA) laser system (PDL and Nd:YAG), have recently been studied in this setting. This novel combined laser delivers sequential pulses of 595 nm (PDL) followed by 1064 nm (Nd:YAG) separated by 50 to 2000 milliseconds.[39] The rationale behind this sequential pulsing is that the initial pulse of 595-nm light (at subpurpuric doses) induces methemoglobin formation within the treated capillaries.[39] Methemoglobin has a significant absorption peak at approximately 1064 nm, which theoretically should increase capillary absorption of the sequentially fired 1064-nm pulse.[39] This combined 595-nm/1064-nm laser treatment has been shown to result in a greater depth of vascular coagulation.[42] It is also reportedly safe and effective treatment of recalcitrant CM.[43]

Alexandrite Laser

The alexandrite 755-nm laser has been reported effective in treating hypertrophic or resistant CM. According to the theory of selective photothermolysis, the deeper vessels in hypertrophic CM may also be specifically targeted with the more deeply penetrating 755-nm laser that has selectivity for deoxyhemoglobin as well as oxyhemoglobin.[44] Due to the depth of penetration, there is a significant risk of scarring. Investigators of one study state that this laser should be used judiciously by an experienced operator.[44] They also underscore the importance of attaining and maintaining the correct endpoint when treating CM with this deeply penetrating laser to achieve maximum benefit while avoiding deep dermal burns that could cause scarring.[45]

Intense Pulsed Light

Over the past several years, many studies have been published reporting the safety and efficacy of IPL in the treatment of CM and PDL treatment–resistant CM.[46–49] The IPL emits a noncoherent light source, which theoretically may match a broader range of vessel sizes (ie, broader range of absorption coefficients and thermal relaxation times) within CM.[50] In several studies, patients showed a good response to IPL and even tended to prefer this treatment because it is associated with less purpura and fewer complications.[46] In the only randomized control trial comparing the efficacy of PDL to IPL, however, PDL performed significantly better with 70% of patients reaching good or excellent clearance versus 30% of patients treated with the IPL.[51]

Photodynamic Therapy

PDT is a new modality that shows some initial promise in the treatment of CM. PDT involves either topical or intracirculatory exposure to an exogenous chromophore into the dilated capillaries of the CM. The most widely used chromophores are the porphyrin precursors, such as hepatoporphyrin and benzoporphyrin (both have been administered intravenously) and aminolavulinic acid, which is

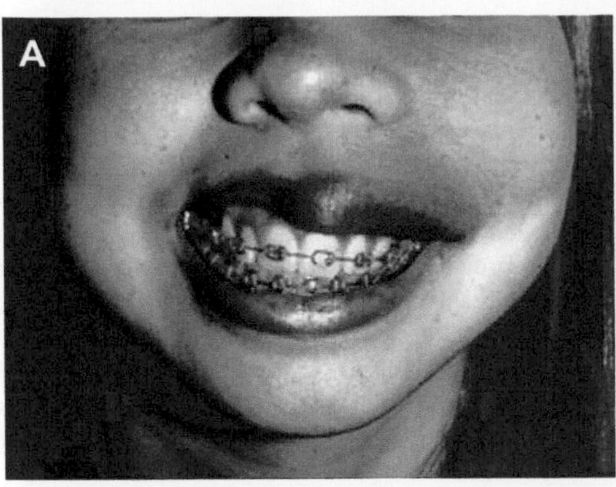

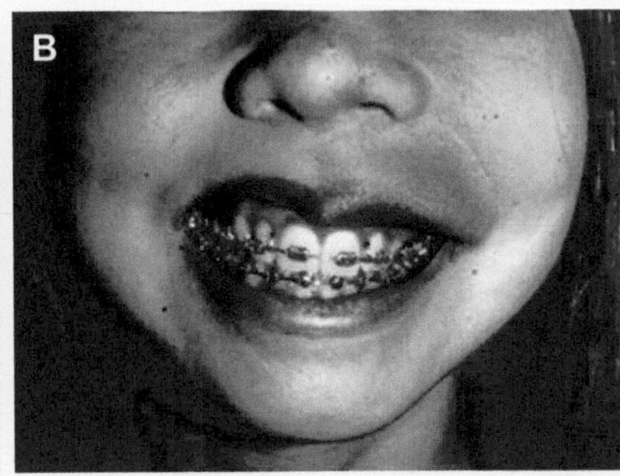

Fig. 5. Adolescent female with SWS and upper labial hypertrophy (*A*). One year after labial reduction by transverse mucosal incision (*B*). (*Courtesy of* John Mulliken, MD.)

topically administered.[32] Several large studies from China have been published that report effective treatment of CM with systemic photosensitizers followed by exposure to the copper vapor laser (which emits two wavelengths of light at 510.6 and 578.2 nm).[52–54] There are currently no large case series or studies on the efficacy and safety of systemic PDT from North American institutions. One study from the United Kingdom, however, reported no significant difference in outcome with topical aminolavulinic acid followed by PDL when compared with PDL alone.[55] More research into the safety and efficacy of both topical and systemic PDT in the management of CM is needed.

Antiangiogenic Therapies

Another emerging therapy in the management of CM is the concomitant use of PDL and topical agents, which inhibit angiogenesis or neovascularization. There is one pilot study demonstrating modest efficacy in several patients treated with PDL and imiquimod.[56] Imiquimod is an immunomodulatory agent that is used in the treatment of many skin conditions from viral HPV infection to cutaneous malignancies. It is known to inhibit neovascularization, which is the basis for assessing a potential role in the treatment of CM.[32,56–58]

Rapamycin, an inhibitor of angiogenesis via the mammalian target of rapamycin pathway that downregulates hypoxia-inducible factor and vascular endothelial growth factor,[57,58] is currently being investigated in in vitro and in vivo studies. It may prove effective as a topical agent in conjunction with PDL in the future. More studies are needed to demonstrate safety and efficacy in the management of CM in the future.

Surgical management

In most cases of uncomplicated CM, surgical intervention is not required. In patients with associated soft tissue and bony overgrowth (as seen in many patients with SWS), however, adjunctive surgical management can be helpful in restoring normal anatomy (**Fig. 5**). In a recent investigation of SWS and associated overgrowth, 60% of patients noted some form of facial enlargement.[18] Hypertrophy of the lip, cheek, or forehead were most commonly reported. Skeletal overgrowth of the maxilla, mandible, or an affected extremity were also frequently observed.[18] Many of these patients (36%) with overgrowth had surgical procedures, the majority of which were to remove/excise excess tissue.[18] Pyogenic granulomas can sometimes arise within the setting of CM. These need to be excised or treated with electrodessication and curettage because they do not resolve spontaneously and in most cases are complicated by repeated bleeding and discomfort.

REFERENCES

1. Metzker A, Shamir R. Butterfly-shaped mark: a variant form of nevus flammeus simplex. Pediatrics 1990;85(6):1069–71.
2. Guggisberg D, Hadj-Rabia S, Viney C, et al. Skin markers of occult spinal dysraphism in children: a review of 54 cases. Arch Dermatol 2004;140(9):1109–15.
3. Wright DR, Frieden IJ, Orlow SJ, et al. The misnomer "macrocephaly-cutis marmorata telangiectatica congenita syndrome": report of 12 new cases and support for revising the name to macrocephaly-capillary malformations. Arch Dermatol 2009;145(3):287–93.
4. Gonzalez ME, Burk CJ, Barbouth DS, et al. Macrocephaly-capillary malformation: a report of three cases and review of the literature. Pediatr Dermatol 2009;26(3):342–6.

5. Ben-Amitai D, Davidson S, Schwartz M, et al. Sacral nevus flammeus simplex: the role of imaging. Pediatr Dermatol 2000;17(6):469–71.
6. Cordoro KM, Speetzen LS, Koerper MA, et al. Physiologic changes in vascular birthmarks during early infancy: mechanisms and clinical implications. J Am Acad Dermatol 2009;60(4):669–75.
7. Swerlick RA, Cooper PH. Pyogenic granuloma (lobular capillary hemangioma) within port-wine stains. J Am Acad Dermatol 1983;8(5):627–30.
8. Rajan N, Natarajan S. Impetiginized eczema arising within a port-wine stain of the arm. J Eur Acad Dermatol Venereol 2006;20(8):1009–10.
9. Haggstrom AN, Lammer EJ, Schneider RA, et al. Patterns of infantile hemangiomas: new clues to hemangioma pathogenesis and embryonic facial development. Pediatrics 2006;117(3):698–703.
10. Mulliken JB, Glowacki J. Classification of pediatric vascular lesions. Plast Reconstr Surg 1982;70(1):120–1.
11. Tallman B, Tan OT, Morelli JG, et al. Location of port-wine stains and the likelihood of ophthalmic and/or central nervous system complications. Pediatrics 1991;87(3):323–7.
12. Baselga E. Sturge-Weber syndrome. Semin Cutan Med Surg 2004;23(2):87–98.
13. Pascual-Castroviejo I, Pascual-Pascual S, Velazquez-Fragua R, et al. Sturge-Weber syndrome: study of 55 patients. Can J Neurol Sci 2008;35(3):301–7.
14. Comi AM. Sturge-Weber syndrome and epilepsy: an argument for aggressive seizure management in these patients. Expert Rev Neurother 2007;7(8):951–6.
15. Hennedige AA, Quaba AA, Al-Nakib K. Sturge-Weber syndrome and dermatomal facial port-wine stains: incidence, association with glaucoma, and pulsed tunable dye laser treatment effectiveness. Plast Reconstr Surg 2008;121(4):1173–80.
16. Bourgeois M, Crimmins DW, de Oliveira RS et al. Surgical treatment of epilepsy in Sturge-Weber syndrome in children. J Neurosurg 2007;106(Suppl 1):20–8.
17. Nelson JS, Geronemus RG. Redarkening of port-wine stains 10 years after laser treatment. N Engl J Med 2007;356(26):2745–6 [author reply: 2746].
18. Greene AK, Taber SF, Ball KL, et al. Sturge-Weber syndrome: soft-tissue and skeletal overgrowth. J Craniofac Surg 2009;20(suppl 1):617–21.
19. Hershkovitz D, Bercovich D, Sprecher E, et al. RASA1 mutations may cause hereditary capillary malformations without arteriovenous malformations. Br J Dermatol 2008;158(5):1035–40.
20. Boon LM, Mulliken JB, Vikkula M. RASA1: variable phenotype with capillary and arteriovenous malformations. Curr Opin Genet Dev 2005;15(3):265–9.
21. Revencu N, Boon LM, Mulliken JB, et al. Parkes Weber syndrome, vein of Galen aneurysmal malformation, and other fast-flow vascular anomalies are caused by RASA1 mutations. Hum Mutat 2008;29(7):959–65.
22. Kienast AK, Hoeger PH. Cutis marmorata telangiectatica congenita: a prospective study of 27 cases and review of the literature with proposal of diagnostic criteria. Clin Exp Dermatol 2009;34(3):319–23.
23. Vogel AM, Paltiel HJ, Kozakewich HPW, et al. Iliac artery stenosis in a child with cutis marmorata telangiectatica congenita. J Pediatr Surg 2005;40(7):e9–12.
24. Fujita M, Darmstadt GL, Dinulos JG. Cutis marmorata telangiectatica congenita with hemangiomatous histopathologic features. J Am Acad Dermatol 2003;48(6):950–4.
25. Maari C, Frieden IJ. Klippel-Trénaunay syndrome: the importance of "geographic stains" in identifying lymphatic disease and risk of complications. J Am Acad Dermatol 2004;51(3):391–8.
26. Huiras EE, Barnes CJ, Eichenfield LF, et al. Pulmonary thromboembolism associated with Klippel-Trenaunay syndrome. Pediatrics 2005;116(4):e596–600.
27. Ulrich S, Fischler M, Walder B, et al. Klippel-Trenaunay syndrome with small vessel pulmonary arterial hypertension. Thorax 2005;60(11):971–3.
28. Minkis K, Geronemus RG, Hale EK. Port wine stain progression: a potential consequence of delayed and inadequate treatment? Lasers Surg Med 2009;41(6):423–6.
29. Chapas AM, Eickhorst K, Geronemus RG. Efficacy of early treatment of facial port wine stains in newborns: a review of 49 cases. Lasers Surg Med 2007;39(7):563–8.
30. van der Horst CM, Koster PH, de Borgie CA, et al. Effect of the timing of treatment of port-wine stains with the flash-lamp-pumped pulsed-dye laser. N Engl J Med 1998;338(15):1028–33.
31. Troilius A, Wrangsjö B, Ljunggren B. Potential psychological benefits from early treatment of port-wine stains in children. Br J Dermatol 1998;139(1):59–65.
32. Cordisco MR. An update on lasers in children. Curr Opin Pediatr 2009;21(4):499–504.
33. Lam SM, Williams EF. Practical considerations in the treatment of capillary vascular malformations, or port wine stains. Facial Plast Surg 2004;20(1):71–6.
34. Tan E, Vinciullo C. Pulsed dye laser treatment of port-wine stains: a review of patients treated in Western Australia. Med J Aust 1996;164(6):333–6.
35. Wimmershoff MB, Wenig M, Hohenleutner U, et al. [Treatment of port-wine stains with the flash lamp pumped dye laser. 5 years of clinical experience]. Hautarzt 2001;52(11):1011–5 [in German].

36. Owens WW, Lang PG. Herpes simplex infection and colonization with Pseudomonas aeruginosa complicating pulsed-dye laser treatment. Arch Dermatol 2004;140(6):760–1.
37. Strauss RM, Sheehan-Dare R. Local molluscum contagiosum infection as a side-effect of pulsed-dye laser treatment. Br J Dermatol 2004;150(5):1047–9.
38. Chen T, Frieden IJ. Development of extensive flat warts after pulsed dye laser treatment of a port-wine stain. Dermatol Surg 2007;33(6):734–5.
39. Jasim ZF, Handley JM. Treatment of pulsed dye laser-resistant port wine stain birthmarks. J Am Acad Dermatol 2007;57(4):677–82.
40. Yang MU, Yaroslavsky AN, Farinelli WA, et al. Long-pulsed neodymium:yttrium-aluminum-garnet laser treatment for port-wine stains. J Am Acad Dermatol 2005;52(3 Pt 1):480–90.
41. Kono T, Frederick Groff W, Chan HH, et al. Long-pulsed neodymium:yttrium-aluminum-garnet laser treatment for hypertrophic port-wine stains on the lips. J Cosmet Laser Ther 2009;11(1):11–3.
42. Borges da Costa J, Boixeda P, Moreno C, et al. Treatment of resistant port-wine stains with a pulsed dual wavelength 595 and 1064 nm laser: a histochemical evaluation of the vessel wall destruction and selectivity. Photomed Laser Surg 2009;27(4):599–605.
43. Alster TS, Tanzi EL. Combined 595-nm and 1,064-nm laser irradiation of recalcitrant and hypertrophic port-wine stains in children and adults. Dermatol Surg 2009;35(6):914–8 [discussion: 918–9].
44. Izikson L, Nelson JS, Anderson RR. Treatment of hypertrophic and resistant port wine stains with a 755 nm laser: a case series of 20 patients. Lasers Surg Med 2009;41(6):427–32.
45. Izikson L, Anderson RR. Treatment endpoints for resistant port wine stains with a 755 nm laser. J Cosmet Laser Ther 2009;11(1):52–5.
46. Ho WS, Ying SY, Chan PC, et al. Treatment of port wine stains with intense pulsed light: a prospective study. Dermatol Surg 2004;30(6):887–90 [discussion: 890–1].
47. Reynolds N, Exley J, Hills S, et al. The role of the Lumina intense pulsed light system in the treatment of port wine stains—a case controlled study. Br J Plast Surg 2005;58(7):968–80.
48. Raulin C, Schroeter CA, Weiss RA, et al. Treatment of port-wine stains with a noncoherent pulsed light source: a retrospective study. Arch Dermatol 1999; 135(6):679–83.
49. Ozdemir M, Engin B. Mevlitoğlu I. Treatment of facial port-wine stains with intense pulsed light: a prospective study. J Cosmet Dermatol 2008;7(2):127–31.
50. Bjerring P, Christiansen K, Troilius A. Intense pulsed light source for the treatment of dye laser resistant port-wine stains. J Cosmet Laser Ther 2003;5(1): 7–13.
51. Faurschou A, Togsverd-Bo K, Zachariae C, et al. Pulsed dye laser vs. intense pulsed light for port-wine stains: a randomized side-by-side trial with blinded response evaluation. Br J Dermatol 2009; 160(2):359–64.
52. Yuan K, Li Q, Yu W, et al. Comparison of photodynamic therapy and pulsed dye laser in patients with port wine stain birthmarks: a retrospective analysis. Photodiagnosis Photodyn Ther 2008;5(1): 50–7.
53. Yuan K, Li Q, Yu W, et al. Photodynamic therapy in treatment of port wine stain birthmarks—recent progress. Photodiagnosis Photodyn Ther 2009; 6(3-4):189–94.
54. Gu Y, Huang NY, Liang J, et al. [Clinical study of 1949 cases of port wine stains treated with vascular photodynamic therapy (Gu's PDT)]. Ann Dermatol Venereol 2007;134(3 Pt 1):241–4 [in French].
55. Evans AV, Robson A, Barlow RJ, et al. Treatment of port wine stains with photodynamic therapy, using pulsed dye laser as a light source, compared with pulsed dye laser alone: a pilot study. Lasers Surg Med 2005;36(4):266–9.
56. Chang C, Hsiao Y, Mihm MC, et al. Pilot study examining the combined use of pulsed dye laser and topical Imiquimod versus laser alone for treatment of port wine stain birthmarks. Lasers Surg Med 2008;40(9):605–10.
57. Kimel S, Svaasand LO, Kelly KM, et al. Synergistic photodynamic and photothermal treatment of port-wine stain? Lasers Surg Med 2004;34(2):80–2.
58. Phung TL, Oble DA, Jia W, et al. Can the wound healing response of human skin be modulated after laser treatment and the effects of exposure extended? Implications on the combined use of the pulsed dye laser and a topical angiogenesis inhibitor for treatment of port wine stain birthmarks. Lasers Surg Med 2008;40(1):1–5.

Management of Lymphatic Malformations

Arin K. Greene, MD, MMSc[a,*], Chad A. Perlyn, MD, PhD[b], Ahmad I. Alomari, MD, MSc[a,c]

KEYWORDS

- Lymphatic malformation • Sclerotherapy • Treatment
- Vascular anomaly • Vascular malformation

CLINICAL FEATURES

Lymphatic malformation (LM) results from an error in the embryonic development of the lymphatic system. Sprouting lymphatics may become separated from the primitive lymph sacs or main lymphatic channels; alternatively, lymphatic tissue may form in an abnormal location.[1] Clinically, LM is characterized by the size of the malformed channels: microcystic, macrocystic, or combined (microcystic/macrocystic).[2,3] Macrocystic lesions are defined as cysts large enough to be treated by sclerotherapy. Because the lymphatic and venous systems share a common embryologic origin, phlebectasia can occur in association with LM.[4–6] LM usually is noted at birth. A small or deep lesion, however, may not become evident until late childhood or adolescence when the lesion has grown large enough to cause a visible deformity or symptoms. LM is most commonly located on the head and neck; other frequent sites include the axilla, chest, and perineum. Lesions are soft and compressible. The overlying skin may be normal, have a bluish hue, or contain pink vesicles that can appear similar to a capillary malformation. Primary lymphedema is also a LM that usually presents in infancy or adolescence and most commonly involves the lower extremity.[7,8] LM is particularly problematic because it is progressive; it slowly expands over time and recurs after treatment.

LM typically causes a deformity and psychosocial morbidity, especially when it involves the head and neck. The 2 most common complications are bleeding and infection. Bleeding results from abnormal venous channels in the malformation or from small arteries in the septi. Intralesional bleeding occurs in up to 35% of LMs causing bluish discoloration, pain, or swelling.[9] LM is prone to infection because the malformed lymphatics are less able to clear foreign material and contribute to antibody production; proteinaceous fluid and blood in the cysts also favor bacterial growth. Infection complicates as many as 71% of lesions and can progress rapidly to sepsis.[9] Poor dental hygiene predisposes to infection of cervicofacial malformations. Similarly, buttock or pelvic LM may be infected by translocation of gut flora. Cutaneous vesicles can bleed, cause malodorous drainage, and serve as a portal for bacteria. Osseous LMs can cause bony destruction. Swelling caused by bleeding, infection, or viral illness may obstruct vital structures.

Two-thirds of patients with cervicofacial LM require tracheostomy to maintain the airway.[9] Secondary bony overgrowth is another complication; the mandible is most commonly involved, and patients can develop an open-bite and

Disclosures: none.
[a] Department of Plastic and Oral Surgery, Vascular Anomalies Center, Children's Hospital Boston, Harvard Medical School, 300 Longwood Avenue, Boston, MA 02115, USA
[b] Florida International University College of Medicine, Miami Children's Hospital, 13400 SW 120th Street, Miami, FL 33186, USA
[c] Department of Radiology, Vascular Anomalies Center, Children's Hospital Boston, Harvard Medical School, 300 Longwood Avenue, Boston, MA 02115, USA
* Corresponding author.
E-mail address: arin.greene@childrens.harvard.edu

Clin Plastic Surg 38 (2011) 75–82
doi:10.1016/j.cps.2010.08.006
0094-1298/11/$ – see front matter

malocclusion. Jaw contouring or orthognathic procedures are required in three-fourths of patients with cervicofacial LM.[9] Oral lesions can cause macroglossia, and vesicles are associated with bleeding, pain, poor oral hygiene, and caries.[10] Thoracic or abdominal LM may lead to pleural, pericardial, or peritoneal chylous effusions. Intestinal LM can present as chronic malabsorption. Periorbital LM causes proptosis (45%), ptosis (52%), and amblyopia (33%); ultimately 40% of patients have a permanent reduction in vision and 7% become blind in the affected eye.[11] Upper extremity LM can significantly limit function, and the brachial plexus may be involved if the lesion is located in the axilla.[12] LM may be diffuse or multifocal (involving multiple noncontiguous areas); patients can have splenic involvement, chylous effusions, or osteolytic bone lesions.

DIAGNOSIS

Ninety percent of LMs are diagnosed by history and physical examination.[2,3] Small, superficial lesions do not require further diagnostic workup. However, large or deep LMs are evaluated by magnetic resonance imaging (MRI) to (1) confirm the diagnosis, (2) define the extent and type of malformation, and (3) plan treatment. MRI sequences are obtained with fat suppression, and gadolinium helps differentiate LM from venous malformation (VM).[13] LM appears as a cystic lesion (macrocystic, microcystic, combined) with septations of variable thickness. Because LM has a high water content, it is hyperintense on T2-weighted sequences.[14] After treatment, though, scar tissue causes LM to become less hyperintense.[13] On T1-weighted images LM shows enhancement of the wall and septa unlike VM, which has heterogeneous patchy enhancement. Macrocystic lesions often have fluid levels because of intracystic blood or protein.[13–15] Microcystic LM has more ill-defined borders and greater enhancement than macrocystic lesions. Unlike VM, LM is more likely to appear infiltrative.

Although ultrasonography (US) is not as informative as MRI, sedation in children is not required. US may provide diagnostic confirmation, document intralesional bleeding, and differentiate between macrocystic and microcystic lesions. US findings for macrocystic LM include anechoic cysts with internal septations, often with debris or fluid-fluid levels.[13] Microcystic LM has ill-defined echogenic masses with diffuse involvement of adjacent tissues. Computed tomography and plain films are occasionally useful to delineate osseous involvement, particularly if resection is planned. Lymphedema can be diagnosed by lymphoscintigraphy.

Histologic confirmation of LM is rarely necessary because lesions are diagnosed by history, physical examination, and imaging. Histopathology is relatively nonspecific; LM shows abnormally walled vascular spaces with eosinophilic protein-rich fluid, and collections of lymphocytes.[16] Immunostaining with the lymphatic markers D2-40 and LYVE-1 are positive.[16] Biopsy may be indicated if imaging is equivocal or if a malignant process is suspected.

MANAGEMENT

Nonoperative

LM is a benign condition, and intervention is not mandatory; small or asymptomatic lesions may be observed. Intralesional bleeding is treated conservatively with pain medication, rest, and occasionally prophylactic antibiotics because bleeding may predispose to infection. An infected LM often cannot be controlled with oral antibiotics, and intravenous antimicrobial therapy usually is required. Patients with more than 3 infections in 1 year are given daily prophylactic antibiotics. Because LM is at risk for infection, good oral hygiene should be maintained and patients should avoid incidental trauma. Lymphedema is managed by layered, custom-fitted compression garments as well as pneumatic compression.

Operative

Intervention for LM is reserved for symptomatic lesions that cause pain or significant deformity, or threaten vital structures. Most children do not require treatment at the time of diagnosis. Because LM slowly expands, however, patients may become symptomatic and seek intervention in childhood or adolescence. Less commonly, an LM involving an anatomically sensitive area or causing a deformity necessitates management as early as infancy. For example, a lesion obstructing the airway or visual axis requires urgent intervention. If possible, treatment may be postponed until after 12 months of age when the risk of anesthesia is lowest.[17–20] Intervention for a lesion causing a visible deformity should be considered before 3.5 years to limit psychological morbidity; at this age long-term memory and self-esteem begin to form.[21–23] Some parents, however, may elect to wait until the child is older and able to make the decision to proceed with operative intervention, especially if the deformity is minor.

Sclerotherapy

Sclerotherapy is first-line management for large or problematic macrocystic/combined LM. Sclerotherapy involves aspiration of the cysts followed by the injection of an inflammatory substance, which causes scarring of the cyst walls to each other. Although sclerotherapy does not remove the LM, it effectively shrinks the lesion (**Fig. 1**). Sclerotherapy has superior efficacy and a lower complication rate than resection; it is 4 times more likely to be successful and has one-tenth the morbidity.[24] Long-term control of LM also is favorable; more than 90% of patients treated with OK-432 do not have a regrowth of their lesion 3 years following treatment.[24] Resection of macrocystic LM generally is not indicated unless (1) the lesion is symptomatic and sclerotherapy is no longer possible because all of the macrocysts have been treated, or (2) resection may be curative because the lesion is small and well localized.

Several sclerosants may be used to treat LM: doxycycline, sodium tetradecyl sulfate (STS), ethanol, bleomycin, and OK-432 (killed group *Streptococcus pyogenes*). The authors prefer doxycycline because it is very effective (83% reduction in size) and safe.[13,25,26] In addition, doxycycline theoretically may prevent infectious complications. Almost all macrocystic LMs have an excellent response; improvement for combined LMs is superior for lesions with a greater macrocystic composition.[24,27] A solution of 10 mg/mL is injected, and up to 50 mL (500 mg) may be used for infants and small children; older children and adults may be treated with as much as 100 mL (1000 mg).[28] STS is another effective agent; it probably has a higher complication rate than doxycycline. Bleomycin causes minimal swelling and is considered for lesions in difficult anatomic areas (eg, airway) or for LMs not responsive to other agents. Bleomycin may have some benefit

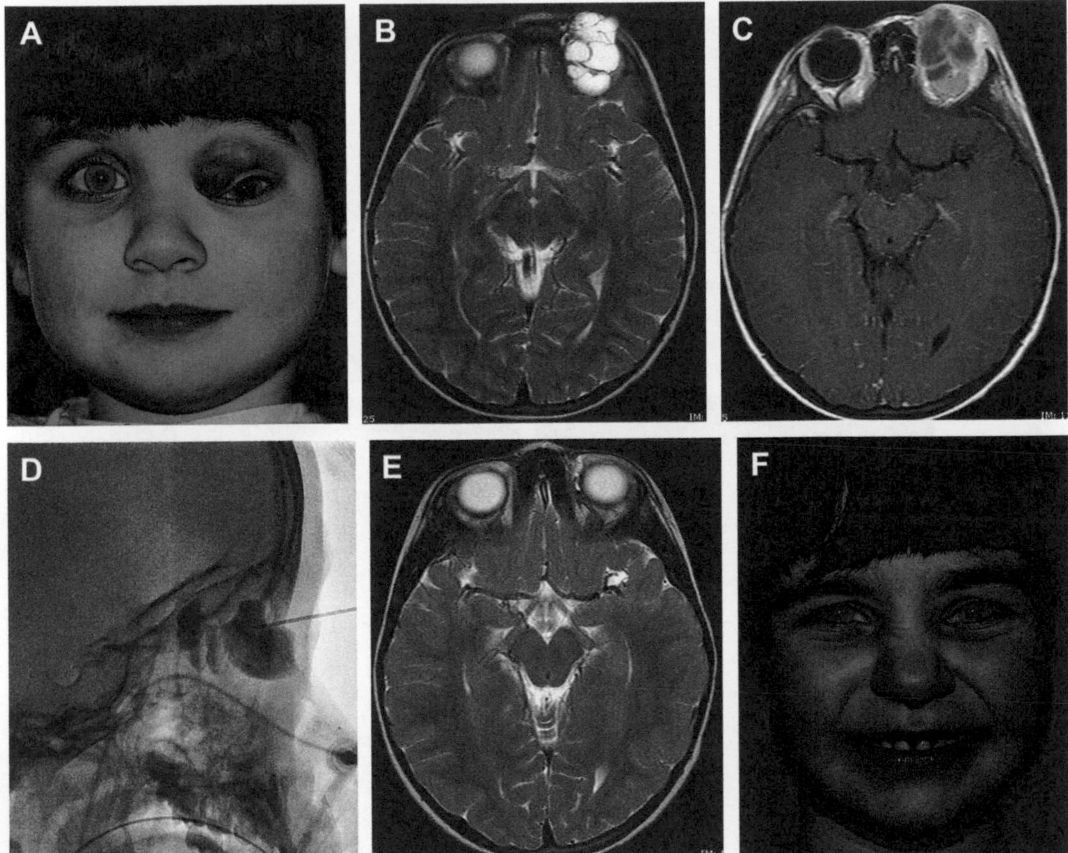

Fig. 1. Management of macrocystic LM. (*A*) A 3-year-old girl with a LM of the left orbit causing exotropia and ptosis. (*B*) Axial T2 MR shows a large hyperintense lesion with multiple, thin internal septations in the superolateral compartment of the orbit. (*C*) Postcontrast T1 MR depicts septal enhancement. There are 2 different signal intensities owing to fluid-fluid levels from intralesional bleeding. (*D*) Fluoroscopic image after needle aspiration and the injection of opacified doxycycline. (*E*) Posttreatment MR demonstrates almost complete resolution of the LM. (*F*) The patient is asymptomatic 4 months after sclerotherapy.

for microcystic lesions that are not amenable to resection.[29] Ethanol is an effective sclerosant but has the highest complication rate. It can be used for small lesions, but large volumes should be avoided to reduce the risk of local and systemic toxicity. Ethanol can injure nerves and, thus, should not be used in proximity to important structures (eg, facial nerve). However, with careful use and avoidance of extravasation, ethanol can be used safely for unresponsive lesions. OK-432 recently has been shown to be effective: 94% and 63% of patients with macrocystic or combined lesions, respectively, have greater than a 60% reduction in size with minimal morbidity.[24] Patients with microcystic LM do not respond to OK-432.[24] OK-432, however, is not widely available.

Small lesions, particularly in adolescents and adults, may be treated in the office without image guidance; 3% STS is diluted with saline to inject a 1% solution. Most patients, especially children, are managed under general anesthesia. Lesions are treated using US with or without fluoroscopy.[24] Contrast can be injected to determine the anatomy of complex lesions, but contrast injection is not usually required. The volume of contrast used to opacify the lesion is less than the amount of sclerosant that is subsequently delivered. After

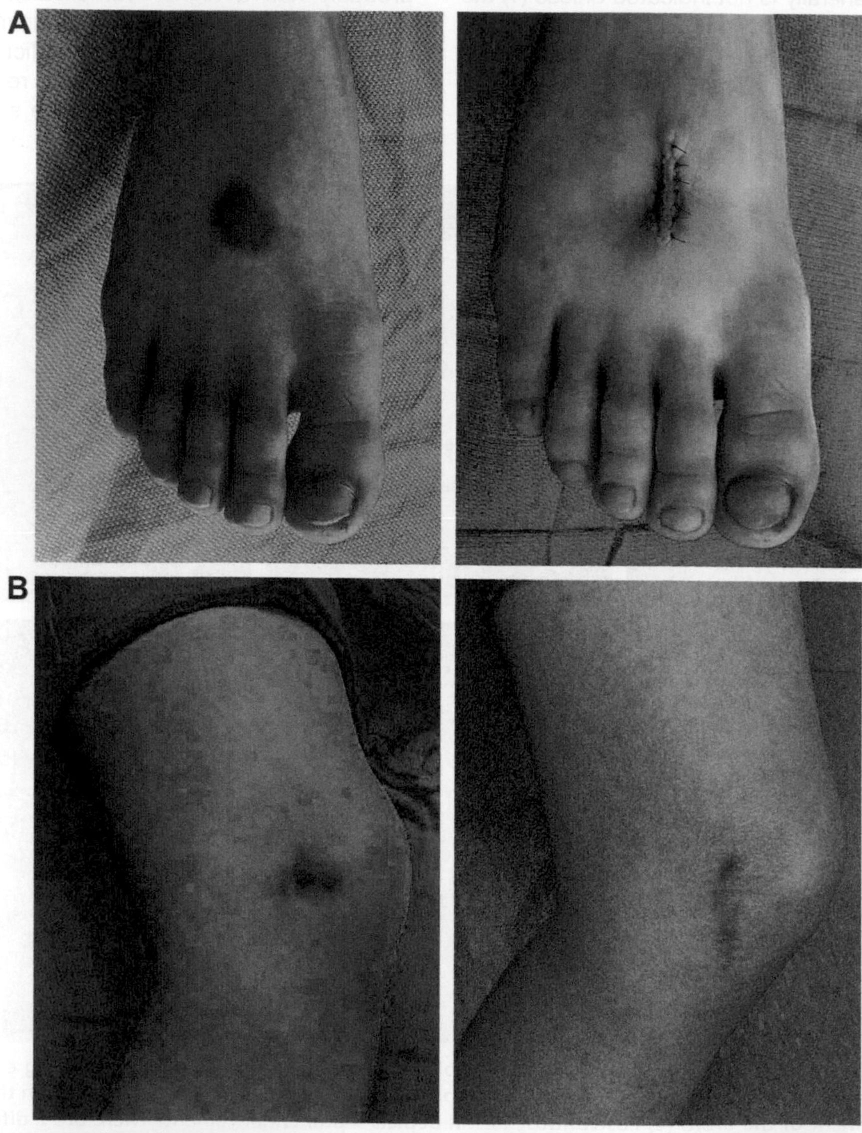

Fig. 2. Management of localized LM. (*A*) A 12-year-old boy with a painful, bleeding, microcystic LM of the foot. (*B*) A 10-year-old girl with a well-localized, combined macro/microcystic LM of her knee causing pain and bleeding. There was no recurrence 1 year after resection.

aspirating fluid from the cyst, the sclerosant is injected. Large cysts occasionally require pigtail catheter placement and sequential drainage and injection over several days. Resolution of macrocysts may occur within days, but may take up to 6 to 8 weeks. Depending on the size of the malformation, and whether there is a residual macrocystic component, additional injections every 6 to 8 weeks may be necessary.

Posttreatment edema progresses for 24 to 48 hours after the procedure. Except for young infants and airway lesions, most patients are discharged home the same day. Dexamethasone is not administered routinely. Posttreatment edema, especially around the airway, may necessitate close monitoring in the intensive care unit; occasionally prolonged intubation or tracheostomy is required. Orbital injections, even with minor extravasation, can cause orbital compartment syndrome, and patients are examined postoperatively by an ophthalmologist. Because LM is at risk for infection, patients are given perioperative antibiotics.

The most common complication of sclerotherapy is skin ulceration (<5%), which is more likely with superficial lesions and when ethanol is used.[13,28] Ulceration is managed with local wound care; the wound is allowed to heal secondarily. STS and doxycycline are not associated with significant systemic adverse effects. In contrast, ethanol can cause central nervous system depression, pulmonary hypertension, hemolysis, thromboembolism, and arrhythmias.[13] Transient (5%) or permanent (2.5%) nerve injury is rare after ethanol sclerotherapy, and has not been noted to occur with doxycycline or STS.[30] LM may reexpand over time; 9% recur within 3 years after OK-432 treatment and most enlarge with longer follow-up.[24,31] Consequently, patients often need repeat sclerotherapy over the course of their lifetime. If a problematic LM recurs and macrocysts are no longer present, then resection is the next treatment option.

Resection

Extirpation of LM can be associated with significant morbidity: major blood loss, iatrogenic injury, and deformity.[9,10,12] For example, resection of cervicofacial LM can injure the facial nerve (76%) or hypoglossal nerve (24%).[9] Excision is usually subtotal because LM involves multiple tissue planes and important structures; recurrence is common (35%–64%).[31–33] Even after complete extirpation, at least 17% of lesions reexpand.[31] Consequently, sclerotherapy is the preferred treatment for macrocystic/combined lesions. Nonproblematic microcystic lesions can be observed. Resection is reserved for (1) small, well-localized LM (microcystic or macrocystic) that may be completely excised for cure (**Fig. 2**), (2) symptomatic microcystic LM (**Fig. 3**), and (3) symptomatic macrocystic/combined LM that no longer can be managed with sclerotherapy because all macrocysts have been treated. When considering resection, the postoperative scar/deformity after removal of the LM should be weighed against the preoperative appearance of the lesion.

Because significant blood loss can occur during extirpation, local anesthetic with epinephrine is administered and resection of an extremity lesion is performed using a tourniquet. A localized LM may be excised and the wound edges reapproximated without complex reconstruction. For diffuse malformations, staged resection of defined anatomic regions is recommended. Subtotal excisions of problematic areas, such as bleeding vesicles or an overgrown lip, should be performed rather than an attempt at complete removal, which would result in a worse deformity than the malformation.

LM involving the head and neck may be resected using a coronal (forehead, orbit), tarsal

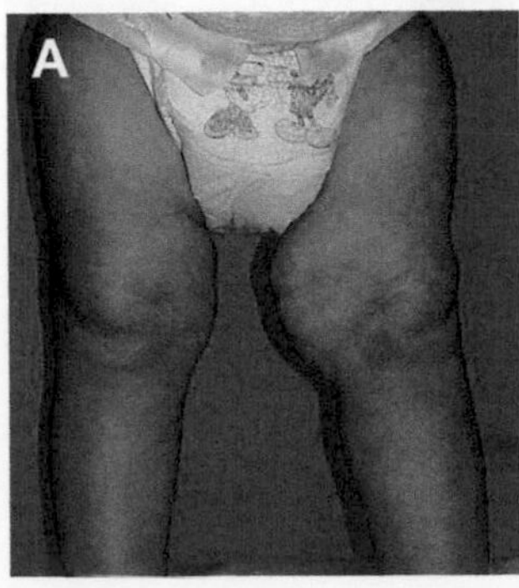

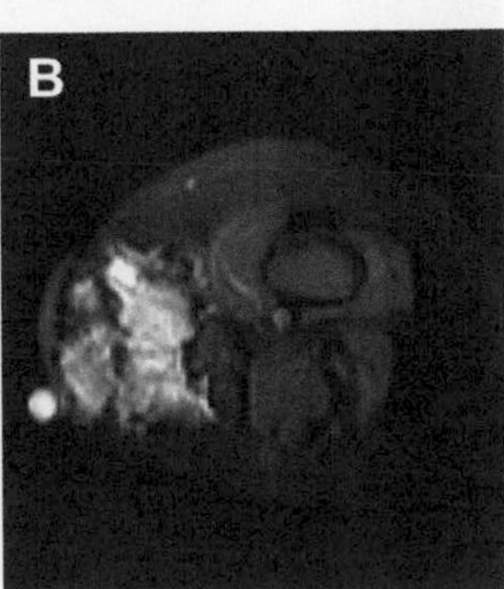

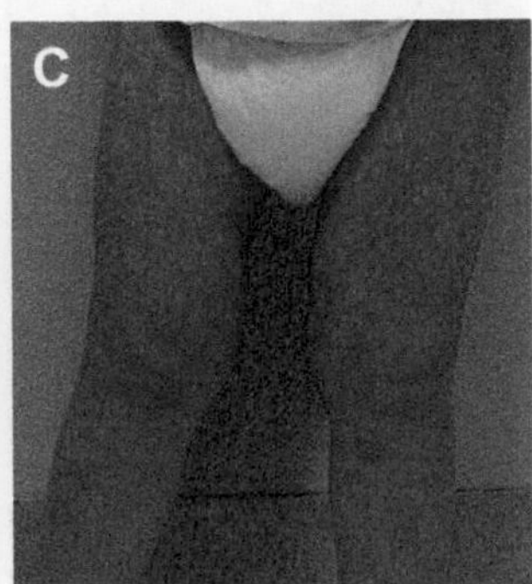

Fig. 3. Management of microcystic LM. (*A*) An 18-month-old boy with a LM of the left lower extremity interfering with ambulation and clothing. (*B*) T2 axial MR shows primarily microscystic LM not amenable to sclerotherapy. (*C*) There was no recurrence 18 months after resection.

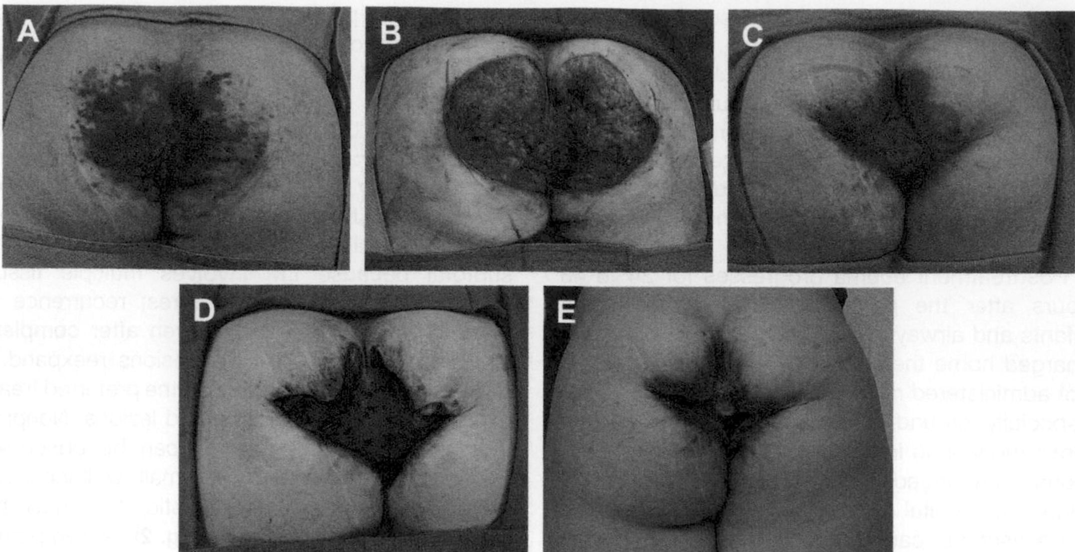

Fig. 4. Operative management of extensive LM. (*A*) An 11-year-old boy presents with chronic bleeding, pain, and discharge. He had previous subtotal resections in infancy complicating local flap closure. (*B*) After resection of involved skin and subcutaneous tissue the wound is allowed to heal secondarily. (*C*) Twelve months postoperatively the area of LM is decreased and replaced by scar. Bleeding, pain and discharge are significantly improved. (*D*) Second-stage excision and healing by secondary intention. (*E*) Two months postoperatively the wound continues to contract and the patient is asymptomatic.

(eyelid), preauricular-melolabial-transoral (cheek), or transverse mucosal (lip) incision. A radical neck approach is required for cervical LM with preservation of important structures. Macroglossia may require tongue reduction to return the tongue to the oral cavity or to correct an open-bite deformity; reexpansion is common. Bony overgrowth is corrected by osseous contouring and malocclusion may require orthognathic correction, usually at the time of skeletal maturity (16 years in women, 18 years in men). Most wounds are amenable to linear closure by advancing skin flaps. Skin grafts may be necessary for wound closure, but there is a risk of vesicles recurring at the edges of the graft. Alternatively, wounds may be allowed to heal

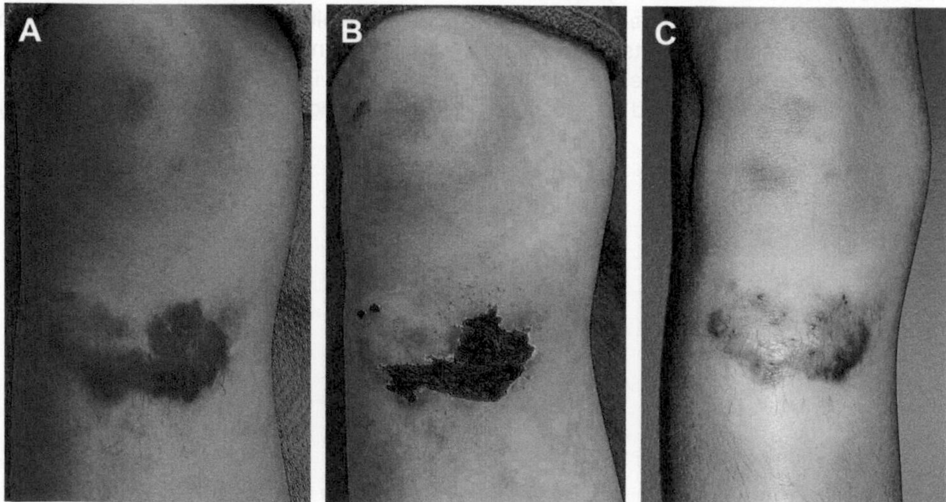

Fig. 5. Management of cutaneous microcystic LM with carbon dioxide laser. (*A*) An 8-year-old girl with a diffuse, superficial LM causing bleeding, pain, and discharge. (*B*) Carbon dioxide laser ablation of lymphatic vesicles. (*C*) Nine months after treatment the patient is asymptomatic.

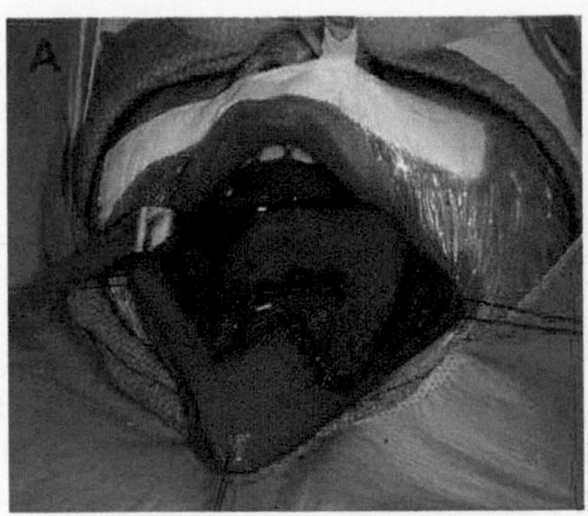

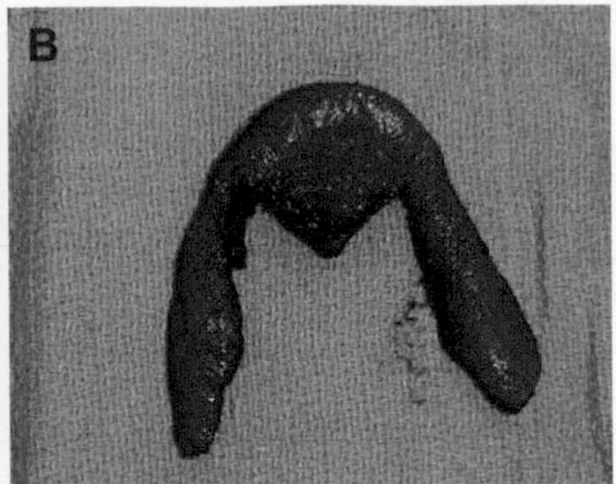

Fig. 6. Surgical management of microcystic LM of the tongue causing macroglossia. (*A*) Intraoperative view showing the "W" resection pattern. (*B*) Excised specimen.

secondarily; the increased scar may help minimize recurrence (**Fig. 4**). Postoperative drainage, seroma, and infection may be minimized using drains and compression garments following the procedure. First-line operative intervention for patients with significant morbidity from lymphedema who have failed maximal nonoperative treatment is suction-assisted lipectomy (SAL) of the suprafascial compartment.[34,35] Patients with severe disease are best managed by staged-skin/subcutaneous excision if significant skin excess is expected following SAL.[36]

Bleeding or leaking vesicles may be managed by carbon dioxide laser photoevaporation, sclerotherapy, or resection. Resection is an option for localized disease because the wound can be closed by direct approximation of tissues. However, vesicles often recur through the scar. Large areas of vesicular bleeding or leakage are best managed by carbon dioxide laser or sclerotherapy; alternatively, wide resection and skin graft coverage is required (**Fig. 5**). Microcystic vesicles involving the oral cavity respond well to radiofrequency ablation.[37] Patients and families are counseled that LM can expand following any intervention and, thus, additional treatments may be required in the future.

Management of LM of the tongue can be particularly challenging. For acute tongue enlargement, patients are admitted for airway observation, antibiotics, and corticosteroids. Although sclerotherapy, radioablation, and laser may effectively treat the surface of the tongue, surgical reduction may be required for severe macroglossia.[37–40] The authors prefer the "W" resection technique, which reduces the tongue anteriorly and laterally away from the neurovascular structures (**Fig. 6**). Stay sutures are placed at the tip and sides of the tongue. The tongue is pulled forward and the lower teeth are palpated. A mark is made at this point, which represents the most posterior aspect of the resection. The "W" pattern is drawn, marking the central wedge and lateral areas that are excised. The corresponding pattern is then outlined on the ventral surface. Starting dorsally, a scalpel is used to incise the mucosa and dissection is carried down partially through the muscle using electrocautery. The procedure is then repeated on the ventral surface. The specimen, resembling a W, is removed, and the central wedge and lateral walls are closed. A nasal feeding tube is placed intraoperatively and is not removed until the child is tolerating oral intake. Patients usually remain intubated following the procedure and are extubated when the postoperative edema has improved.

REFERENCES

1. Young AE. Pathogenesis of vascular malformations. In: Mulliken JB, Young AE, editors. Vascular birthmarks: hemangiomas and malformations. Philadelphia (PA): Saunders; 1988. p. 107–13.
2. Mulliken JB, Glowacki J. Hemangiomas and vascular malformations in infants and children: a classification based on endothelial characteristics. Plast Reconstr Surg 1982;69:412–22.
3. Finn MC, Glowacki J, Mulliken JB. Congenital vascular lesions: clinical application of a new classification. J Pediatr Surg 1983;18:894–900.
4. Sabin F. On the origin of the lymphatic system from the veins and the development of the lymph hearts and thoracic duct in the pig. Am J Anat 1902;1:367–89.
5. Kaipainen A, Korhonen J, Mustonen T, et al. Expression of the fms-like tyrosine kinase 4 gene becomes restricted to lymphatic endothelium during development. Proc Natl Acad Sci U S A 1995;92:3566–70.
6. Wigle JT, Oliver G. Prox 1 function is required for the development of the murine lymphatic system. Cell 1999;98:769–78.
7. Smeltzer DM, Stickler GB, Schirger A. Primary lymphedema in children and adolescents: a follow-up study and review. Pediatrics 1985;76:206–18.

8. Limaye N, Boon LM, Vikkula M. From germline towards somatic mutations in the pathophysiology of vascular anomalies. Hum Mol Genet 2009;18:65–75.
9. Padwa BL, Hayward PG, Ferraro NF, et al. Cervicofacial lymphatic malformation: clinical course, surgical intervention, and pathogenesis of skeletal hypertrophy. Plast Reconstr Surg 1995;95:951–60.
10. Edwards PD, Rahbar R, Ferraro NF, et al. Lymphatic malformation of the lingual base and oral floor. Plast Reconstr Surg 2005;115:1906–15.
11. Greene AK, Burrows PE, Smith L, et al. Periorbital lymphatic malformation: clinical course and management in 42 patients. Plast Reconstr Surg 2005;115:22–30.
12. Upton J, Coombs CJ, Mulliken JB, et al. Vascular malformations of the upper limb: a review of 270 patients. J Hand Surg Am 1999;24:1019–35.
13. Choi DJ, Alomari AI, Chaudry G, et al. Neurointerventional management of low-flow vascular malformations of the head and neck. Neuroimaging Clin N Am 2009;19:199–218.
14. Burrows RE, Laor T, Paltiel H, et al. Diagnostic imaging in the evaluation of vascular birthmarks. Dermatol Clin 1998;16:455–88.
15. Paltiel H, Burrows PE, Kozakewich HP, et al. Soft-tissue vascular anomalies: utility of US for diagnosis. Radiology 2000;214:747–54.
16. Florez-Vargas A, Vargas SO, Debelenko LV, et al. Comparative analysis of D2-40 and LYVE-1 immunostaining in lymphatic malformations. Lymphology 2008;41:103–10.
17. Tiret L, Nivoche Y, Hatton F, et al. Complications related to anesthesia in infants and children. Br J Anaesth 1988;61:263–9.
18. Cohen MM, Cameron CB, Duncan PG. Pediatric anesthesia morbidity and mortality in the perioperative period. Anesth Analg 1990;70:160–7.
19. Tay CL, Tan GM, Ng SA. Critical incidents in paediatric anaesthesia: an audit of 1000 anaesthetics in Singapore. Paediatr Anaesth 2001;11:711–8.
20. Murat I, Constant I, Maudhuy H. Perioperative anaesthetic morbidity in children: database of 24,165 anaesthetics over a 30-month period. Paediatr Anaesth 2004;14:158–66.
21. Charlesworth R. The toddler: affective development. In: Charlesworth R, editor. Understanding child development. 6th edition. Clifton Park (NY): Delmar Learning; 1994. p. 304.
22. Santrock JW. The self and identity. In: Santrock JW, editor. Child development. 7th edition. Columbus (OH): McGraw-Hill; 1996. p. 378–85.
23. Neisser U. Memory development: new questions and old. Developmental Review 2004;24:154.
24. Smith MC, Zimmerman B, Burke DK, et al. Efficacy and safety of OK-432 immunotherapy of lymphatic malformations. Laryngoscope 2009;119:107–15.
25. Burrows PE, Mitri RK, Alomari A, et al. Percutaneous sclerotherapy of lymphatic malformations with doxycycline. Lymphat Res Biol 2008;6:209–16.
26. Nehra D, Jacobson L, Barnes P, et al. Doxycycline sclerotherapy as primary treatment of head and neck lymphatic malformations in children. J Pediatr Surg 2008;43:451–60.
27. Alomari AI, Karian VE, Lord DJ, et al. Percutaneous sclerotherapy for lymphatic malformations: a retrospective analysis of patient-evaluated improvement. J Vasc Interv Radiol 2006;17:1639–48.
28. Burrows PE, Mason KP. Percutaneous treatment of low flow vascular malformations. J Vasc Interv Radiol 2004;15:431–45.
29. Bai Y, Jia J, Huang XX, et al. Sclerotherapy of microcystic lymphatic malformations in oral and facial regions. J Oral Maxillofac Surg 2009;67:251–6.
30. Berenguer B, Burrows PE, Zurakowski D, et al. Sclerotherapy of craniofacial venous malformations: complications and results. Plast Reconstr Surg 1999;104:1–11.
31. Alqahtani A, Nguyen LT, Flageole H, et al. 25 years' experience with lymphangiomas in children. J Pediatr Surg 1999;34:1164–8.
32. Saijo M, Munro IR, Mancer K. Lymphangioma. A long-term follow-up study. Plast Reconstr Surg 1975;56:642–51.
33. Fliegelman LJ, Friedland D, Brandwein M, et al. Lymphatic malformation: predictive factors for recurrence. Otolaryngol Head Neck Surg 2000;123:706–10.
34. Brorson H, Svensson H. Liposuction combined with controlled compression therapy reduces arm lymphedema more effectively than controlled compression therapy alone. Plast Reconstr Surg 1998;102:1058–67.
35. Greene AK, Slavin SA, Borud L. Treatment of lower extremity lymphedema with suction-assisted lipectomy. Plast Reconstr Surg 2006;118:118e–21e.
36. Miller TA, Wyatt LE, Rudkin GH. Staged skin and subcutaneous excision for lymphedema: a favorable report of long-term results. Plast Reconstr Surg 1998;102:1486–98.
37. Grimmer JF, Mulliken JB, Burrows PE, et al. Radiofrequency ablation of microcystic lymphatic malformation in the oral cavity. Arch Otolaryngol Head Neck Surg 2006;132:1251–6.
38. Wiegand S, Eivazi B, Zimmermann AP, et al. Microcystic lymphatic malformations of the tongue: diagnosis, classification, and treatment. Arch Otolaryngol Head Neck Surg 2009;135:976–83.
39. Boardman SJ, Cochrane LA, Roebuck D, et al. Multimodality treatment of pediatric lymphatic malformations of the head and neck using surgery and sclerotherapy. Arch Otolaryngol Head Neck Surg 2010;136:270–6.
40. Perkins JA. Overview of macroglossia and its treatment. Curr Opin Otolaryngol Head Neck Surg 2009;17:460–5.

Management of Venous Malformations

Arin K. Greene, MD, MMSc[a,*], Ahmad I. Alomari, MD, MSc[b]

KEYWORDS

- Glomuvenous • Sclerotherapy • Treatment
- Vascular anomaly • Vascular malformation
- Venous malformation • Verrucous hemangioma

CLINICAL FEATURES

Venous malformation (VM) results from an error in vascular morphogenesis; veins are dilated with thin walls and abnormal smooth muscle.[1] Consequently, lesions expand, flow stagnates, and clotting occurs. Although a VM is present at birth, it may not become evident until childhood or adolescence when it has grown large enough to cause a visible deformity or symptoms. Lesions are blue, soft, and compressible; hard calcified phleboliths may be palpable. VMs may range from small localized skin lesions to diffuse malformations involving multiple tissue planes and vital structures.

VMs are typically sporadic and solitary in 90% of patients; 50% of patients have a somatic mutation in the endothelial receptor TIE2.[2,3] Angiopoietins, the ligands for TIE2, are involved in angiogenesis; the mutation uncouples endothelial cells and pericytes altering venous development.[3,4] Sporadic VMs are usually larger than 5 cm (56%); single (99%); and located on the head/neck (47%), extremities (40%), or trunk (13%).[2] Almost all lesions involve the skin, mucosa, or subcutaneous tissue; 50% of the lesions also affect deeper structures (ie, muscle, bone, joints, viscera).[2]

Approximately 10% of patients with VM have multifocal familial lesions, either glomuvenous malformation (GVM) (8.0%) or cutaneomucosal VM (CMVM) (2.0%).[2,5] GVM is an autosomal dominant condition with abnormal smooth muscle–like glomus cells along the ectatic veins and is caused by a loss-of-function mutation in the glomulin gene.[6,7] Lesions are typically multiple (70%), small (two-thirds are <5 cm), and located in the skin and subcutaneous tissue. GVM involves the extremities (76%), trunk (14%), or head/neck (10%). GVM is more painful than typical VM, especially on palpation.[7] It is reported that 17% of patients develop new lesions over time.[7] CMVMs are small multifocal mucocutaneous anomalies caused by a gain-of-function mutation in the TIE2 receptor.[4] The condition is autosomal dominant and less common than GVM. Lesions are small (76% of the lesions are <5 cm); multiple (73%); and located on the head/neck (50%), extremity (37%), or trunk (13%).[2] Unlike GVMs, CMVMs are not painful on palpation.[2] Cerebral cavernous malformation (CCM) is a rare familial disorder with VM involving the brain and spinal cord; patients may also have hyperkeratotic skin lesions.[5,8] The disorder results from mutations in CCM1/KRIT1, CCM2, and CCM3 genes, and patients are at risk for developing new intracranial malformations and hemorrhage.[9–11]

Blue rubber bleb nevus syndrome (BRBNS) is a rare condition with multiple small (<2 cm) VMs

Disclosures: None.

[a] Department of Plastic and Oral Surgery, Vascular Anomalies Center, Children's Hospital Boston, Harvard Medical School, 300 Longwood Avenue, Boston, MA 02115, USA
[b] Department of Radiology, Vascular Anomalies Center, Children's Hospital Boston, Harvard Medical School, 300 Longwood Avenue, Boston, MA 02115, USA
* Corresponding author.
E-mail address: arin.greene@childrens.harvard.edu

Clin Plastic Surg 38 (2011) 83–93
doi:10.1016/j.cps.2010.08.003
0094-1298/11/$ – see front matter

involving the skin, soft tissue, and gastrointestinal tract.[12–14] Morbidity is primarily associated with gastrointestinal bleeding requiring long-term blood transfusions. Diffuse phlebectasia of Bockenheimer is an eponym occasionally used for an extensive extremity VM involving the skin, subcutaneous tissue, muscle, and bone.[15] Sinus pericranii is a venous anomaly of the scalp or face with transcalvarial communication with the dural sinus. Verrucous hemangioma (VH) most closely resembles a hyperkeratotic VM (verrucous VM), although some histologic features are similar to an involuted infantile hemangioma.[16] Lesions range from 2 to 8 cm and are located on an extremity (91%) or the trunk (9%).[16] VH involves the skin and subcutis, becomes more hyperkeratotic over time, and is frequently associated with bleeding. VMs may also be a part of a combined malformation, particularly lymphatic, because lymphatics arise from veins embryologically.[1,17–19] Phlebectasia, a distinct venous anomaly, has 3 major forms: (1) sporadic (also called congenital varicosity), (2) associated with lymphatic malformation (LM), and (3) syndromic (eg, Klippel-Trénaunay syndrome).[20]

Complications of VMs depend on the extent and location of the anomaly. Lesions often cause psychosocial morbidity because of their appearance. Patients can have pain and swelling from dependent positioning or secondary to thrombosis and phlebolith formation. Head and neck VMs may present with mucosal bleeding or progressive distortion, leading to airway or orbital compromise. Extremity VMs can cause leg length discrepancy, hypoplasia due to disuse atrophy, pathologic fracture, hemarthrosis, and degenerative arthritis.[21] VMs of muscle may result in fibrosis and subsequent pain and disability.[22] Patients with phlebectasia, particularly when it communicates with the deep venous system through large perforators, are at risk for thrombosis and pulmonary embolism. Gastrointestinal VMs can cause bleeding and chronic anemia. Stagnation within a large VM results in a localized intravascular coagulopathy (LIC) and thromboses. A VM is especially problematic because it is progressive; it enlarges over time, particularly during adolescence; and often reexpands after treatment. Consequently, most patients who present with asymptomatic lesions will ultimately require intervention.

DIAGNOSIS

At least 90% of VMs are diagnosed by history and physical examination.[23,24] The primary differential diagnosis is LM. Patients should be queried about a family history of similar lesions, especially if GVM or CMVM is suspected. Unlike sporadic VMs, familial lesions are usually smaller, multiple, and superficial; GVM is painful on palpation. If the diagnosis is equivocal, a hand-held Doppler will rule out a fast-flow lesion and dependent positioning will cause a VM to enlarge.

Small superficial VMs do not require further diagnostic workup. However, large or deeper lesions are evaluated by magnetic resonance imaging (MRI) or ultrasonography (US) to (1) confirm the diagnosis, (2) define the extent of the malformation, and (3) plan treatment. To adequately assess a vascular anomaly, MRI sequences are obtained with fat suppression and contrast. VMs are hyperintense on T2-weighted images, except for phleboliths, which demonstrate a low-intensity signal on both T1- and T2-weighted sequences. Abnormal arterial flow is not present.[25] VMs can appear less intense after treatment because of scar tissue.[25] VMs enhance heterogeneously after gadolinium administration. Magnetic resonance venography delineates the deep venous system in extremity lesions. US is a good alternative for some localized VMs and does not require sedation in young children. US findings include compressible anechoic to hypoechoic spaces, with septations that show no flow on color Doppler and are separated by more solid regions of variable echogenicity.[26] Phleboliths are hyperechoic, with acoustic shadowing.[27] Computed tomography is occasionally indicated to assess an osseous VM. Intralesional venography is not usually needed for confirming the diagnosis but is essential before sclerosant injection. Phlebectasia is initially imaged with US to demonstrate the dilated incompetent veins and large perforators. Histopathologic diagnosis of VM is rarely necessary but may be indicated if findings of imaging are equivocal.

MANAGEMENT

Nonoperative

Patients with GVM or CMVM are counseled about the risk of developing new lesions as well as the autosomal dominant inheritance pattern. The natural history of VM is explained, including the possibility of expansion and phlebothrombosis. Because VMs are at a greatest risk for expansion in adolescence, sex hormones may be involved in its pathogenesis. Consequently, the authors recommend progesterone-only oral contraceptives for women with problematic lesions because estrogen has more potent proangiogenic activity than progesterone.[28–31] Patients with a large extremity VM are prescribed custom-fitted compression garments to reduce blood stagnation and thus minimize expansion, LIC, phleboliths, and pain.[32–34]

Patients with recurrent pain secondary to phlebothrombosis are given prophylactic aspirin, 81 mg daily, to prevent thrombosis. Patients with an extensive VM are evaluated by a hematologist. Large lesions are at risk for coagulation of stagnant blood, stimulation of thrombin, and conversion of fibrinogen to fibrin. Fibrinolysis results in LIC.[34] Levels of plasma D dimers and fibrin split products are elevated, whereas levels of fibrinogen; factors V, VIII, and XIII; and antithrombin are low.[34] Prothrombin time and activated partial thromboplastin time are normal.[34] The chronic consumptive coagulopathy can cause either thrombosis (phleboliths) or bleeding (hemarthrosis, hematoma, intraoperative blood loss).[34]

Significant bleeding or life-threatening thrombosis is rare. Almost all patients with VMs are not at risk for thromboemboli because VMs do not affect the deep venous system and thrombosed lesions are sequestered from larger veins. However, patients with phlebectasia or extensive venous anomalies involving the deep venous system are at risk for thromboemboli. Low-molecular-weight heparin (LMWH) is considered for patients with significant LIC or for those who are at risk for disseminated intravascular coagulation.[35] Individuals who develop a serious thrombotic event require long-term anticoagulation. Usually, heparin is given for a short term, and the patient is transitioned to warfarin. An inferior or superior vena caval filter is considered for patients with contraindications to anticoagulation or for those who have thromboembolic events despite anticoagulation.[34]

Operative

Intervention for VM is reserved for symptomatic lesions that cause pain or deformity or threaten vital structures. VM is a benign condition, and nonproblematic lesions can be observed. Many children do not require treatment at the time of diagnosis. However, because a VM slowly expands, patients may become symptomatic and seek intervention in childhood or adolescence. Less commonly, a VM involving an anatomically sensitive area or causing gross deformity necessitates management as early as infancy. If possible, intervention may be postponed until after 12 months of age when the risk of anesthesia is lowest.[36–39] Therapy for lesions causing a visible deformity should be considered before the age of 3.5 years to limit psychological morbidity; at this age, long-term memory and self-esteem begin to form.[40–42] Some parents, however, elect to wait until the child is older and able to make the decision to proceed with operative intervention, especially if the deformity is minor. However, as lesions enlarge with age, they may become more difficult to treat.

Sclerotherapy

The first-line treatment of problematic VMs is sclerotherapy, which is generally safer and more effective than resection.[43] Sclerotherapy involves the injection of a sclerosant into the malformation, which then causes cellular destruction, thrombosis, and intense inflammation. Scarring leads to shrinkage of the lesion (**Fig. 1**). Good to excellent results are obtained in 75% to 90% of patients, including reduction in the size of the malformation and alleviation of the symptoms (**Fig. 2**).[27,43,44] Often, multiple treatments are required, spaced approximately 6 weeks apart. Diffuse malformations (ie, Bockenheimer-type VM) are managed by targeting specific symptomatic areas because the lesion is too extensive to treat at one time. Sclerotherapy is continued until symptoms are alleviated or vascular spaces are no longer present to inject. Although sclerotherapy effectively reduces the size of the lesion and improves symptoms, it does not remove the malformation. Consequently, patients can continue to have a mass or visible deformity after treatment, which may be improved by resection. In addition, VMs usually reexpand after sclerotherapy, and patients often require additional interventions over the course of their lifetime. For example, after 6 months of treatment with sodium tetradecyl sulfate (STS), 45% of patients have partial recanalization.[45]

The authors' preferred sclerosants are STS and absolute ethanol (95%–98%). Other sclerosants include polidocanol (Aetoxisclerol), alcoholic solution of zein (Ethibloc), bleomycin, sodium morrhuate, or ethanolamine oleate. STS is most commonly used, and the authors mix 10 mL of 3% STS (maximum dose is 0.5 mL/kg) with 2 mL of ethiodized oil (Ethiodol) and 10 mL (or more) of air. The mixture is then repeatedly forced back and forth between 2 syringes attached to a 3-way stopcock to produce a foaming solution, which increases efficacy.[27] Ethanol is probably more toxic to the VM than STS, but it has to be used carefully because of potential local and systemic complications. The ethanol dose should not exceed 0.5 to 1 mL/kg (maximum of 30–60 mL). Because ethanol can cause nerve damage, care should be taken when it is used adjacent to important structures (eg, facial nerve). Small lesions, particularly in adolescents and

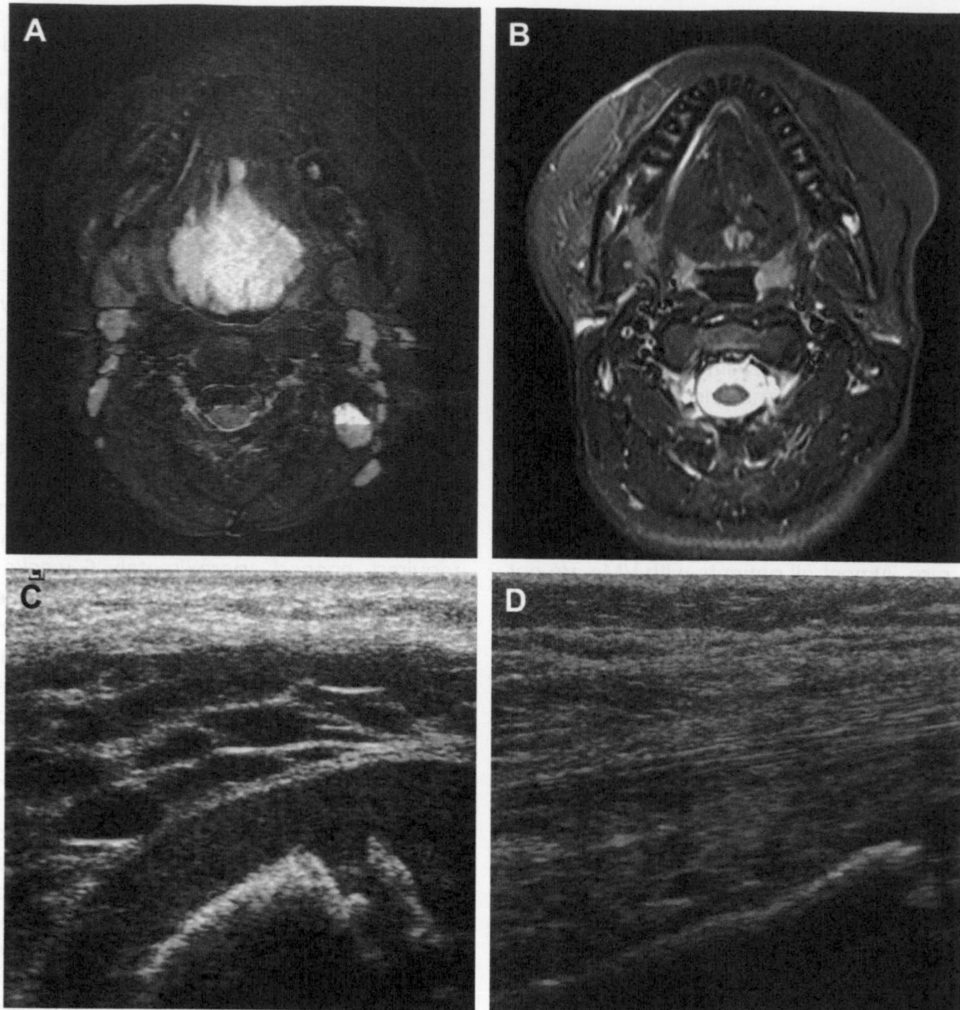

Fig. 1. Effects of sclerotherapy on VM. (*A*) Axial T2 MRI with fat saturation showing a VM of the tongue in a 13-year-old girl. (*B*) Resolution of the VM 3 years after treatment. (*C*) Sonographic image of a large VM of the knee showing compressible venous spaces. (*D*) The venous spaces are replaced by scar tissue 2 months after sclerotherapy.

adults, may be treated in the office without image guidance; the authors dilute 3% STS with saline to inject a 1% solution.

Whenever possible, the malformation is documented with serial photographs. Most patients, especially children, are managed under general anesthesia. For large VMs, a Foley catheter is placed to monitor the urine output. High-quality US and fluoroscopic imaging are instrumental in performing sclerotherapy. The VM is first cannulated with US guidance using small needles (20–22 gauge). After confirming venous return, diluted contrast is injected under digital subtraction angiography (or fluoroscopy) to determine the anatomy of the lesion and its relation to the adjacent venous drainage system. Multiple injections into different portions of the VM are often needed. For extremity lesions, the authors initially obtain an ascending venogram and confirm the patency and morphology of the deep venous system. Extravasation should be excluded before sclerosant injection; otherwise the access is adjusted or abandoned. The volume of contrast injected to opacify the lesion approximates the amount of sclerosant that will be subsequently delivered. Typically, a contrast agent (Ethiodol) or air/carbon dioxide is mixed with the sclerosant to allow fluoroscopic or sonographic monitoring. If venous drainage is noted to be large and rapid, the outflow is occluded with external pressure or a tourniquet. Preventing the rapid distribution of the sclerosant into the systemic circulation

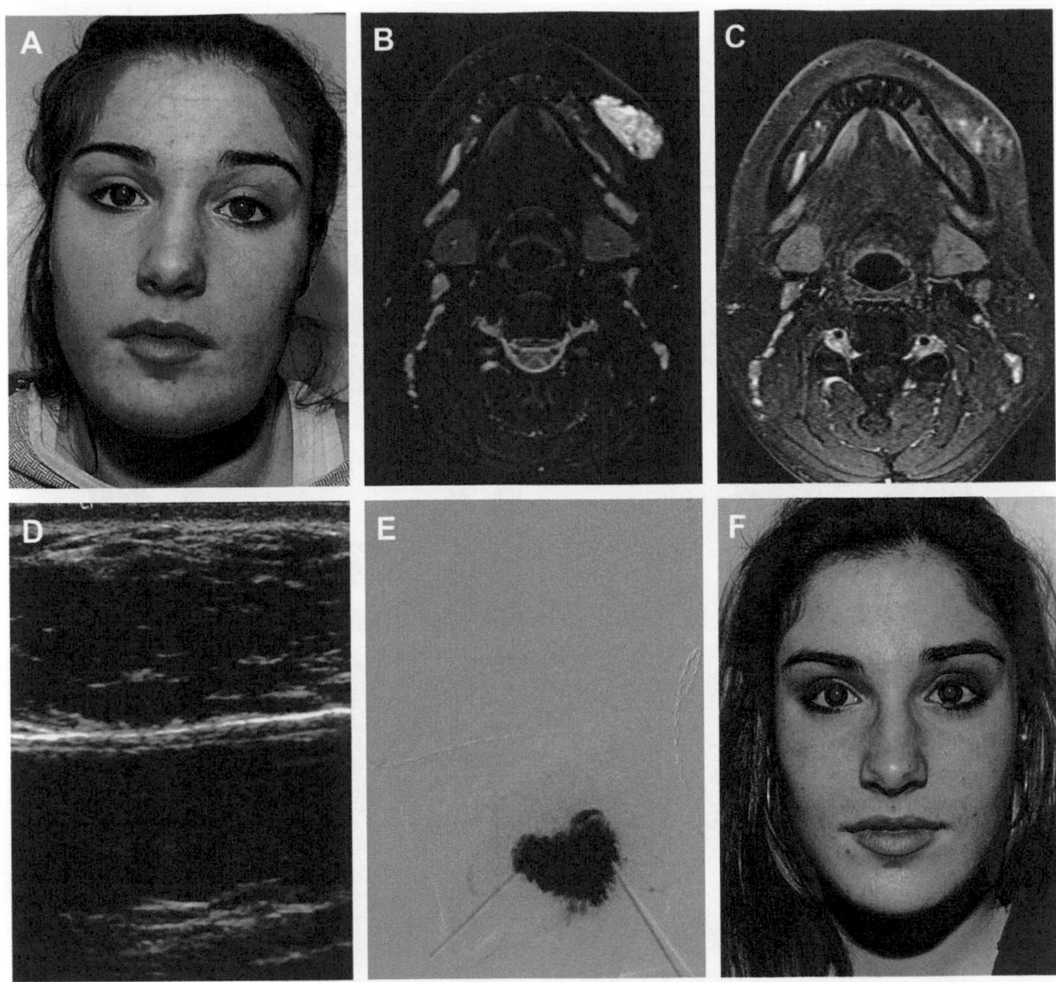

Fig. 2. Management of VM with sclerotherapy. (*A*) A 15-year-old girl with an enlarging lesion of the left cheek. (*B*) Axial T2 MRI with fat saturation shows a localized VM involving the cheek. (*C*) Axial T1 MRI illustrates heterogeneous enhancement of the lesion with contrast. (*D*) US shows compressible hypoechoic venous spaces outlined by echogenic walls. (*E*) Intralesional venogram of a spongiform venous lesion with a minor draining vein. (*F*) Resolution of cheek asymmetry 2 months after sclerotherapy with sodium tetradecyl sulfate.

improves the containment of the agent inside the VM and minimizes systemic complications. Rarely, operative intervention, platinum coils, or a liquid polymer (Onyx, ev3 Neurovascular, Irvine, CA, USA) is required to close large venous outflow channels before sclerotherapy to protect important areas (eg, ophthalmic veins, sinus pericranii).[27]

Early responses to sclerotherapy are swelling, irritation of the overlying skin, and bruising. The most common local complication is skin blistering and ulceration (<5%).[43,44] Ulceration is more common if the VM involves the dermis or when ethanol is used. Wounds are allowed to heal secondarily and are managed with topical antibiotics or dressing changes, depending on the depth of the wound. Transient or permanent nerve injury can occur after ethanol sclerotherapy, which is likely caused by extravasation.[43] Extravasation of the sclerosant into muscle can cause atrophy and contracture.[44] Posttreatment edema progresses for 48 hours. Except for high-risk individuals, most patients are discharged home the same day. Corticosteroids and antibiotics are not regularly administered perioperatively. Posttreatment swelling in certain anatomic areas may necessitate close monitoring. Patients with airway lesions are admitted to the intensive care unit; occasionally, prolonged intubation or tracheostomy is required. Orbital injections can cause orbital compartment syndrome, and patients are examined by an ophthalmologist immediately after the procedure. Excessive intrafascial treatment of deep extremity lesions can cause compartment

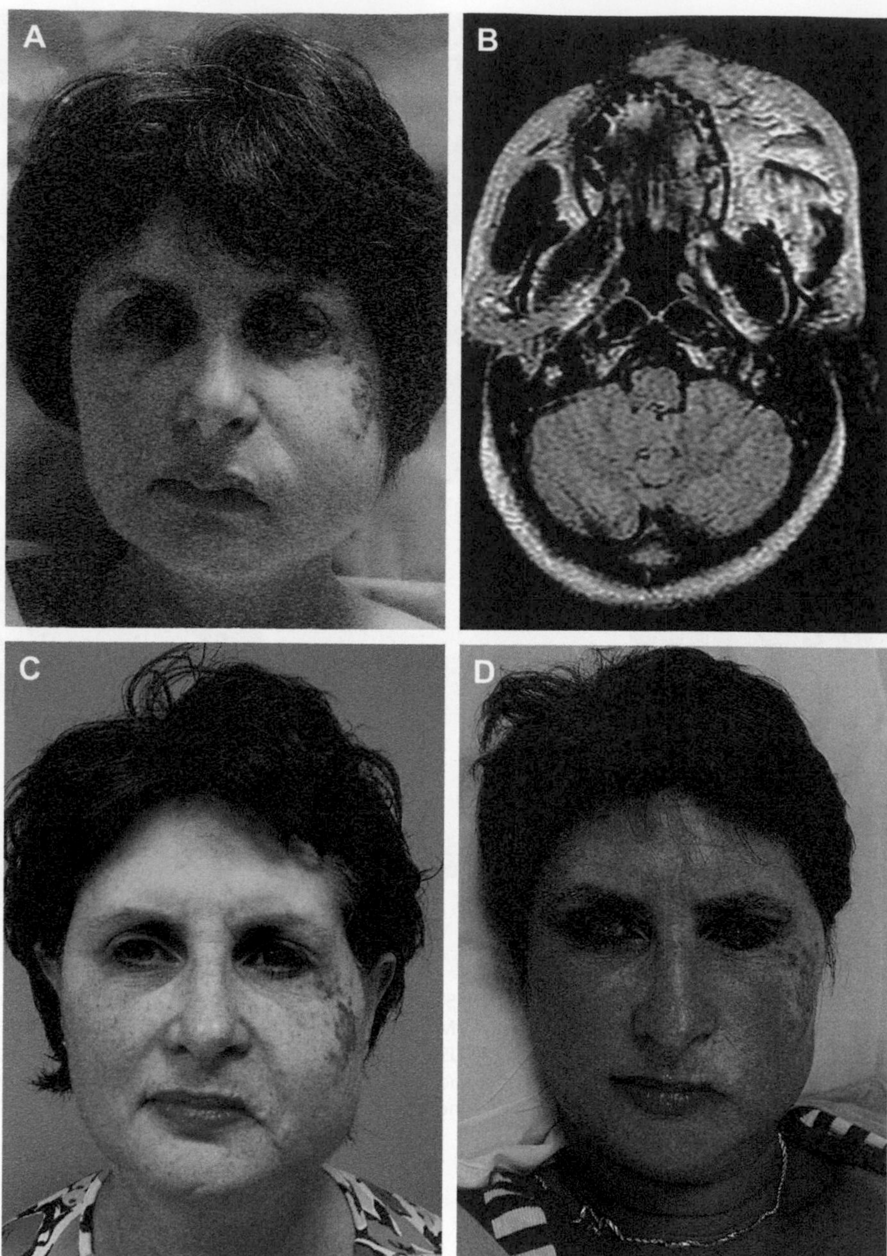

Fig. 3. Management of diffuse VM with sclerotherapy and subtotal resection. (*A*) A 54-year-old woman with an enlarging VM of the left side of the face causing progressive visual obstruction, pain, and deformity. She had been treated with sclerotherapy and radiation as a child. (*B*) Axial T2 MRI shows diffuse involvement of the left side of the face. (*C*) Twelve months after subtotal resection of the fibrotic malformation of the cheek, not amenable to sclerotherapy, through a transbuccal incision. Intraoperatively, her upper lip, eyelids, oral mucosa, and superficial cheek were also treated with sclerotherapy (1% STS). (*D*) Twelve months after additional sclerotherapy to the upper lip, oral mucosa, and cheek, done in the office with local anesthesia.

syndrome if extravasation of the sclerosant occcurs.[27]

Systemic adverse events from sclerotherapy, including hemolysis, hemoglobinuria, and oliguria, are more common when large lesions are managed with a significant volume of a sclerosant. To prevent renal injury, patients are administered 5% dextrose in water containing 75 mEq/L of sodium bicarbonate to alkalinize the urine; maintenance fluid is doubled for the first 4 hours after treatment. Oliguria is successfully managed with 1 small dose of diuretic. Patients with low fibrinogen levels who are at risk of thromboembolism may be given LMWH (0.5 mg/kg/dose twice daily to a maximum of 30 mg twice daily) 14 days before and after the procedure. Large ethanol volumes have been associated with additional systemic toxicity, including central nervous system depression, pulmonary hypertension, hemolysis, thromboembolism, and arrhythmias.[27] Clinical and sonographic examinations assess the response to treatment and any residual disease.

Resection

Extirpation of VMs can be associated with significant morbidity, such as major blood loss, iatrogenic injury, and deformity. In contrast to sclerotherapy, resection is not favorable because (1) the entire lesion can rarely be removed, (2) the excision may cause a deformity worse than the malformation, (3) the risk of recurrence is high because abnormal channels adjacent to the lesion are not treated, and (4) the risk of blood loss and iatrogenic injury is high. Resection should be considered for (1) small well-localized VMs that can be completely removed or (2) persistent symptoms after completion of sclerotherapy (patent channels are not accessible for further injection) (**Fig. 3**). When considering resection, the postoperative scar/deformity left after removal of the VM should be weighed against the preoperative appearance of the lesion.

Almost all patients with VMs should undergo sclerotherapy several months before operative intervention to facilitate the resection, improve the outcome, and lower the recurrence rate (**Fig. 4**). After adequate sclerotherapy, the VM is replaced by a scar, and thus the risk of blood loss, iatrogenic injury, and recurrence is reduced. In addition, fibrosis facilitates resection and reconstruction. Even after a VM has been sclerosed, major blood loss can occur during extirpation. Some small well-localized VMs may be removed without preoperative sclerotherapy. If a patient is

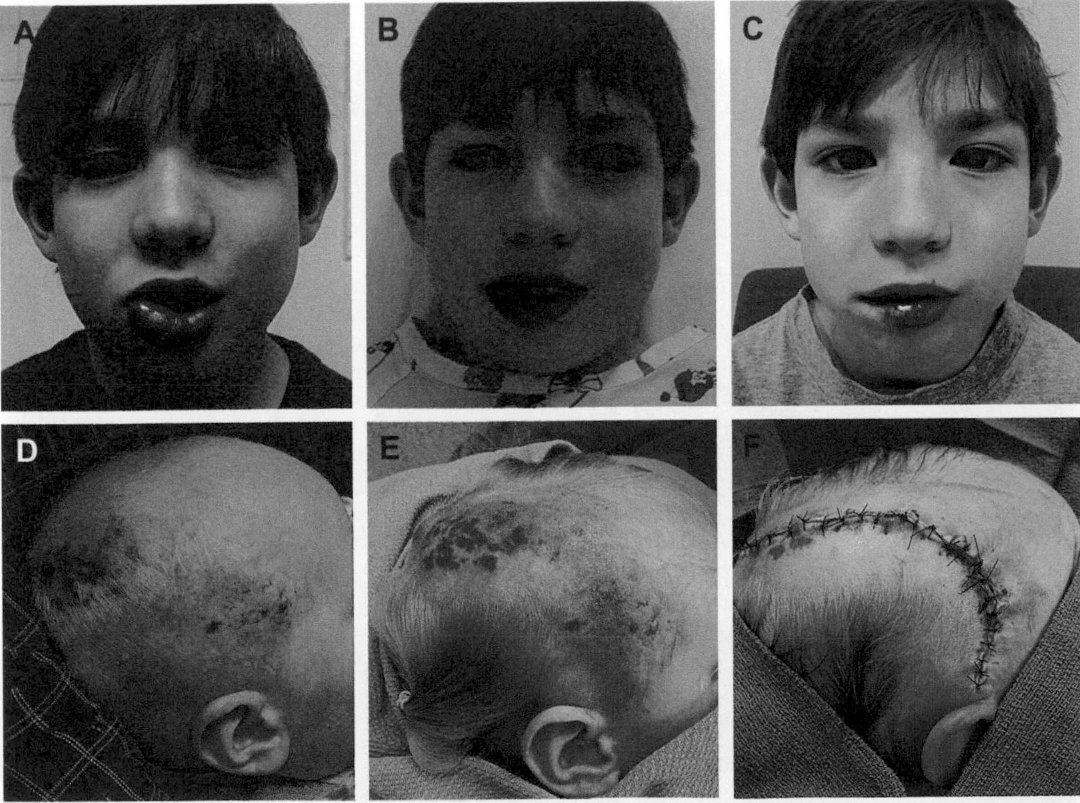

Fig. 4. Management of VM with sclerotherapy followed by resection. (*A*) A 5-year-old boy with an enlarging VM of the lower lip. (*B*) Reduction of the VM after 3 sessions of sclerotherapy with STS. Further sclerotherapy was not possible because venous spaces had been replaced by fibrosis. (*C*) Improved contour 6 weeks after resection of residual VM and scar tissue using a transverse mucosal incision. (*D*) A 7-month-old girl with a VM of the scalp. (*E*) Reduction of the lesion after 3 STS treatments. Additional sclerotherapy was not possible because accessible venous spaces had been obliterated. (*F*) The scalp after resection of the residual VM and scar tissue.

receiving long-term anticoagulation, it is held for 24 hours perioperatively (12 hours before and after the intervention) to prevent bleeding complications.[27,34] If fibrinogen levels are low on the day of the procedure, cryoprecipitate is occasionally administered. Because GVMs are usually small and less amenable to sclerotherapy, the first-line therapy for symptomatic lesions is often resection (**Fig. 5**). VH is not amenable to sclerotherapy, and the only treatment is resection (**Fig. 6**). Because VH is often large and located on the lower extremity, staged serial excision or reconstruction with a skin graft is frequently required. Nd:YAG photocoagulation may be an adjuvant to sclerotherapy for the management of difficult airway lesions.[46] Gastrointestinal VMs with chronic bleeding, anemia, and transfusion requirements are typically managed by resection. Solitary lesions are treated by endoscopic banding or sclerotherapy.[14] Multifocal VMs (ie, BRBNS) require removal of as many lesions as possible through multiple enterotomies, instead of bowel resection, to preserve the intestinal length.[14] About 90% of patients do not have recurrent bleeding after resection of all individual VMs of the bowel.[14] Diffuse problematic colorectal VMs may require colectomy, anorectal mucosectomy, and endorectal pull-through.[47]

Head and neck VMs are removed by coronal (forehead, orbit), tarsal (eyelid), preauricular-melolabial-transoral (cheek), or transverse mucosal (lip) incision. Because significant blood loss can occur during extirpation, a local anesthetic with epinephrine is administered and resection of an extremity lesion is performed using a tourniquet. Postoperative compression reduces bleeding and swelling. Rarely, a localized VM may be excised and the wound edges reapproximated without complex reconstruction. For diffuse malformations, staged resection of defined regions is recommended. In problematic areas, such as bleeding vesicles or an overgrown lip, a subtotal resection should be performed rather than attempting complete excision of a benign lesion, which would result in a deformity worse than the malformation. Patients and families are

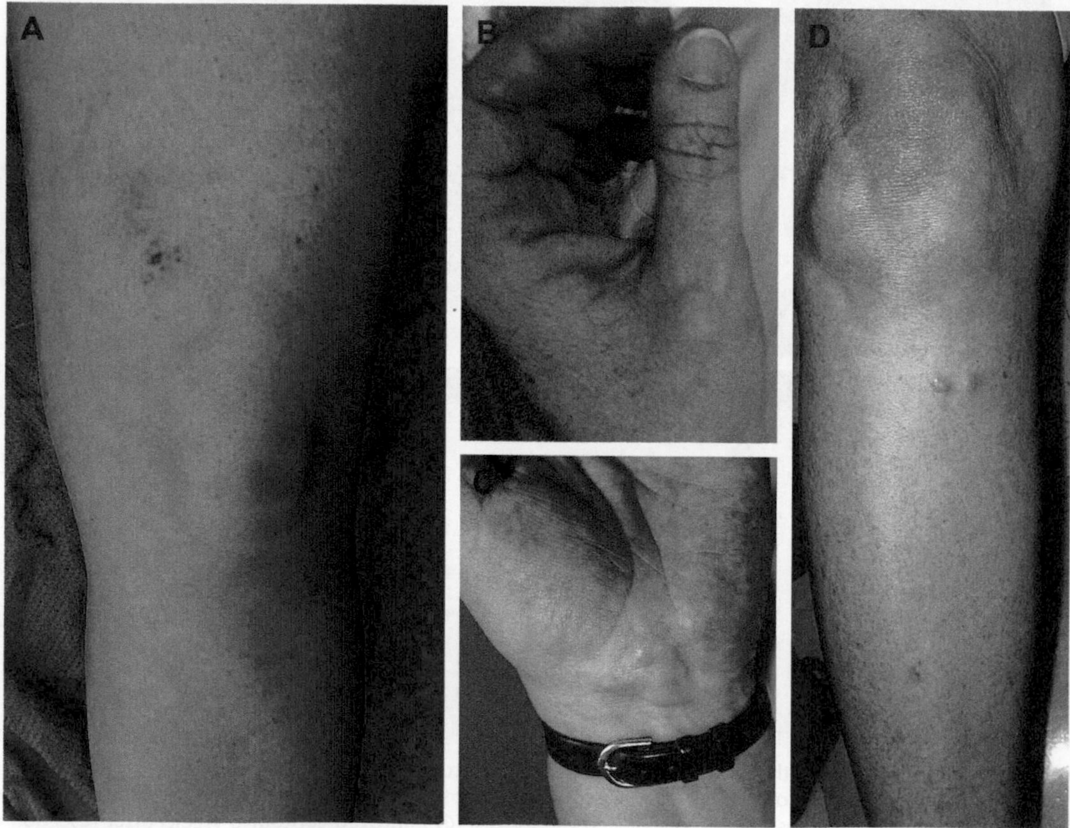

Fig. 5. Management of GVM. (*A*) A 16-year-old girl with a localized painful lesion of the lower extremity, which was resected. Pathology showed GVM. (*B–D*) The patient's mother had asymptomatic GVMs involving the hand and lower extremity, which did not require intervention.

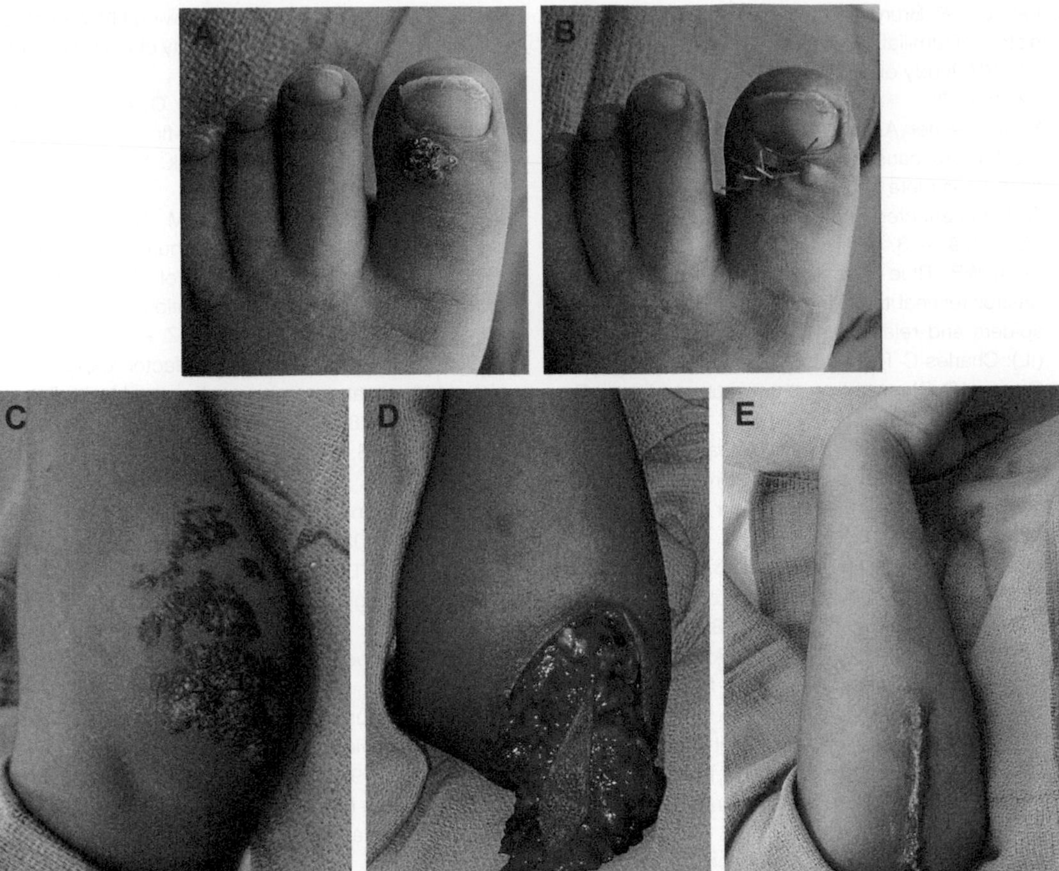

Fig. 6. Management of VH. (*A, B*) A 3-year-old girl with a localized bleeding lesion of the toe, which was excised. (*C–E*) A 9-year-old girl with an extensive bleeding VH of the upper extremity, managed by resection.

counseled that VMs can expand after excision and additional operative intervention may be required in the future.

REFERENCES

1. Young AE. Pathogenesis of vascular malformations. In: Mulliken JB, Young AE, editors. Vascular birthmarks: hemangiomas and malformations. Philadelphia: Saunders; 1988. p. 107–13.
2. Boon LM, Mulliken JB, Enjolras O, et al. Glomuvenous malformation (glomangioma) and venous malformation: distinct clinicopathologic and genetic entities. Arch Dermatol 2004;140:971–6.
3. Limaye N, Wouters V, Uebelhoer M, et al. Somatic mutations in angiopoietin receptor gene TEK cause solitary and multiple sporadic venous malformations. Nat Genet 2009;41:118–24.
4. Vikkula M, Boon LM, Carraway KL, et al. Vascular dysmorphogenesis caused by an activating mutation in the receptor tyrosine kinase TIE2. Cell 1996;87:1181–90.
5. Limaye N, Boon LM, Vikkula M. From germline towards somatic mutations in the pathophysiology of vascular anomalies. Hum Mol Genet 2009;18:65–75.
6. Brouillard P, Boon LM, Mulliken JB, et al. Mutations in a novel factor, glomulin, are responsible for glomuvenous malformations ("glomangiomas"). Am J Hum Genet 2002;70:866–74.
7. Brouillard P, Ghassibe M, Penington A, et al. Four common glomulin mutations cause two thirds of glomuvenous malformations ("familial glomangiomas"): evidence for a founder effect. J Med Genet 2005;42:e13.
8. Labauge P, Enjolras O, Bonerandi JJ, et al. An association between autosomal dominant cerebral cavernomas and a distinctive hyperkeratotic cutaneous vascular malformation in 4 families. Ann Neurol 1999;45:250–4.
9. Laberge-le Couteulx S, Jung HH, Labauge P, et al. Truncated mutations in CCM1, encoding KRIT1, cause cavernous angiomas. Nat Genet 1999;23:189–93.

10. Labauge P, Brunereau L, Levy C, et al. The natural history of familial cerebral cavernomas: a retrospective MRI study of 40 patients. Neuroradiology 2000; 42:327–32.
11. Pagenstecher A, Stahl S, Sure U, et al. A two-hit mechanism causes cerebral cavernous malformations: complete inactivation of CCM1, CCM2 or CCM3 in affected endothelial cells. Hum Mol Genet 2009;18:911–8.
12. Bean WB. Blue rubber-bleb nevi of the skin and gastrointestinal tract. In: Bean WB, editor. Vascular spiders and related lesions of the skin. Springfield (IL): Charles C Thomas; 1958. p. 17–185.
13. Oranje AP. Blue rubber bleb nevus syndrome. Pediatr Dermatol 1986;3:304–10.
14. Fishman SJ, Smithers CJ, Folkman J, et al. Blue rubber bleb nevus syndrome: surgical eradication of gastrointestinal bleeding. Ann Surg 2005;241: 523–8.
15. Kubiena HF, Liang MG, Mulliken JB. Genuine diffuse phlebectasia of Bockenheimer: dissection of an eponym. Pediatr Dermatol 2006;23:294–7.
16. Tennant LB, Mulliken JB, Perez-Atayde AR, et al. Verrucous hemangioma revisited. Pediatr Dermatol 2006;23:208–15.
17. Sabin FR. On the origin of the lymphatic system from the veins and the development of the lymph hearts and thoracic duct in the pig. Am J Anat 1902;1: 367–89.
18. Kaipainen A, Korhonen J, Mustonen T, et al. Expression of the fms-like tyrosine kinase 4 gene becomes restricted to lymphatic endothelium during development. Proc Natl Acad Sci U S A 1995;92:3566–70.
19. Wigle JT, Oliver G. Prox 1 function is required for the development of the murine lymphatic system. Cell 1999;98:769–78.
20. Alomari AI. Characterization of a distinct syndrome that associates complex truncal overgrowth, vascular, and acral anomalies: a descriptive study of 18 cases of CLOVES syndrome. Clin Dysmorphol 2009;18:1–7.
21. Upton J, Coombs CJ, Mulliken JB, et al. Vascular malformations of the upper limb: a review of 270 patients. J Hand Surg Am 1999;24:1019–35.
22. Hein KD, Mulliken JB, Kozakewich HP, et al. Venous malformations of skeletal muscle. Plast Reconstr Surg 2002;110:1625–35.
23. Mulliken JB, Glowacki J. Hemangiomas and vascular malformations in infants and children: a classification based on endothelial characteristics. Plast Reconstr Surg 1982;69:412–22.
24. Finn MC, Glowacki J, Mulliken JB. Congenital vascular lesions: clinical application of a new classification. J Pediatr Surg 1983;18:894–900.
25. Burrows RE, Laor T, Paltiel H, et al. Diagnostic imaging in the evaluation of vascular birthmarks. Dermatol Clin 1998;16:455–88.
26. Paltiel H, Burrows PE, Kozakewich HPW, et al. Soft-tissue vascular anomalies: utility of US for diagnosis. Radiology 2000;214:747–54.
27. Choi DJ, Alomari AI, Chaudry G, et al. Neurointerventional management of low-flow vascular malformations of the head and neck. Neuroimaging Clin N Am 2009;19:199–218.
28. Johannisson E, Oberholzer M, Swahn ML, et al. Vascular changes in the human endometrium following the administration of the progesterone antagonist RU 486. Contraception 1989;39:103–17.
29. Hyder SM, Huang JC, Nawaz Z, et al. Regulation of vascular endothelial growth factor expression by estrogens and progestins. Environ Health Perspect 2000;108:785–90.
30. Heryanto B, Rogers PA. Regulation of endometrial endothelial cell proliferation by oestrogen and progesterone in the ovariectomized mouse. Reproduction 2002;123:107–13.
31. Kayisli UA, Luk J, Guzeloglu-Kayisli O, et al. Regulation of angiogenic activity of human endometrial endothelial cells in culture by ovarian steroids. J Clin Endocrinol Metab 2004;89:5794–802.
32. Enjolras O, Ciabrini D, Mazoyer E, et al. Extensive pure venous malformations in the upper or lower limb: a review of 27 cases. J Am Acad Dermatol 1997;36:219–25.
33. Mazoyer E, Enjolras O, Laurian C, et al. Coagulation abnormalities associated with extensive venous malformations of the limbs: differentiation from Kasabach-Merritt syndrome. Clin Lab Haematol 2002;24:243–51.
34. Adams DM, Wentzel MS. The role of the hematologist/oncologist in the care of patients with vascular anomalies. Pediatr Clin North Am 2008;55:339–55.
35. Dompmartin A, Acher A, Thibon P, et al. Association of localized intravascular coagulopathy with venous malformations. Arch Dermatol 2008;144:873–7.
36. Tiret L, Nivoche Y, Hatton F, et al. Complications related to anesthesia in infants and children. Br J Anaesth 1988;61:263–9.
37. Cohen MM, Cameron CB, Duncan PG. Pediatric anesthesia morbidity and mortality in the perioperative period. Anesth Analg 1990;70:160–7.
38. Tay CL, Tan GM, Ng SA. Critical incidents in paediatric anaesthesia: an audit of 1000 anaesthetics in Singapore. Paediatr Anaesth 2001;11:711–8.
39. Murat I, Constant I, Maudhuy H. Perioperative anaesthetic morbidity in children: database of 24165 anaesthetics over a 30-month period. Paediatr Anaesth 2004;14:158–66.
40. Charlesworth R. The toddler: affective development. In: Understanding child development. 6th edition. Clifton Park (NY): Delmar Learning; 1994. p. 304.
41. Santrock JW. The self and identity. In: Child development. 7th edition. Columbus (OH): McGraw-Hill; 1996. p. 378–85.

42. Neisser U. Memory development: new questions and old. Dev Rev 2004;24:154.
43. Berenguer B, Burrows PE, Zurakowski D, et al. Sclerotherapy of craniofacial venous malformations: complications and results. Plast Reconstr Surg 1999;104:1–11.
44. Burrows PE, Mason KP. Percutaneous treatment of low flow vascular malformations. J Vasc Interv Radiol 2004;15:431–45.
45. Yamaki T, Nozaki M, Sakurai H, et al. Prospective randomized efficacy of ultrasound-guided foam sclerotherapy compared with ultrasound-guided liquid sclerotherapy in the treatment of symptomatic venous malformations. J Vasc Surg 2008;47: 578–84.
46. Ohlms LA, Forsen J, Burrows PE. Venous malformations of the pediatric airway. Int J Pediatr Otorhinolaryngol 1996;37:99–114.
47. Fishman SJ, Shamberger RC, Fox VL, et al. Endorectal pull-through abates gastrointestinal hemorrhage from colorectal venous malformations. J Pediatr Surg 2000;35:982–4.

Management of Arteriovenous Malformations

Arin K. Greene, MD, MMSc[a,*], Darren B. Orbach, MD, PhD[b]

KEYWORDS

- Arteriovenous malformation • AVM • Capillary malformation
- CM-AVM • Embolization • PTEN

Arteriovenous malformation (AVM) results from an error in vascular development during embryogenesis. An absent capillary bed causes shunting of blood directly from the arterial to venous circulation through a fistula (direct connection of an artery to a vein) or nidus (abnormal channels bridging the feeding artery to the draining veins).[1] AVM may develop because primitive arteriovenous shunts fail to undergo apoptosis; AVM is 20 times more common in the central nervous system, where apoptosis is rare.[2] Genetic abnormalities cause certain types of familial AVMs. Hereditary hemorrhagic telangiectasia is attributable to mutations in endoglin and activin receptor–like kinase 1 (ALK-1), which affect transforming growth factor-beta (TGF-β) signaling.[3–5] Capillary malformation–arteriovenous malformation (CM-AVM) results from a mutation in RASA1.[6] Patients with PTEN mutations also can develop arteriovenous anomalies.[7]

ARTERIOVENOUS MALFORMATION

Clinical Features

The most common site of extracranial AVM is the head and neck, followed by the limbs, trunk, and viscera.[8] Although present at birth, AVM may not become evident until childhood. Lesions have a pink-red cutaneous stain, are warm, have a palpable thrill or bruit, and may be initially mistaken for a capillary malformation or hemangioma. Arteriovenous shunting reduces capillary oxygen delivery causing ischemia; patients are at risk for pain, ulceration, bleeding, and congestive heart failure. AVM also may cause disfigurement, destruction of tissues, and obstruction of vital structures. High-pressure shunting of blood can cause venous hemorrhage, and rupture of arteries may occur in weakened areas, such as aneurysms. Arterial bleeding most commonly occurs at skin or mucosal surfaces from erosion into a superficial component of the lesion.

Although AVM is considered a quiescent lesion, as evidenced by endothelial turnover,[9] it is not a static malformation; it progresses over time and recurs after treatment. Although the presence of an AVM may be troublesome, it is the *expansion* of the lesion that is the primary cause of morbidity. AVM worsens over time, and can be classified according to the Schobinger staging system (**Table 1**).[10] AVM may enlarge because of increased blood flow causing collateralization, dilatation of vessels (especially venous ectasia), and thickening of adjacent arteries and veins.[1,11] Latent arteriovenous shunts may open, stimulating hypertrophy of surrounding vessels from increased pressure.[1,10,12] Alternatively, aneurysms may increase the size of these lesions.[13,14]

Disclosures: none.

[a] Department of Plastic and Oral Surgery, Vascular Anomalies Center, Children's Hospital Boston, Harvard Medical School, 300 Longwood Avenue, Boston, MA 02115, USA
[b] Department of Radiology, Vascular Anomalies Center, Children's Hospital Boston, Harvard Medical School, 300 Longwood Avenue, Boston, MA 02115, USA
* Corresponding author. Department of Plastic and Oral Surgery, Vascular Anomalies Center, Children's Hospital Boston, Harvard Medical School, 300 Longwood Avenue, Boston, MA 02115.
E-mail address: arin.greene@childrens.harvard.edu

Clin Plastic Surg 38 (2011) 95–106
doi:10.1016/j.cps.2010.08.005
0094-1298/11/$ – see front matter

Table 1
Schobinger staging of AVM

Stage	Clinical Findings
I (Quiescence)	Warm, pink-blue, shunting on Doppler
II (Expansion)	Enlargement, pulsation, thrill, bruit, tortuous veins
III (Destruction)	Dystrophic skin changes, ulceration, bleeding, pain
IV (Decompensation)	Cardiac failure

Angiogenesis (growth of new blood vessels from preexisting vasculature) and/or vasculogenesis (de novo formation of new vasculature) may be involved in AVM expansion.[15] Although neovascularization may be a primary stimulus for AVM growth, it also could be a secondary event. For example, ischemia, a potent stimulator of angiogenesis, causes enlargement of AVM after proximal arterial ligation or trauma.[1,10,16] Alternatively, increased blood flow because of arteriovenous shunting may promote angiogenesis; vascular endothelial growth factor (VEGF) production and endothelial proliferation are stimulated by elevated blood flow.[17,18] Because both males and females have a twofold risk of progression to a higher Schobinger stage in adolescence, circulating hormones during this period may promote AVM expansion.[15]

Diagnosis

Ninety percent of AVMs are diagnosed by history and physical examination.[9,19] Unlike hemangioma, AVM expands after infancy, and, in contrast to capillary malformation, AVM has fast-flow. Hand-held Doppler examination showing fast-flow aids the clinical diagnosis and can exclude slow-flow vascular anomalies, such as venous or lymphatic malformation. If AVM is suspected, the diagnosis can be confirmed by ultrasonography (US), with color Doppler examination showing fast-flow and shunting. Magnetic resonance imaging (MRI) also is obtained to (1) confirm the diagnosis, (2) determine the extent of the lesion, and (3) plan treatment. To adequately assess a vascular anomaly, MRI with contrast and fat suppression, as well as T2-weighted sequences, is necessary. MRI shows dilated feeding arteries and draining veins, enhancement, and flow-voids.[20] Unlike hemangioma, AVM does not have a significant parenchymal mass. If the diagnosis remains unclear after US and MRI, angiography is performed. Angiography also is indicated if embolization or resection is planned, and can help determine the flow dynamics of the lesion. AVM shows tortuous, dilated, arteries with arteriovenous shunting and enlarged draining veins on angiography.[20] The nidus is angiographically manifest as dysplastic, tortuous, small vessels, with occasionally ill-defined larger contiguous vascular spaces. Computed tomography (CT) may be indicated if the AVM involves bone. Histopathological diagnosis of AVM is rarely necessary, but may be indicated if imaging is equivocal or to rule out malignancy. Biopsy of an AVM may be complicated by bleeding and reactive expansion of the lesion.[15]

Nonoperative Management

For superficial AVMs, patients should apply hydrated-petroleum to prevent desiccation and subsequent ulceration. Compression garments for extremity lesions may reduce pain and swelling, but can also worsen symptoms. If bleeding occurs, it is readily controlled by compression; further intervention is rarely necessary. Because estrogen is proangiogenic and may stimulate AVM progression, we recommend progesterone-only oral contraceptives.[21–24] Although pregnancy has been thought to increase the risk of AVM expansion,[10,25] pregnant women with Stage I lesions do not have an increased rate of progression compared with nonpregnant women.[15] However, pregnancy in women with Stage II–IV AVM has not been studied, and thus we caution women with advanced lesions that pregnancy may exacerbate their malformation.

Operative Management

Indications

Approximately three-fourths of patients with AVM require treatment in childhood or adolescence; the remaining individuals do not need intervention until adulthood.[15] Because AVM is often diffuse, involving multiple tissue planes and important structures, cure is rare. The goal of treatment usually is to *control* the malformation. Intervention is focused on alleviating symptoms (ie, bleeding, pain, ulceration), preserving vital functions (ie, vision, mastication), and improving a deformity. Management options include embolization, resection, or a combination; pharmacologic treatment currently does not exist. Resection offers the best chance for long-term control, but the reexpansion rate is high and extirpation may cause a worse deformity than the malformation. Embolization is not curative, and most AVMs will ultimately reexpand after embolization. Consequently, embolization is most commonly used preoperatively to reduce blood loss during resection, or for palliation of unresectable lesions.[15]

Asymptomatic AVM should be observed unless it can be removed for possible cure with minimal morbidity; embolization or incomplete excision of an asymptomatic lesion may stimulate it to enlarge and become problematic. Intervention is determined by (1) the size and location of the AVM, (2) the age of the patient, and (3) Schobinger stage. Although resection of an asymptomatic Stage I AVM offers the best chance for long-term control or "cure," intervention must be individualized based on the degree of deformity that would be caused by excision and reconstruction.[15] For example, a large Stage I AVM in a nonanatomically important location (ie, trunk, proximal extremity) may be resected without consequence, before it progresses to a higher stage when excision is more difficult and the recurrence rate is greater.[15] Similarly, a small, well-localized AVM in a more difficult location (ie, face, hand) may be removed for possible "cure" before it expands and complete extirpation is no longer possible.

In contrast, a large, asymptomatic AVM located in an anatomically sensitive area, such as the face, is best observed, especially in a young child not psychologically prepared for a major procedure. First, resection and reconstruction may result in a more noticeable deformity or functional problem than the malformation. Second, although the recurrence rate is lower when a Stage I AVM is resected, it is still high and thus even after major resection and reconstruction the malformation may recur. Third, some children (17.4%) do not experience significant long-term morbidity from their AVM until they are adults.[15]

Intervention for Stage II AVMs is similar to Stage I lesions. However, the threshold for treatment is lower if an enlarging lesion is causing a worsening deformity or if functional problems are expected. Stage III and IV AVMs require intervention to control pain, bleeding, ulceration, or congestive heart failure.

Embolization

Embolization involves the delivery of an inert substance, typically through a catheter proximal to the AVM, to occlude blood flow and/or fill a vascular space. Successful embolization requires penetration of the embolic agent to the nidus, ideally to the point of initial venous drainage. Proximal arterial embolization is contraindicated because recanalization occurs and the lesion becomes inaccessible for future embolization.[20]

In addition to the replacement of arterialized blood with an inert embolic substance, ischemia and scarring may further reduce arteriovenous shunting, shrink the lesion, and improve symptoms. Even if significant volume reduction does not occur after embolization, symptoms are improved. For the vast majority of patients, embolization is performed under general anesthesia. Often multiple treatments are required, typically spaced by several weeks.

Because the AVM is not removed, almost all lesions eventually will expand after treatment; most older studies suggest that multiple embolizations do not lower the rate of recurrence,[1,10,15,16,26–29] although newer embolic agents may offer more lasting results. Stage I AVM has a lower recurrence rate than higher-staged lesions. Most recurrences occur within the first year after embolization and 98% reexpand within 5 years; although this may reflect results obtained with older embolic agents.[15] Patients who have not exhibited enlargement 5 years following embolization are more likely to have long-term control.[15] Despite the high likelihood of reexpansion, embolization can effectively palliate an AVM by reducing its size, slowing expansion, and alleviating pain and bleeding (**Fig. 1**). The aim of preoperative embolization is to reduce blood loss during extirpation.

Substances used for embolization may be liquid (n-butyl cyanoacrylate [n-BCA], Onyx, ethanol) or solid (polyvinyl alcohol [PVA] particles, coils). The choice of embolic agent depends on whether embolization is being used as primary treatment or as a preoperative adjunct to excision. For preoperative embolization, temporary occlusive substances (gelfoam powder, PVA, embospheres), which may undergo phagocytosis if left in place over several weeks, are used. Delivery of PVA and embospheres with different particle sizes allows the initial occlusion of small, distal vessels followed by blockage of more proximal branches with larger emboli. Permanent liquid agents capable of permeating the nidus (ethanol, n-BCA, Onyx) are used when embolization is the primary treatment. We prefer Onyx, which is an ethylene-vinyl alcohol copolymer (EV3 Neurovascular, Irvine, CA, USA).[20,30] Onyx precipitates on the surface after contact with blood. A nonadhesive liquid core is maintained, which allows repetitive injection from the same pedicle, each time filling a different AVM compartment. Consequently, Onyx allows more aggressive embolization than other liquid agents of multiple nidal areas from a single catheter position.[20,31] Onyx also causes less inflammation and endothelial damage than n-BCA or alcohol, and resection is facilitated because the vessels are less fragile.[32,33]

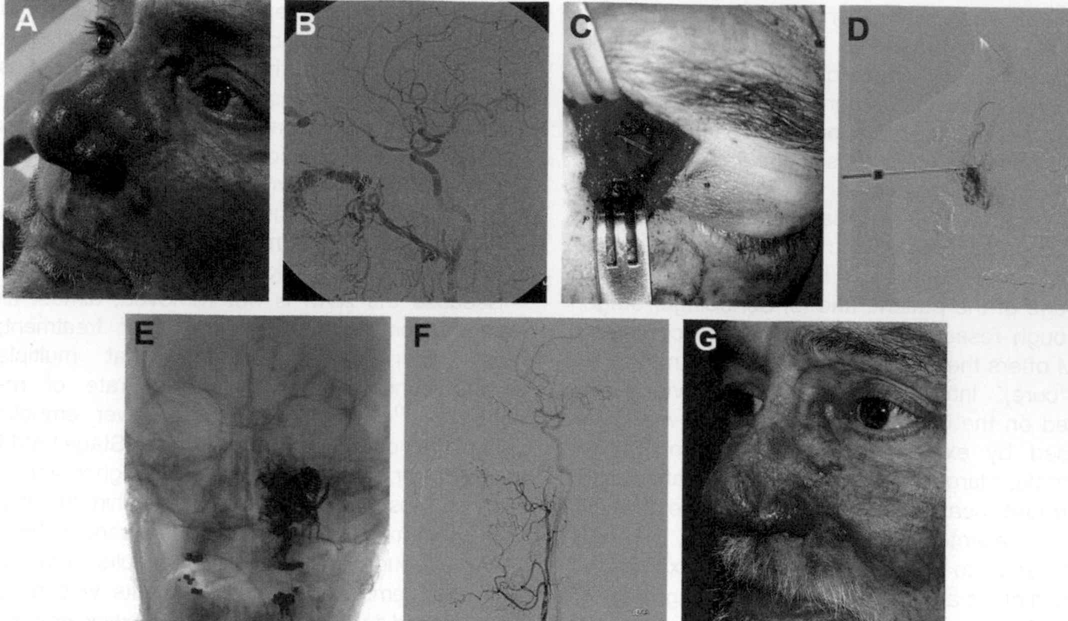

Fig. 1. Management of arteriovenous malformation (AVM) with embolization: (*A*) 51-year-old male with a diffuse AVM of the left cheek, nose, and orbit causing frequent epistaxis. Radical resection and reconstruction would cause a significant deformity and would likely be complicated by recurrence. (*B*) Lateral view of a left common carotid injection demonstrating the main supply to the AVM to be via an enlarged left internal maxillary artery with a dysplastic, fusiform dilatation. The left ophthalmic artery is prominent and provides additional supply to the AVM, causing distal ophthalmic aneurysms near the medial canthus (seen in the clinical photograph). (*C*) Pre-embolization operative occlusion of the feeding vessels from the ophthalmic artery to prevent migration of embolic material into the artery and blindness. (*D*) Direct percutaneous embolization of the nidus. (*E*) Onyx cast of AVM nidus. (*F*) Postembolization angiogram shows nonopacification of nidus. (*G*) Epistaxis has resolved following embolization. Note improvement of ophthalmic aneurysms in medial canthal area.

The most frequent complication of embolization is ulceration, which is more common for superficial lesions. Wounds are allowed to heal secondarily with local wound care. Distal migration of embolic material can cause ischemic injury to uninvolved tissues. Unlike sclerotherapy for slow-flow malformations, posttreatment edema after AVM embolization is rare, unless ethanol is used as the embolic agent. Except for small lesions, most patients are observed overnight in the hospital. If swelling is a significant concern, dexamethasone can be administered perioperatively followed by a 1-week oral corticosteroid taper. Posttreatment swelling may necessitate close monitoring if airway or orbital lesions are embolized; deep extremity lesions are at risk for compartment syndrome. Patients and families are counseled that AVM is likely to reexpand following treatment, and thus additional embolizations may be required in the future.

Sclerotherapy

Sclerotherapy involves the transcutaneous injection of a substance into the malformation, which causes endothelial destruction and thrombosis. Subsequent fibrosis of the vascular space decreases the size of the lesion and improves symptoms. Sclerotherapy is reserved for an AVM that cannot be accessed transarterially, usually because of previous embolization of proximal feeding vessels. Alternatively, a localized AVM may be treated by sclerotherapy as well. The danger in using sclerosants in a high-flow lesion is the potential for the agent to escape into the systemic circulation. Our preferred sclerosants are sodium tetradecyl sulfate (STS) and absolute ethanol. Although ethanol is more effective than STS, it has a higher complication rate. Because ethanol can cause nerve damage, it should be used with great care in proximity to important structures (ie, facial nerve), and the dose should not exceed 1 mL/kg (maximum of 60 mL).

Resection

Resection of AVM has a lower recurrence rate than embolization and is considered for well-localized lesions (**Fig. 2**) or to correct focal deformities (ie, bleeding or ulcerated areas, labial hypertrophy)

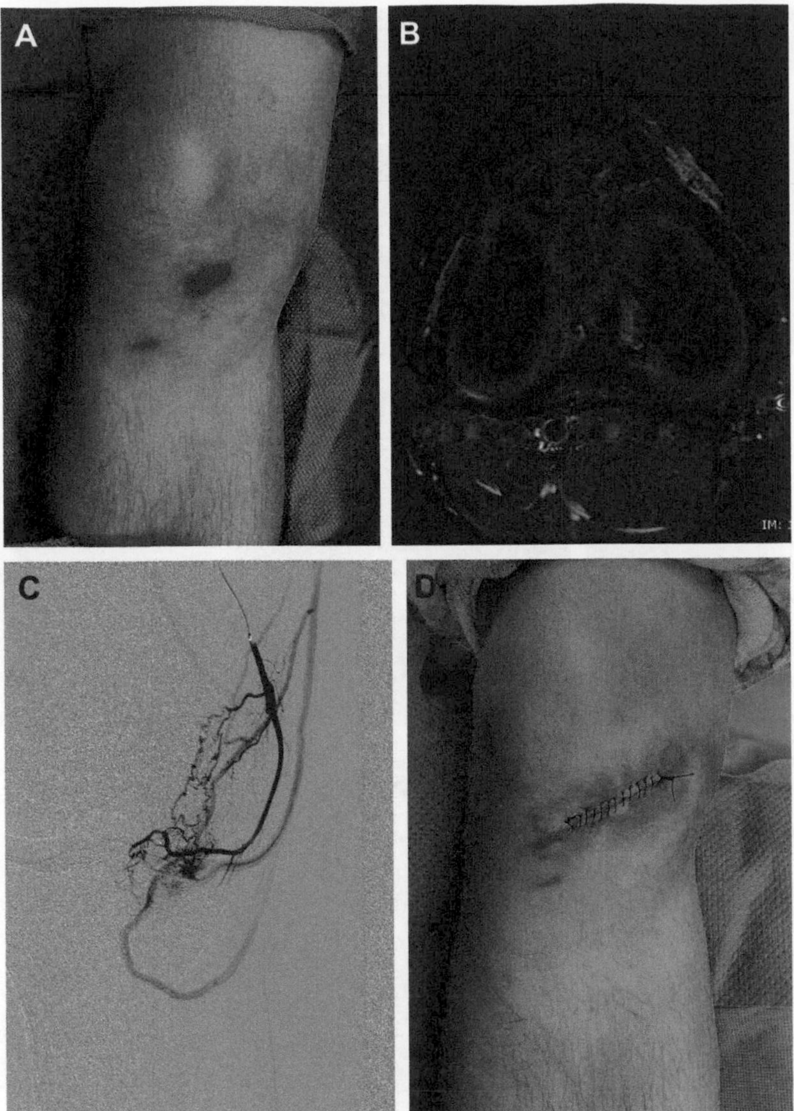

Fig. 2. Management of localized arteriovenous malformation (AVM): (*A*) 15-year-old male with a lesion of the lower extremity since birth. (*B*) Axial T1 MR image with fat suppression showing an enhancing, localized lesion confined to the skin and subcutaneous tissue. (*C*) Angiogram illustrates nidus, arteriovenous shunting, and early opacification of draining veins. (*D*) Resection of AVM and linear closure following preoperative embolization.

(**Figs. 3** and **4**).[15] Wide extirpation and reconstruction of a large, diffuse AVM should be exercised with caution because (1) cure is rare and the recurrence rate is high; (2) the resulting deformity is often worse than the appearance of the malformation; and (3) resection is associated with significant blood loss, iatrogenic injury, and morbidity.

When excision is planned, preoperative embolization will facilitate the procedure by reducing the size of the AVM, minimizing blood loss, and creating scar tissue to aid the dissection. Multiple embolizations, typically spaced several weeks apart, may be required for extensive lesions. Excision should be performed 24 to 72 hours after embolization, before recannalization and angiogenesis restores blood flow to the lesion, especially if particulate agents, such as PVA, were used. To further reduce blood loss, an epinephrine-containing local anesthetic is infused throughout the operative field and a tourniquet is used when removing an extremity lesion. Small, well-localized AVMs or those that cannot be accessed for embolization can be treated by resection alone. Proximal feeding vessels to the AVM should never be ligated because collateralization will stimulate

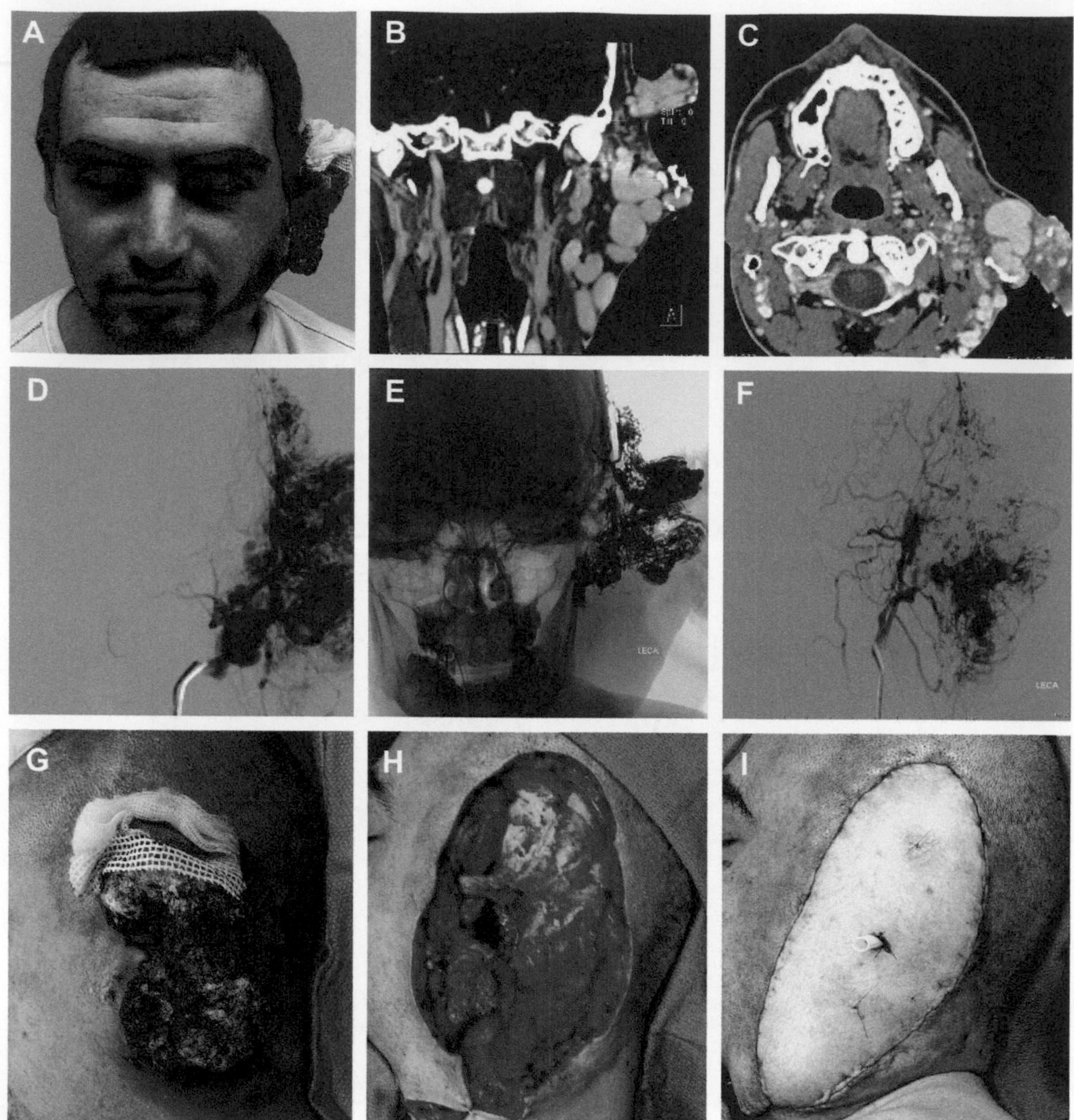

Fig. 3. Management of large arteriovenous malformation (AVM): (*A*) 22-year-old male with a Stage III auricular AVM causing pain, bleeding, and ulceration. (*B, C*) Coronal and axial CT angiograms show large, ectatic vascular structures and soft tissue overgrowth. (*D*) Left external carotid injection illustrates diffuse nidus. (*E*) Onyx casting of nidus following embolization. (*F*) Postembolization angiogram shows decreased opacification of AVM. (*G, H, I*) Following embolization and wide resection, the defect was closed with a free latissimus dorsi myocutaneous flap.

enlargement; access for future embolization also will no longer be possible.

Surgical margins are best determined clinically, by assessing the amount of bleeding from the wound edges.[10] Most defects can be reconstructed by advancing local skin flaps. Skin grafting ulcerated areas has a high failure rate because the underlying tissue is ischemic; excision with regional flap transfer may be required. Free-flap reconstruction permits wide resection and primary closure of complicated defects. Although some investigators have proposed that free tissue transfer may minimize recurrence by reducing hypoxia,[34–38] we and others have not found that free-tissue transfer improves long-term AVM control.[10,15,16,39–41]

Despite subtotal and presumed “complete” extirpation, most AVMs treated by resection recur; serial excisions do not reduce the recurrence rate (**Fig. 5**).[1,15,26,27] Most recurrences occur within the first year after intervention, and 86.6% reexpand within 5 years of resection.[15] Thus, patients who

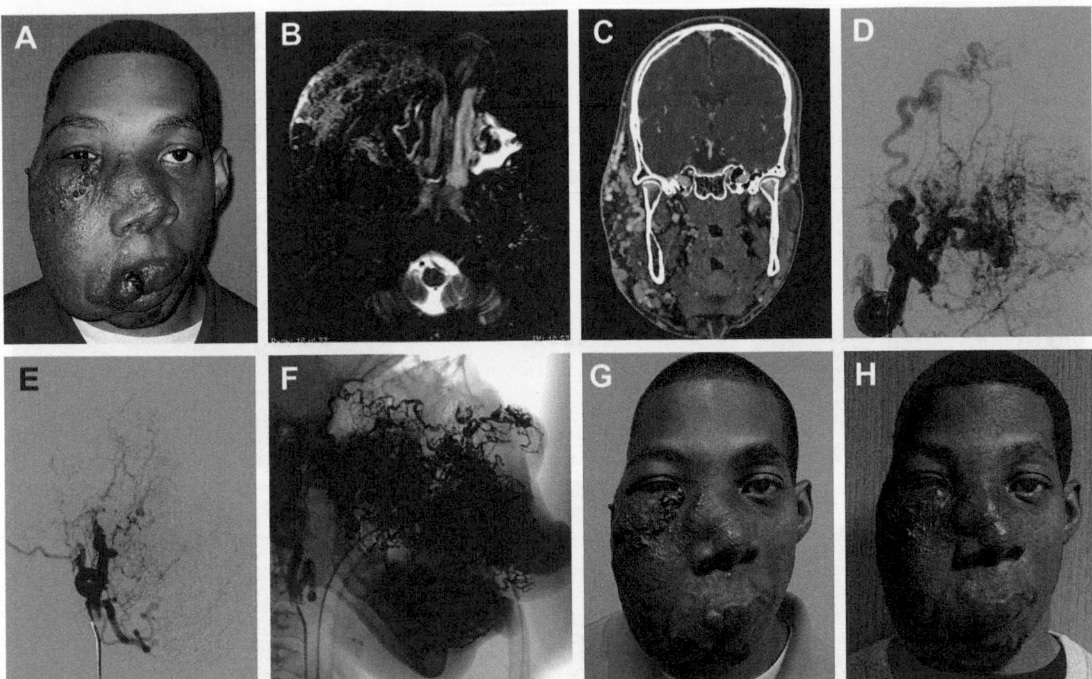

Fig. 4. Management of diffuse arteriovenous malformation (AVM): (*A*) 25-year-old male with a Stage III facial AVM causing a worsening deformity, bleeding, pain, and ulceration. Because the lesion involved all structures of the face (including orbit, maxilla, and mandible), complete extirpation was not possible. He was managed with embolization and subtotal resection of the symptomatic ulcerated and bleeding areas. (*B*) Axial T2 MR image showing diffuse signal abnormality and overgrowth of the right face. (*C*) Coronal CT angiogram illustrates prominent, diffuse vascular anomaly with soft tissue enlargement. (*D*) Angiogram showing diffuse nidus involving the right face. (*E*) Nonopacification of most of the AVM nidus following embolization. (*F*) Onyx cast in AVM nidus. (*G*) Healed lip ulceration and resolution of bleeding following 6 embolizations. (*H*) Improved appearance following subtotal resection of the upper lip and cheek. Twenty-four months postoperatively he has not had recurrent pain, bleeding, or ulceration.

have not exhibited recurrence 5 years following intervention are more likely to have long-term control of their AVM, although 5.2% will reexpand more than 10 years later.[15] Patients and families are counseled that AVM is likely to recur following resection, and thus intervention may be required in the future.

The causes for AVM expansion following treatment likely are similar to those responsible for its natural progression: collateralization, dilation of vessels, and/or production of new vasculature. AVM is stimulated by therapy; both embolization and excision cause trauma, which is well-known to incite enlargement.[1,10,16] These interventions create a proangiogenic environment because they cause local hypoxia and the production of angiogenic factors (hypoxia-inducible factor-1, basic fibroblast growth factor, vascular endothelial growth factor, matrix metalloproteinases) from platelets, neutrophils, and macrophages.[42–48] Although the mechanisms for AVM expansion are unknown, pharmacotherapy might be possible because it is not a quiescent lesion. For example, angiogenesis inhibitors or hormone antagonists could potentially slow the natural progression of AVM, reducing the need for intervention. Similarly, if a drug could control recurrence, then the efficacy of embolization and resection would be improved. Although not a cure, pharmacotherapy might allow patients to live with a "dormant" AVM, similar to the antiangiogenic strategy for controlling cancer.[49]

CAPILLARY MALFORMATION–ARTERIOVENOUS MALFORMATION

Clinical Features

The prevalence of capillary malformation–arteriovenous malformation (CM-AVM) is estimated to be 1 in 100,000 Caucasians.[6,50] Patients have atypical capillary malformations (CMs) that are small, multifocal, round, pinkish-red, and surrounded by a pale halo (50%).[6,50] An individual may have as many as 53 CMs, ranging in size from 1 to 15 cm in diameter, although 6% of patients have only a solitary lesion.[50] Thirty percent of

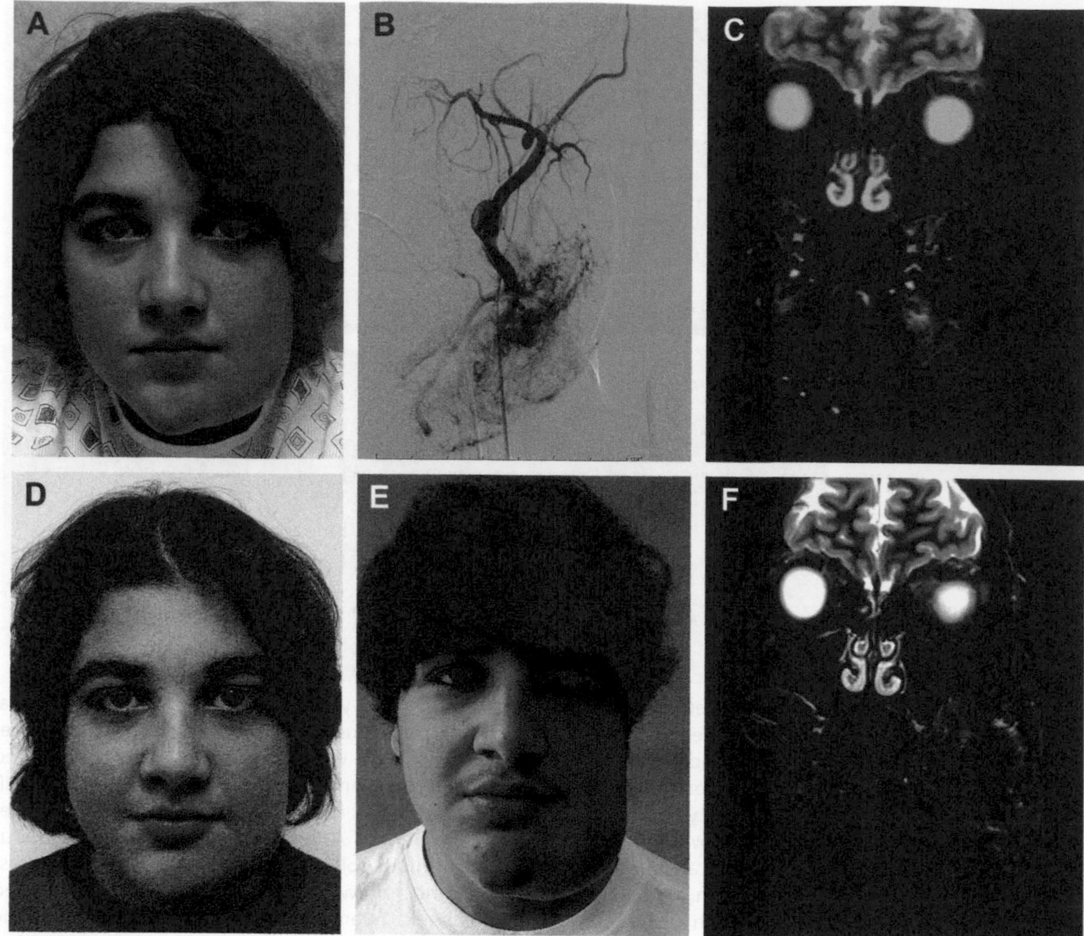

Fig. 5. Recurrence of arteriovenous malformation (AVM) following treatment: (*A*) 11-year-old male with an AVM of the left face before treatment. Workup for PTEN mutation was negative. (*B*) Angiogram illustrates diffuse arteriovenous shunting. (*C*) Preoperative coronal T2 MR with fat suppression showing overgrowth of the left face with an adipose component. (*D*) Improved contour 12 weeks following preoperative embolization and subtotal resection. (*E*) AVM has expanded 2 years postoperatively. (*F*) Coronal T2 MR shows increased soft tissue overgrowth and flow-voids.

individuals also have an AVM: Parkes-Weber syndrome (PWS) (12%), extracerebral AVM (11%), or intracerebral AVM (7%).[50] PWS describes a diffuse AVM of an overgrown extremity with an overlying CM.[8,51] Intracranial lesions are associated with vein of Galen aneurysmal malformations, seizures, hydrocephalus, congestive heart failure, and developmental delay.[50] Radiographically, AVMs appear similar to nonfamilial lesions.[50] An association between CM-AVM and spinal arteriovenous lesions (AVM and AVF) recently has been reported.[52] Five percent of patients have benign or malignant tumors, most commonly involving the nervous system (neurofibroma, optic glioma, vestibular schwannoma).[50]

CM-AVM is caused by a loss-of-function mutation in the *RASA1* gene, which encodes p120RasGAP. This protein inhibits RAS p21 control of cellular proliferation, survival, and differentiation.[6] CM-AVM is an autosomal dominant condition with high penetrance (98%), although phenotypic heterogeneity is common within families. For example, one individual may exhibit multifocal CMs, whereas another family member may have a solitary CM as well as a large AVM.[6,50] Not all patients with CM-AVM clinically will show a *RASA1* mutation, suggesting that unknown mutations in *RASA1* or other genes may result in the same phenotype.[50]

Diagnosis

Diagnosis is made by history and physical examination. The presence of multifocal CMs, especially with a positive family history, suggests CM-AVM (**Fig. 6**). The CMs appear round, pinkish-red, and usually are surrounded by a halo. Doppler examination often shows fast-flow, which is not present in sporadic CM.

Management

A patient presenting with multiple CMs, especially with a family history of similar lesions, should be evaluated for possible AVMs on physical examination. Although the CM is rarely problematic, associated AVMs can cause significant morbidity. Because patients with CM-AVM are at risk for intracranial and spinal fast-flow lesions, MRI of the brain and/or spine should be considered.[53] Exploratory imaging of other anatomic areas is not necessary because extracranial AVMs have not been found to involve the viscera.[50] Patients with PWS should be followed by a cardiologist to monitor for signs of congestive heart failure.[50] In addition, orthopedic evaluation is necessary to follow patients with PWS for a leg-length discrepancy. A shoe lift may be indicated to prevent limping and scoliosis; femoral epiphysiodesis may be required in adolescence. Patients are counseled about the risk of transmitting the gene to their offspring.

PTEN-ASSOCIATED VASCULAR ANOMALY

Clinical Features

The PTEN (phosphatase and tensin homolog) gene encodes a tumor suppressor lipid phosphatase involved in the phosphoinositide-3 kinase pathway; it mediates cell-cycle arrest and apoptosis.[54] Patients with PTEN mutations have PTEN hamartoma-tumor syndrome (PHTS). This autosomal dominant condition had previously been referred to as Cowden syndrome or Bannayan-Riley-Ruvalcaba syndrome (BRRS).[7,55] Males and females are equally affected, and approximately one-half (54%) of patients have a unique fast-flow vascular anomaly with

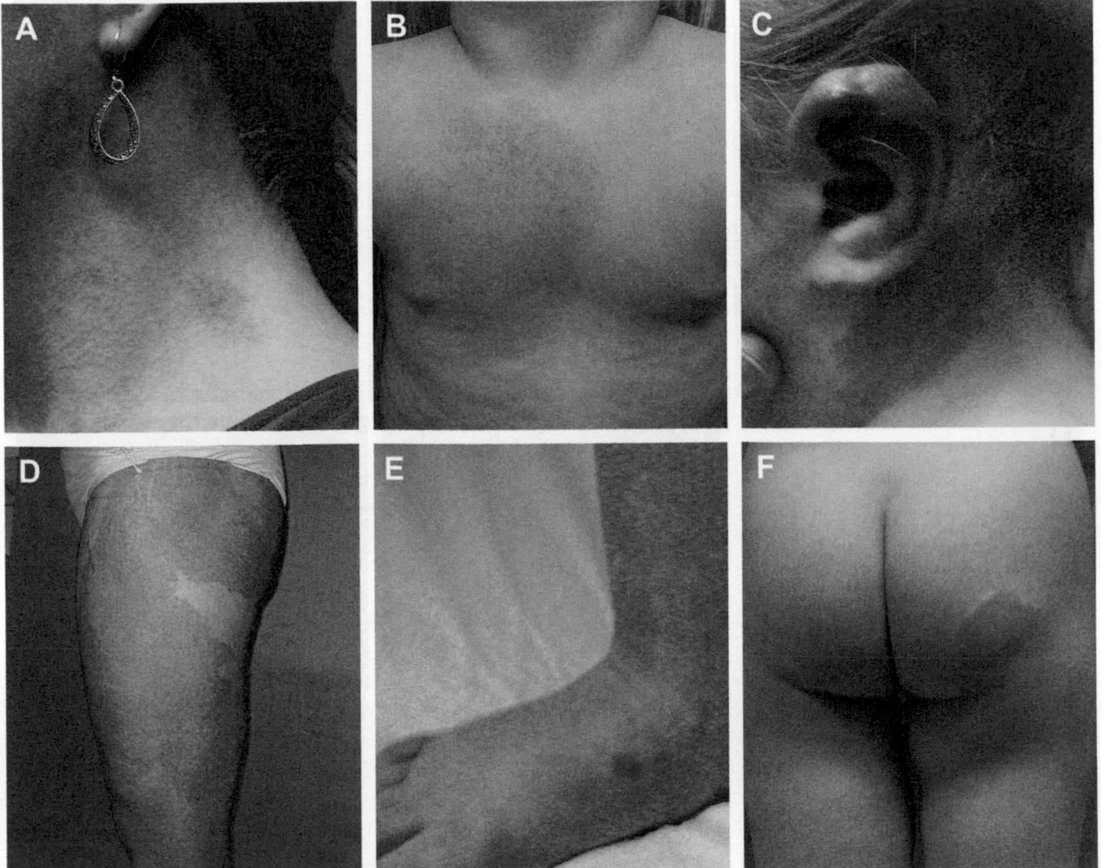

Fig. 6. Capillary malformation-arteriovenous malformation (CM-AVM): (*A, D*) 35-year-old female with a fast-flow stain of the neck and Parkes-Weber syndrome of the left lower extremity; (*B, E*) 5-year-old daughter has fast-flow stains over her chest and right foot; (*C, F*) 2-year-old daughter has a Stage 2 AVM of the ear and fast-flow stains of the neck and buttock.

arteriovenous shunting, referred to as a PTEN-associated vascular anomaly (PTEN-AVA).[7] Patients may have multiple PTEN-AVAs (57%), and 85% are intramuscular.[7]

Diagnosis

Suspicion of a PTEN-AVA usually is initiated after reviewing the MRI or angiographic study of a patient thought to have an AVM. Unlike typical AVM, PTEN-AVA can be multifocal, associated with ectopic adipose tissue, and have disproportionate, segmental dilation of the draining veins.[7,20] Intramuscular lesions replace the architecture with disorganized fat, in contrast with nonsyndromic muscular AVMs that cause symmetric overgrowth without adipose tissue.[7] If a patient is suspected of having a PTEN-AVA based on imaging characteristics, a physical examination is performed. Patients with PHTS have macrocephaly (>97th percentile), and all males have penile freckling.[7] In addition, PHTS is associated with mental retardation/autism (19%), thyroid lesions (31%), or gastrointestinal polyps (30%).[7] Biopsy may aid the diagnosis of a PTEN-AVA. Histopathology shows skeletal muscle infiltration with adipose tissue, fibrous bands, and lymphoid aggregates. In addition, tortuous arteries with transmural muscular hyperplasia and clusters of abnormal veins with variable smooth muscle are present.[7] Genetic testing is confirmative, although a germline mutation is not found in 9% of families clinically diagnosed with PHTS.[56]

Management

Patients who present to our Vascular Anomalies Center with fast-flow lesions consistent with a PTEN-AVA are evaluated for possible PHTS. Head circumference is measured and males are examined for penile freckling. If physical examination is consistent with PHTS, molecular testing is

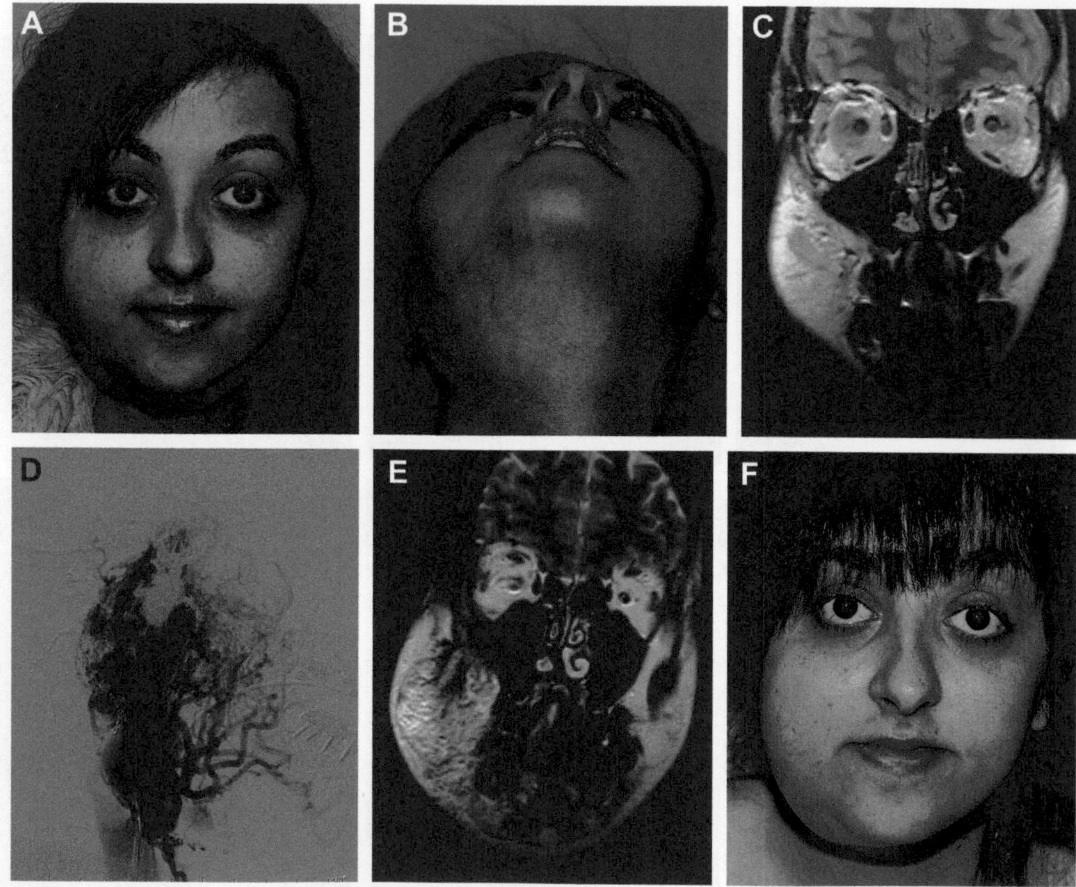

Fig. 7. Management of PTEN-associated vascular anomaly (PTEN-AVA): (*A, B*) 20-year-old female positive for PTEN mutation with an enlarging right cheek and submandibular mass. (*C*) Coronal T2 MR shows soft tissue overgrowth with signal consistent with fat. (*D*) Angiogram illustrates dramatic enlargement of feeding arteries and diffuse arteriovenous shunting without a discrete nidus. (*E*) After embolization, coronal T2 MR shows worsening soft tissue overgrowth and flow-voids. (*F*) Enlarging lesion at age 21, following 3 embolization treatments.

obtained because the mutation is associated with multiple benign and malignant tumors, which require surveillance. Patients are followed closely for the presence of tumors, particularly endocrine and gastrointestinal malignancies. Families are counseled about the risk of transmitting the mutation to their offspring. Symptomatic lesions are managed similarly to nonsyndromic AVM, with embolization or resection (**Fig. 7**). It is our experience that the recurrence rate after these interventions is even higher than for nonsyndromic AVM, possibly because the loss of the tumor suppressor protein favors a more proliferative environment.

REFERENCES

1. Young AE, Mulliken JB. Arteriovenous malformations. In: Mulliken JB, Young AE, editors. Vascular birthmarks: hemangiomas and malformations. Philadelphia: Saunders; 1988. p. 228–45.
2. Gomes MM, Bernatz PE. Arteriovenous fistulae: a review and ten-year experience at the Mayo Clinic. Mayo Clin Proc 1970;45:81–102.
3. Li DY, Sorensen LK, Brooke BS, et al. Defective angiogenesis in mice lacing endoglin. Science 1999;284:1534–7.
4. Urness LD, Sorensen LK, Li DY. Arteriovenous malformations in mice lacing activin receptor-like kinase-1. Nat Genet 2000;26:328–31.
5. Thomas B, Eyries M, Montagne K, et al. Altered endothelial gene expression associated with hereditary haemorrhagic telangiectasia. Eur J Clin Invest 2007;37:580–8.
6. Eerola I, Boon LM, Mulliken JB, et al. Capillary malformation-arteriovenous malformation: a new clinical and genetic disorder cased by RASA1 mutations. Am J Hum Genet 2003;73:1240–9.
7. Tan WH, Baris HN, Burrows PE, et al. The spectrum of vascular anomalies in patients with PTEN mutations: implications for diagnosis and management. J Med Genet 2007;44:594–602.
8. Mulliken JB, Fishman SJ, Burrows PE. Vascular anomalies. Curr Probl Surg 2000;37:517–84.
9. Mulliken JB, Glowacki J. Hemangiomas and vascular malformations in infants and children: a classification based on endothelial characteristics. Plast Reconstr Surg 1982;69:412–22.
10. Kohout MP, Hansen M, Pribaz JJ, et al. Arteriovenous malformations of the head and neck: natural history and management. Plast Reconstr Surg 1998;102:643–54.
11. Holman E. The physiology of an arteriovenous fistula. Am J Surg 1955;89:1101–8.
12. Braverman IM, Keh A, Jacobson BS. Ultrastructure and three-dimensional organization of the telangiectases of hereditary hemorrhagic telangiectasia. J Invest Dermatol 1990;95:422–7.
13. Turjman F, Massoud TF, Vinuela F, et al. Correlation of the angioarchitectural features of cerebral arteriovenous malformations with clinical presentation of hemorrhage. Neurosurgery 1995;37:856–60.
14. Friedlander RM. Arteriovenous malformations of the brain. N Engl J Med 2007;356:2704–12.
15. Liu AS, Mulliken JB, Zurakowski D, et al. Extracranial arteriovenous malformations: natural progression and recurrence after treatment. Plast Reconstr Surg 2010;125:1185–94.
16. Wu JK, Bisdorff A, Gelbert F, et al. Auricular arteriovenous malformation: evaluation, management, and outcome. Plast Reconstr Surg 2005;115:985–95.
17. Masuda H, Zhuang YJ, Singh TM, et al. Adaptive remodeling of internal elastic lamina and endothelial lining during flow-induced arterial enlargement. Arterioscler Thromb Vasc Biol 1999;19:2298–307.
18. Karunanyaka A, Tu J, Watling A, et al. Endothelial molecular changes in a rodent model of arteriovenous malformation. J Neurosurg 2008;109:1165–72.
19. Finn MC, Glowacki J, Mulliken JB. Congenital vascular lesions: clinical application of a new classification. J Pediatr Surg 1983;18:894–900.
20. Wu IC, Orbach DB. Neurointerventional management of high-flow vascular malformations of the head and neck. Neuroimaging Clin N Am 2009;19:219–40.
21. Johannisson E, Oberholzer M, Swahn ML, et al. Vascular changes in the human endometrium following the administration of the progesterone antagonist RU 486. Contraception 1989;39:103–17.
22. Hyder SM, Huang JC, Nawaz Z, et al. Regulation of vascular endothelial growth factor expression by estrogens and progestins. Environ Health Perspect 2000;108:785–90.
23. Heryanto B, Rogers PA. Regulation of endometrial endothelial cell proliferation by oestrogen and progesterone in the ovariectomized mouse. Reproduction 2002;123:107–13.
24. Kayisli UA, Luk J, Guzeloglu-Kayisli O, et al. Regulation of angiogenic activity of human endometrial endothelial cells in culture by ovarian steroids. J Clin Endocrinol Metab 2004;89:5794–802.
25. Esplin MS, Varner MW. Progression of pulmonary arteriovenous malformation during pregnancy: case report and review of the literature. Obstet Gynecol Surv 1997;52:248–53.
26. Szilagyi DE, Smith RF, Elliott JP, et al. Congenital arteriovenous malformations of the limbs. Arch Surg 1976;111:423–9.
27. Flye MW, Jordan BP, Schwartz MZ. Management of congenital arteriovenous malformations. Surgery 1983;94:740–7.
28. Burrows PE, Mulliken JB, Fishman SJ, et al. Pharmacological treatment of a diffuse arteriovenous malformation of the upper extremity in a child. J Craniofac Surg 2009;20:597–602.

29. Fleetwood IG, Steinberg K. Arteriovenous malformations. Lancet 2009;359:863–73.
30. Taki W, Yonekawa Y, Iwata H, et al. A new liquid material for embolization or arteriovenous malformations. AJNR Am J Neuroradiol 1990;11:163–8.
31. Mounayer C, Hammami N, Piotin M, et al. Nidal embolization of brain arteriovenous malformations using Onyx in 94 patients. AJNR Am J Neuroradiol 2007;28:518–23.
32. Duffner F, Ritz R, Bornemann A, et al. Combined therapy of cerebral arteriovenous malformations: histological differences between a non-adhesive liquid embolic agent and n-butyl 2-cyanoacrylate (NBCA). Clin Neuropathol 2002;21:13–7.
33. Akin ED, Perkins E, Ross IB. Surgical handling characteristics of an ethylene vinyl alcohol copolymer compared with N-butyl cyanoacrylate used for embolization of vessels in an arteriovenous malformation resection model in swine. J Neurosurg 2003;98:366–70.
34. Hurwitz DJ, Kerber CW. Hemodynamic considerations in the treatment of arteriovenous malformations of the face and scalp. Plast Reconstr Surg 1981;67:431–4.
35. Dompmartin A, Labbe D, Barrellier MT, et al. Use of a regulating flap in the treatment of a large arteriovenous malformation of the scalp. Br J Plast Surg 1998;51:561–3.
36. Tark KC, Chung S. Histologic change of arteriovenous malformations of the face and scalp after free flap transfer. Plast Reconstr Surg 2000;106:87–93.
37. Koshima I, Nanba Y, Tsutsui T, et al. Free perforator flap for the treatment of defects after resection of huge arteriovenous malformations in the head and neck regions. Ann Plast Surg 2003;51:194–9.
38. Hong JP, Choi JW, Chang H, et al. Reconstruction of the face after resection of arteriovenous malformations using anterolateral thigh perforator flap. J Craniofac Surg 2005;16:851–5.
39. Yamamoto Y, Ohura T, Minakawa H, et al. Experience with arteriovenous malformations treated with flap coverage. Plast Reconstr Surg 1994;94:476–82.
40. Upton J, Coombs CJ, Mulliken JB, et al. Vascular malformations of the upper limb: a review of 270 patients. J Hand Surg Am 1999;24:1019–35.
41. Hartzell LD, Stack BC Jr, Yuen J, et al. Free tissue reconstruction following excision of head and neck arteriovenous malformations. Arch Facial Plast Surg 2009;11:171–7.
42. Shweiki D, Itin A, Soffer D, et al. Vascular endothelial growth factor induced by hypoxia may mediate hypoxia-initiated angiogenesis. Nature 1992;359:843–5.
43. Pierce GF, Tarpley JE, Yanagihara D, et al. Platelet derived growth factor (BB homodimer), transforming growth factor-beta 1, and basic fibroblast growth factor in dermal wound healing. Neovessel and matrix formation and cessation of repair. Am J Pathol 1992;140:1375–88.
44. Nissen NN, Polverini PJ, Koch AE, et al. Vascular endothelial growth factor mediates angiogenic activity during the proliferative phase of wound healing. Am J Pathol 1998;152:1445–52.
45. McCourt M, Wang JH, Sookhai S, et al. Proinflammatory mediators stimulate neutrophil-directed angiogenesis. Arch Surg 1999;134:1325–31.
46. Lingen MW. Role of leukocytes and endothelial cells in the development of angiogenesis in inflammation and wound healing. Arch Pathol Lab Med 2001;125:67–71.
47. Sure U, Battenberg E, Dempfle A, et al. Hypoxia-inducible factor and vascular endothelial growth factor are expressed more frequently in embolized than in nonembolized cerebral arteriovenous malformations. Neurosurgery 2004;55:663–9.
48. Kadirvel R, Dai D, Ding YH, et al. Endovascular treatment of aneurysms: healing mechanisms in a swine model are associated with increased expression of matrix metalloproteinases, vascular cell adhesion molecule-1, and vascular endothelial growth factor, and decreased expression of tissue inhibitors of matrix metalloproteinases. AJNR Am J Neuroradiol 2007;28:849–56.
49. Folkman J. Angiogenesis: an organizing principle for drug discovery? Nat Rev Drug Discov 2007;6:273–86.
50. Revencu N, Boon LM, Mulliken JB, et al. Parkes Weber syndrome, vein of galen aneurismal malformation, and other fast-flow vascular anomalies are caused by RASA1 mutations. Hum Mutat 2008;29:959–65.
51. Parkes Weber F. Hemangiectatic hypertrophy of limbs—congenital phlebarteriectasis and so-called congenital varicose veins. Br J Child Dis 1918;15:13–7.
52. Thiex R, Mulliken JB, Revencu N, et al. A novel association between RASA1 mutations and spinal arteriovenous anomalies. AJNR Am J Neuroradiol 2010;31(4):775–9.
53. Limaye N, Boon LM, Vikkula M. From germline towards somatic mutations in the pathophysiology of vascular anomalies. Hum Mol Genet 2009;18:65–75.
54. Sansal I, Sellers WR. The biology and clinical relevance of the PTEN tumor suppressor pathway. J Clin Oncol 2004;22:2954–63.
55. Eng C. PTEN: one gene, many syndromes. Hum Mutat 2003;22:183–98.
56. Marsh DJ, Coulon V, Lunetta KL, et al. Mutation spectrum and genotype-phenotype analyses in Cowden disease and Bannayan-Zonana syndrome, two hamartoma syndromes with germline PTEN mutation. Hum Mol Genet 1998;7:507–15.

Management of Combined Vascular Malformations

Ann M. Kulungowski, MD, Steven J. Fishman, MD*

KEYWORDS

- Capillary-arteriovenous fistula
- Capillary-arteriovenous malformation
- Capillary-lymphatico-venous malformation
- CLOVES syndrome • Klippel-Trénaunay syndrome
- Parkes Weber syndrome

Historically, combined vascular malformations have been named after the physician who is credited with the most memorable description of the condition. Unfortunately, the eponyms are often misused and offer little insight into the underlying pathogenesis.[1] We, therefore, favor a more anatomic description of the malformations and name them according to the anomalous vascular channels present. Like single-channel-type vascular malformations, combined lesions are also categorized as slow-flow and fast-flow lesions. Many of the combined vascular malformations are associated with soft tissue and skeletal hypertrophy.

CAPILLARY-LYMPHATICO-VENOUS MALFORMATION

The first reports of patients with a slow-flow capillary-lymphatico-venous malformation (CLVM) were published in the nineteenth century by Hilaire, Trélat, and Monod.[2,3] It was not until 1900 that this constellation of findings was considered more than mere coincidence. French physicians, Maurice Klippel and Paul Trénaunay,[4] were the first to recognize Klippel-Trénaunay syndrome as a distinct entity.[5] They proposed the main characteristics of the syndrome were a localized vascular nevus, congenital or early infantile varicosities, and hypertrophy of tissue occurring in the same body part. They also recognized the variability in the severity of symptoms. For more than 100 years, the well-worn eponym, Klippel-Trénaunay syndrome, has been used to describe patients with CLVM. It is often incorrectly called "Klippel-Trénaunay-Weber syndrome" suggesting a relation to Parkes Weber syndrome, a fast-flow malformation consisting of a capillary-arteriovenous malformation (CAVM) in association with limb hypertrophy.[6,7]

Etiology and Genetics

CLVM has an equal gender distribution and occurs sporadically. No chromosomal localization or linkage with a causative gene has been identified.[5] The pathogenesis is also not understood, but several theories have been proposed. Klippel and Trénaunay[4] suggested that the mechanism responsible was a congenital spinal cord abnormality that altered autonomic control of capillaries causing increased blood flow to the skin, soft tissue, and bone with resultant hypertrophy. Perturbations in vasculogenesis during the specific stages of embryonic development with localized overgrowth as the hemodynamic consequence have also been theorized. The angiogenic factor gene, *AGGF1*, has been suggested as a candidate susceptibility gene.[8,9] Additional conjectures include paradominant inheritance, genetic mosaicism, and a polygenic hypothesis.[5]

Department of Surgery, Vascular Anomalies Center, Children's Hospital Boston, Harvard Medical School, 300 Longwood Avenue, Boston, MA 02115, USA
* Corresponding author.
E-mail address: steven.fishman@childrens.harvard.edu

Clin Plastic Surg 38 (2011) 107–120
doi:10.1016/j.cps.2010.08.009

CLVM occurring in two members of the same family has not been observed in our center.

Clinical Features

CLVM is usually diagnosed at birth. The classic presentation is an infant who presents with an enlarged lower extremity with lateral capillary malformations (CMs), lymphatic vesicles, and visible varicosities. CLVM can be suspected on antenatal imaging due to the presence of an enlarged limb. Severe cases are more likely to be detected antenatally. The diagnosis of CLVM cannot easily be confirmed until delivery since congenital lymphedema, Parkes Weber, CLOVES, and Proteus syndromes are included in the differential diagnosis.

Morphologic variability is the norm in patients with CLVM (**Fig. 1**). A single-center review of 252 patients documented involvement of the lower extremity (88%), upper extremity (29%), and trunk (23%).[10] The deformity can range from barely perceptible capillary staining with mild soft tissue overgrowth to a grotesquely deformed limb. Soft tissue and skeletal hypertrophy of the involved limb predominate, but in 10% of patients, the affected extremity may be short or hypotrophic.[1] Because hemihypertrophy is often a component of CLVM, many patients undergo ultrasonographic screening for Wilms tumor. Patients with CLVM, however, are not at increased risk for Wilms tumor and do not require screening.[11]

Expansion of CLVM tends to be commensurate with the growth of the child. The CMs are often multiple, occurring predominantly on the lateral side of the extremity, buttock, or thorax. The CM is macular in a newborn and tends to darken with time. Lymphatic malformations (LMs) present as lymphedema or lymphatic cysts. Lymphatic vesicles typically erupt through the CM. LMs may be found in the buttock/perineum and in the pelvis. Bladder outlet obstruction can result from compression by the vascular malformations. The lymphatic component can also extend through the inguinal canal and into the labia or scrotum masquerading as an inguinal hernia. CLVM of the upper extremity or torso commonly involves the mediastinum or retropleural space.

Venous malformations (VMs) in CLVM are heterogeneous. They can be focal VMs, varicosities, phlebectasias, hypoplastic or aplastic vessels, or veins with absent or incompetent valves. VMs can extend into the perineum, pelvis, and retroperitoneum. VMs are also frequently encountered in the left colon and rectum. As many as 10% of CLVM patients have hematochezia.[12] Rarely, these patients suffer chronic lower gastrointestinal tract bleeding, requiring transfusion. Colectomy, anorectal mucosectomy, and coloanal pull-through may be necessary.[13] Rectal VMs can be associated with ectatic mesenteric veins. Portomesenteric venous thrombosis and resultant portal hypertension have been observed in patients with this pattern.[14]

The presence of persistent embryonic veins ranges from 18% to 65% in patients with CLVM.[10,15,16] The true occurrence is likely higher because not all patients with CLVM undergo imaging. The most common persistent embryonic vessels are the lateral marginal vein (the vein of Servelle) and the sciatic vein. Persistent

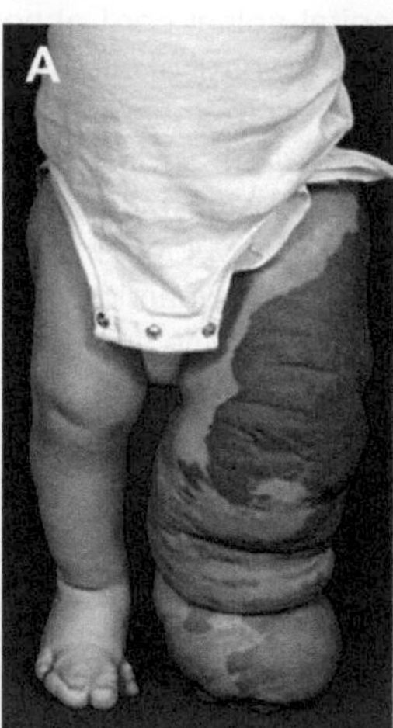

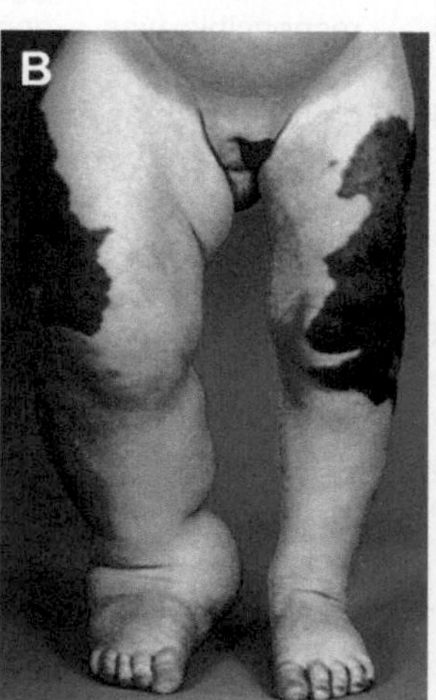

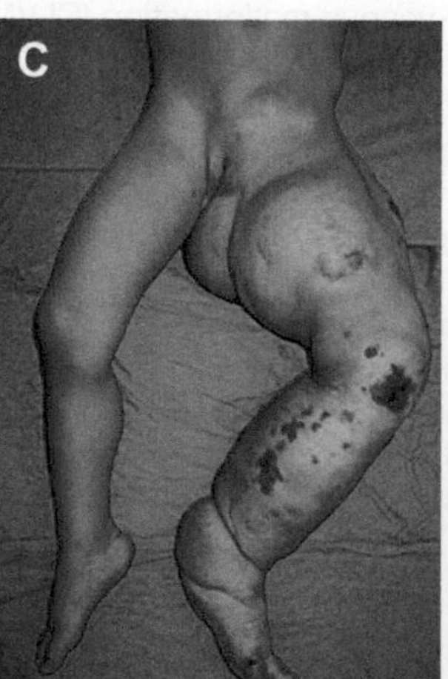

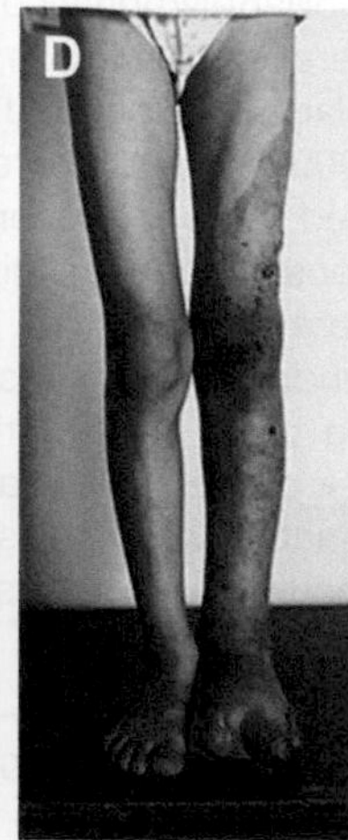

Fig. 1. Morphologic variation of CLVM. (*A*) Unilateral lower extremity CLVM. (*B*) Bilateral lower extremity CLVM with cutaneous lymphatic vesicles. (*C*) Unilateral CLVM with extension into the perineum and buttock. (*D*) Unilateral CLVM with minimal hypertrophy of the involved limb.

embryonic vessels are often associated with hypoplasia or aplasia of the normal named branches of the deep venous system. The lateral marginal vein originates in the lateral aspect of the foot and travels proximally underneath the CM, although its course can be variable (**Fig. 2**). The lateral marginal vein may not be visible in some patients because of soft tissue overgrowth but can be easily recognized by light palpation of a compressible cord-like structure in the lower leg and/or thigh.[17] The lateral marginal vein is usually thick walled and incompetent; the embryonic veins can be valveless.[18] The lateral marginal vein often has associated incompetent collateral and perforator veins, especially around the knee. Several recognized termination sites of the lateral vein include the profunda femoral, external or internal iliac, popliteal, and greater saphenous veins as well as the inferior vena cava (IVC).[18,19] The persistent sciatic vein arises from the popliteal vein, or nearby tributaries, traverses the sciatic notch, and terminates at the internal iliac vein.[20]

Soft tissue and bony hypertrophy range in severity from mild to severe. In some patients, only the subcutis is overgrown, whereas others have overgrowth of predominantly fatty tissues within or between the muscles as well. Imaging shows whether the hypertrophied components are predominantly extrafascial, intrafascial, or both. This finding is important when considering surgical debulking procedures. Bony hypertrophy may affect all bones in an extremity or can be limited to specific structures. Other limb findings seen in CLVM include macrodactyly, syndactyly, clinodactyly, polydactyly, ectrodactyly, and metatarsus varus.[18]

Imaging

We usually do not obtain baseline imaging in asymptomatic infants with CLVM, especially in the first 6 months of life. High-quality images require anesthesia in young infants and children. We prefer to delay imaging in infants unless there is an urgent indication such as bladder outlet obstruction, severe hematochezia, or surgical planning.

Plain film radiography is used to evaluate bony deformities and to follow limb length

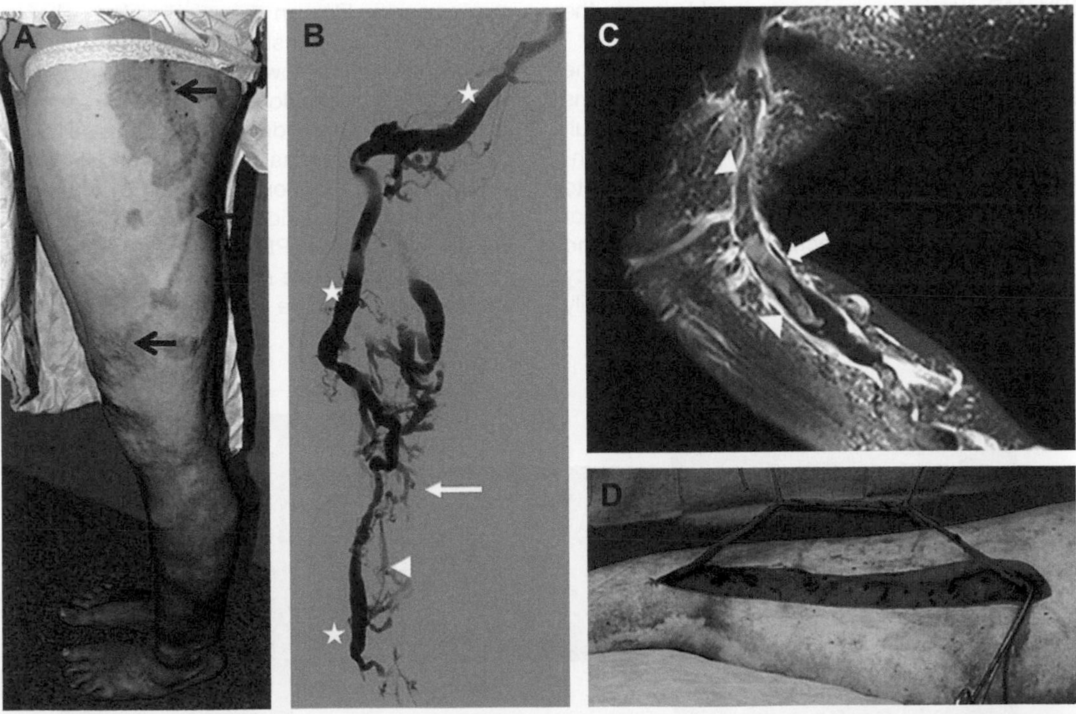

Fig. 2. Lateral marginal vein. (*A*) CLVM with a prominent lateral marginal vein (*arrows*). (*B*) Ascending venogram of a lower extremity (*arrow* marks the knee joint). Marginal vein is depicted (*stars*) in the lateral calf and thigh. The vein has numerous tributaries communicating with deep veins (*arrowhead*). The vein drains into the iliac vein in the pelvis (*superior star*). (*C*) Sagittal magnetic resonance image of a lower extremity in a patient with CLVM. An ectatic marginal vein (*arrowheads*) containing a nonocclusive intraluminal thrombus (*arrow*) is present. (*D*) Excision of the lateral marginal vein in the thigh.

discrepancies (LLDs). Duplex ultrasonography can help determine the presence of persistent embryonic veins as well as hypoplasia and aplasia of the deep venous system. Duplex ultrasonography provides morphologic information about the size of veins, perforators, and reflux. Because of its portability, Doppler ultrasonography can be performed as an adjunct to physical examination in the office setting. Focal VMs and LMs may be further characterized by ultrasonography. The use of ultrasonography is limited for larger lesions because of its inability to determine the exact size, extent, and tissue composition.[21]

Magnetic resonance imaging (MRI) and MR venography (MRV) provide the foundation for describing type, location, and extent of the vascular malformation components of CLVM (**Fig. 3**). Soft tissue and bony overgrowth are also depicted. Macrocystic LMs are usually seen in the pelvis and thigh, whereas microcystic LMs predominate in the abdominal wall, buttock, and distal extremity. LMs can be localized to the subcutaneous tissues or can extend into the intramuscular compartments. MRV delineates the extremity veins and demonstrates the anomalous venous channels. The veins of the trunk, pelvis, rectum, and mesentery are readily shown by MRV. MR arteriography is not useful because the arteries are normal in CLVM.

Venography may be useful for mapping the venous drainage and delineating malformations during sclerotherapy (see **Fig. 2**). It can be difficult to opacify the deep venous system with this technique because contrast preferentially flows into the capacious superficial channels. The use of tourniquets, direct puncture, ascending and descending phelobography, and dependency optimizes visualization.[22] Venography is generally performed only when an intervention is planned to avoid unnecessary morbidity.

Special Issues

A team of specialists is often necessary to manage patients with CLVM. Some of the more common manifestations of this disease include superficial thrombophlebitis, deep venous thrombosis (DVT), pulmonary thromboembolism (PE), infection, pain, and depression. Parental and patient education should start in infancy and continue into adulthood.

Persistent embryonic and phlebectatic veins can be troublesome to patients. These veins can be associated with pain, edema, sensation of heaviness, bleeding, and ulceration. Superficial thrombophlebitis has a frequency between 15% and 50%.[10,23] The organized thrombus may calcify and form phleboliths which can be a source of discomfort. Treatment consists of non-narcotic analgesics, anti-inflammatory medications, and limb elevation. Low-dose aspirin (81 mg) can be used to minimize phlebothromboses. If phlebothromboses recur, sclerotherapy can be considered.

DVT and PE occur in 4% to 11% of cases of CLVM. Persistent embryonic veins are likely the major source. Flow in these capacious channels is often retrograde or stagnant; thrombosis occurs due to diminished flow. Because these channels may connect anomalously to the femoral or iliac veins or IVC, a dislodged clot may result in PE. Patients with anomalous connections to the femoral or iliac veins or IVC should be considered for pre-emptive ablation or resection to decrease the risk of DVT and PE. This pattern should also be recognized before major invasive procedures, and when present, we recommend the placement

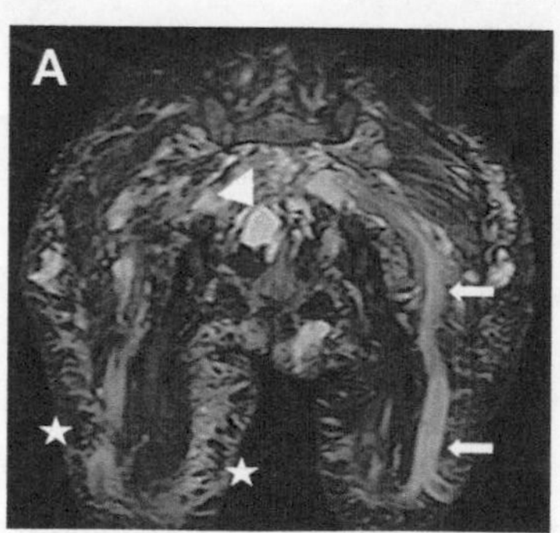

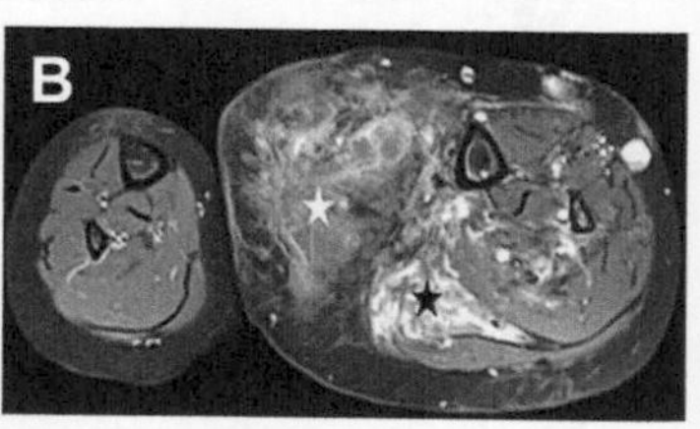

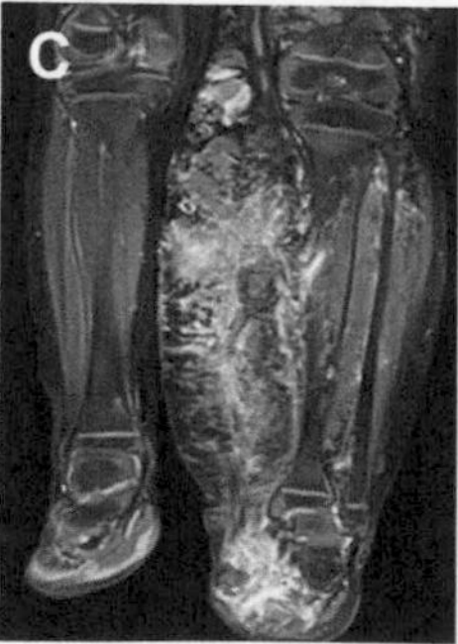

Fig. 3. MRI of lower extremity CLVM. (*A*) Coronal T1-weighted image shows a lateral marginal vein in the left thigh (*arrows*). Macrocystic LMs are seen in the buttocks (*arrowhead*). Microcystic LMs predominate in the thighs (*stars*). (*B*) Postcontrast axial T1-weighted image shows an uninvolved right leg in comparison to an affected left leg. There is predominantly extrafascial hypertrophy of the soft tissue of the left leg (*white star*). Some intrafascial component is seen as well (*black star*). (*C*) Coronal view of soft tissue hypertrophy.

of retrievable IVC filters. Careful pre-placement mapping of the venous drainage of the involved extremities is imperative to ensure that the drainage does not bypass the site of filter placement. In addition, treatment with perioperative prophylactic anticoagulation is recommended in all patients with CLVM. Our general practice is to administer low-molecular-weight heparin (LMWH) preoperatively for 14 days and to continue postoperatively until the patient has returned to full mobility.

Some patients with CLVM, particularly those with an extensive VM component or large embryonic veins, may have altered coagulation profiles due to constant activation of the coagulation cascade. Stagnant blood leads to the production of thrombin and conversion of fibrinogen to fibrin. Fibrinolysis results in elevated levels of fibrin degradation products. These products are measured with D-dimer levels. This process is called localized intravascular coagulopathy.[24] We obtain a baseline coagulation profile (platelet count, prothrombin time, partial thromboplastin time, fibrinogen, and D-dimer level) before any major procedure. LMWH should be administered to those patients with elevated D-dimer levels perioperatively to stabilize their hematologic status.

CLVM patients are susceptible to infection. Chronic lymphedema, poor skin integrity, venous stasis, and open lymphatic vesicles, especially when located on the lower leg or foot, predispose patients to cellulitis. Excellent skin hygiene and proper shoes are essential. Perineal and pelvic involvement also increases the risk of complications. Some patients may present with recurrent bacteremia due to translocation from gut flora. Patients with recurrent cellulitis may require antibiotic prophylaxis.

Chronic pain and depression should not go unrecognized. Pain is a major complaint in 88% of patients.[25] Varicosities, VMs, and ectatic embryonic veins contribute to venous stasis in the affected extremity. Patients report that their legs often ache and feel heavy. Intra-articular vascular malformations are also a source of pain. Multiple factors, such as chronic pain, frequent hospitalizations, and feelings of isolation, contribute to the development of depression. School-aged children and adolescents may be ostracized by their peers because of visible deformities and physical limitations.

Orthopedic consultation is usually necessary to evaluate the need for extremity amputation, management of intra-articular disease, and LLD. Amputation is indicated for lower extremity deformities that would preclude ambulation (**Fig. 4**). The level of amputation depends on the extent of the deformity. Gross foot enlargement that impairs ambulation and the ability to wear shoes requires orthopedic corrective procedures and partial amputations.[26] It is preferable to perform these procedures during infancy. In some instances, VMs have an intra-articular extension, most commonly in the knee joint. Range of motion may be limited because of the pain resulting in the development of flexion contractures. VMs may also cause hemarthroses, arthropathy, and ultimately arthritis. Focused imaging of the joint may show synovial involvement. Sclerotherapy can reduce pain and improve mobility. Simultaneous arthroscopy can be performed to clarify the extent of intra-articular involvement.

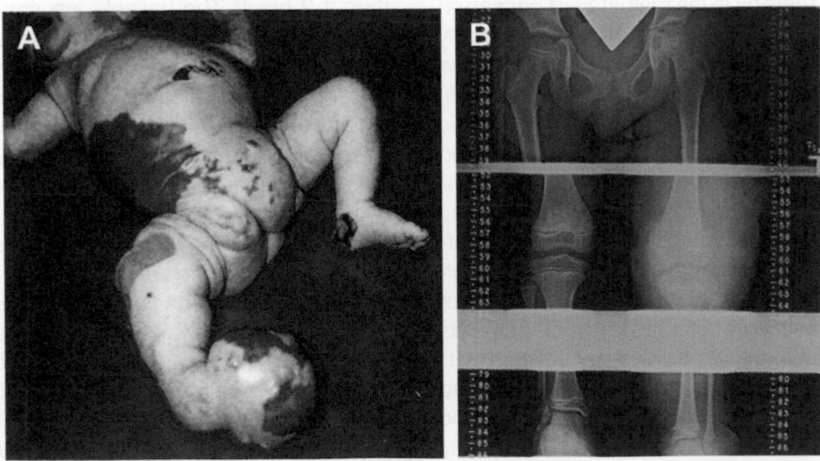

Fig. 4. Orthopedic morbidity. (*A*) Infant with CLVM of the extremity, genitalia, and trunk. Severe limb deformity precludes ambulation and thus requires selective amputation. (*B*) Scanogram shows an LLD (left leg longer than the right).

Subsequent synovectomy may prevent recurrent pain, hemarthrosis, and premature arthritis.

LLD is common in CLVM, occurring in 67% of patients. The average LLD in CLVM is 1.75 cm, ranging from 0.1 to 10.0 cm.[10] The initial assessment should start in infancy. The infant is placed supine on a flat surface, the feet are held in place, and the knees are flexed to 90°. Determination of whether the femur or tibia of the affected limb is longer or shorter can be made in this position. Older patients should be evaluated while standing on a flat floor. Symmetry of the gluteal folds and transverse popliteal skin creases of both legs should be inspected. Suspicion of a LLD warrants radiographic assessment. A standing or supine anteroposterior radiograph of both lower extremities is obtained. Alternatively, a scanogram can be taken in the supine position with a ruler placed between the lower extremities. The hips, knees, and ankles are evaluated (see **Fig. 4**). Regardless of the method, it should be consistent to allow for comparison.

Prediction of LLD in patients with complex combined vascular malformations is challenging. Yearly orthopedic examination to evaluate bone age helps to determine the most appropriate time for corrective orthopedic procedures.[27] Differences less than 0.5 cm require no therapy. Differences between 0.5 and 2.0 cm are managed with internal or external heel lifts. Discrepancies greater than 2 cm in the legs are often treated with epiphysiodesis at the distal femoral and/or proximal tibial growth plates around 11 to 12 years of age.[27] It is not necessary to correct upper extremity LLD.

Nonoperative Management

Compression therapy is the mainstay of conservative treatment in patients with CLVM. We generally do not recommend compression therapy until the child begins to walk; compression is difficult in toddlers, and garments are expensive. Elastic bandages can be used during periods of rapid growth. We recommend routine use of compression therapy by 4 to 5 years of age to minimize swelling from lymphedema, chronic venous insufficiency, and lymphatic vesicles. Compression therapy may improve pain and the sensation of heaviness. The length of the garment depends on the extent of extremity involvement. The greatest tolerated pressure should be used (a good starting point is 30–40 mm Hg). Pneumatic compressive devices are also an option, especially while recumbent or sleeping.

Sclerotherapy is used to treat focal VMs, small varicosities, LMs, and lymphatic vesicles. Small focal VMs can be accessed by direct puncture with injection of the sclerosant under fluoroscopy. Manual compression or tourniquets are used to limit venous drainage and systemic delivery of the sclerosant. Chronic venous stasis ulcers may improve or heal after sclerotherapy. Microfoam sclerotherapy for the treatment of large VMs and phlebectasias has increased in popularity in recent years,[28–30] and several studies have documented improvement in pain and reduction in the size of the malformation.[28–30] The delivery of the sclerosant in microfoam form allows for more precise dosing and prolongs contact time with the endothelial surface.[31] Regardless of the sclerosing agent chosen (alcohol, sodium tetradecyl sulfate, polidocanol), multiple sclerotherapy sessions are often required. Macrocystic LMs can also be treated with sclerotherapy. Cutaneous lymphatic vesicles may be managed with intravesicular sclerotherapy, cauterization, carbon-dioxide laser ablation, or excision.

Early detection of persistent embryonic veins allows for intervention to prevent chronic venous insufficiency, pain, DVT, and PE. Identification of patients with persistent embryonic vessels by a combination of physical examination, screening ultrasonography, and MRI/MRV should be performed in the first five years of life. We recommend that consideration be given to obliteration or removal of persistent embryonic veins with anomalous connections to femoral or iliac veins or the IVC in early childhood because of the risk of DVT and PE (see **Fig. 2**). Endovenous laser ablation (EVLA) is a minimally invasive procedure for the obliteration of persistent embryonic veins of suitable size. Recanalization or recurrent reflux rates of 67% have been observed when the venous diameter is greater than 1.2 cm.[32] The vessels are smallest in childhood and are therefore more amenable to EVLA. Older patients are often not candidates for EVLA because the vessel is too large; hence, it must be resected. Historically, many practitioners have been reluctant to consider surgical excision of the lateral marginal vein when associated with hypoplasia or aplasia of the deep venous system.[16–18,21,25] They feared that removal of the vein would prevent venous outflow from the leg resulting in phlegmasia alba or cerulea dolens. We support prior observations that the lateral marginal vein can be safely removed in the presence of hypoplasia because the hypoplastic veins dilate spontaneously to an almost normal size.[17,33] This rerouting of venous flow also occurs when the lateral marginal vein is ablated or resected in the face of an aplastic deep venous system.[17]

Operative Treatment

Debulking procedures to remove excess girth traditionally have not been recommended due to the possibility of long-term complications from fibrosis and pedal edema.[27] On the contrary, our experience with surgical debulking has been positive. We believe that surgical debulking can be performed safely with minimal long-term morbidity. There is tremendous psychological value for both the patient and family in making a child with CLVM look as "normal" as possible. In our center, debulking is considered to reduce excessive bulk and weight of the lower extremity, trunk, perineum, buttock, and genitalia. Debulking also can benefit those patients with a history of multiple soft tissue infections. The most important factor in deciding whether or not a patient is a candidate for surgical debulking of the extremity is the location of the overgrowth (see **Fig. 3**). We do not recommend debulking of intrafascial overgrowth due to morbidity associated with muscle resection and possible injury to neurovascular structures.

Surgeons must be committed to managing all postoperative complications and to reoperating when necessary. Patients are counseled about the risks of DVT, PE, injury to neurovascular structures, possible need for blood transfusion, and prolonged use of closed suction drains. There is a high likelihood of wound dehiscence, flap necrosis, and infection; the skin flaps are composed of abnormal skin with poor lymphatic drainage and altered circulation. Postoperatively, lymphatic vesicles may appear in or around the scar. We also inform patients about the potential need for multiple-staged resections, especially when the overgrowth is circumferential and extensive.

Because of significant morphologic variation in the presentation of CLVM, each patient's debulking procedure is tailored based on problematic areas. After appropriate counseling and administration of perioperative anticoagulants when indicated, the surgeon must decide which portion of the extremity to debulk. In general, we recommend starting the procedure in the most extensive area; there usually is disproportionate overgrowth of the lateral leg. Some patients have excess soft tissue around their ankle which can make fitting into shoes difficult (**Fig. 5**). Debulking the ankle can be done alone or in combination with a more extensive procedure. Tourniquets may be used when performing a distal extremity operation to minimize blood loss. The use of an intraoperative cell salvage machine can limit blood transfusions.

In order to minimize postoperative wound complications and ensure flap viability, only

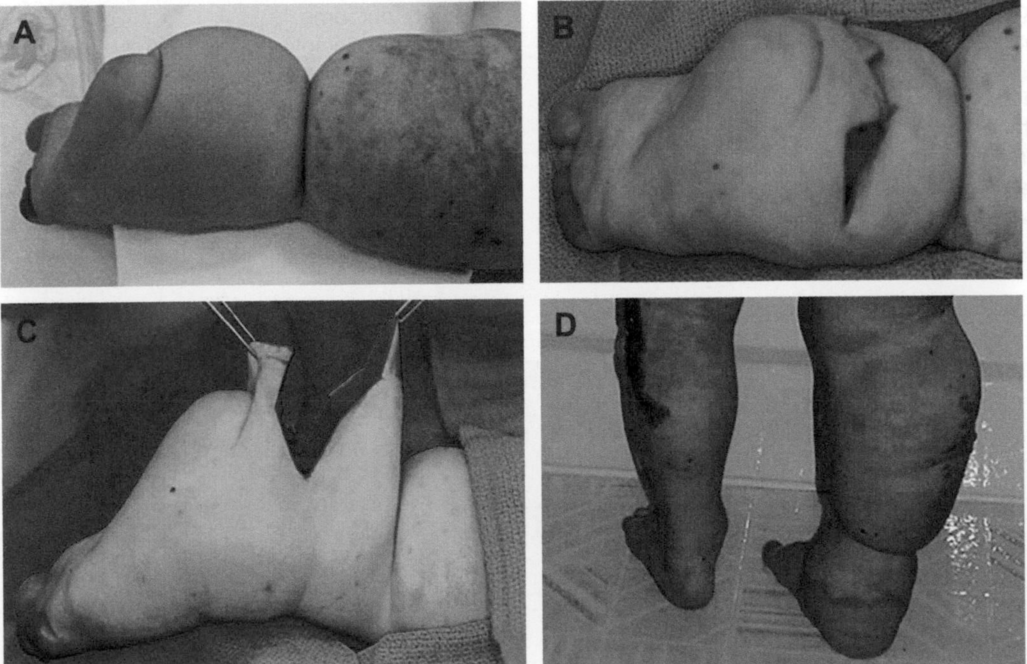

Fig. 5. Surgical correction of soft tissue overgrowth of the ankle to allow use of footwear. (*A*) Preoperative appearance. (*B*) Intraoperative incision. (*C*) Flaps are raised cephalad and caudad. (*D*) Four months postoperation.

a maximum circumference of 180° can be resected at one time when debulking an extremity. A lenticular skin excision design is made when excess skin is present. The use of lenticular excisions can help minimize operative time and blood loss by avoiding unnecessary dissection through tissue which is ultimately removed. When possible, we place the lenticular excision to incorporate skin that is most involved with cutaneous malformation. These principles can be applied to debulking procedures of the trunk and thoracic wall. Dissection is usually not extended into the thorax or mediastinum, unless the patient is symptomatic.

The goal of debulking is to remove as much excess weight and bulk as possible. The skin is incised until the subcutaneous tissue is visualized. Well-vascularized skin flaps are raised (no more than 90° in each direction in an extremity) (**Fig. 6**). In areas where the malformation involves or is adjacent to the dermis, the flap should be made as thin as possible without devascularization. Residual malformation left behind at the time of closure can result in "recurrence" and thickening of the flaps. After raising the flaps, the malformed tissue between the skin and muscle fascia is excised (**Fig. 7**). The fascia is usually left intact to avoid injuring neurovascular structures and the underlying muscle. We recommend the removal of large embryonic veins when encountered (see **Fig. 2**). Often a large amount of excess skin can be removed because the underlying malformation has served as a tissue expander. A moderate amount of tension on the wound is accepted to maximally reduce the size of the limb, realizing that the scar may be slightly wider. Skin flaps are reapproximated over closed suction drains. Drainage can initially be as high as several hundred milliliters per day because the tissue usually has poor lymphatic drainage. Drains should be removed when the drain output decreases to between 10 and 15 mL per day.

Extension of the vascular malformation into the genitalia, buttock, and perineum is common with CLVM. The buttock and perineum are frequently affected by LM, whereas the genitalia may contain LM, VM, or both. These anatomic locations present challenges related to urinary, defecatory, sexual, reproductive, and emotional function. These locations are fortunately concealed during the first few years of life, so there is less social pressure for rapid contour improvement. If there are no functional impairments during infancy, it is often wise to delay intervention until the later stages of development (**Fig. 8**). The genitalia particularly undergo dramatic changes during adolescence. The patient may not be cognizant of these anatomic differences until adolescence when they cause distress. Genital lesions with significant overgrowth can be partially dealt with during childhood. Therapeutic options include compression, sclerotherapy, and resection. Compression therapy of the male genitalia can be beneficial, but it is often limited due to patient discomfort. Sclerotherapy can be used preoperatively to facilitate surgical debulking. However, overzealous excision can be just as disfiguring as the malformation itself. For example, if too much tissue is removed from the labia majora in infancy or childhood, they do not develop during adolescence. Adopt a "less is more" approach in genital debulking procedures in order to achieve the best ultimate outcome.

Several principles guide debulking procedures of the buttocks and perineum. We recommend a preoperative bowel preparation if the resection is in proximity to the anus. The incisions should be planned so that the scar will be in the anticipated location of the infragluteal fold. The intergluteal cleft should never be crossed. Vertical incisions that extend from the buttock to thigh,

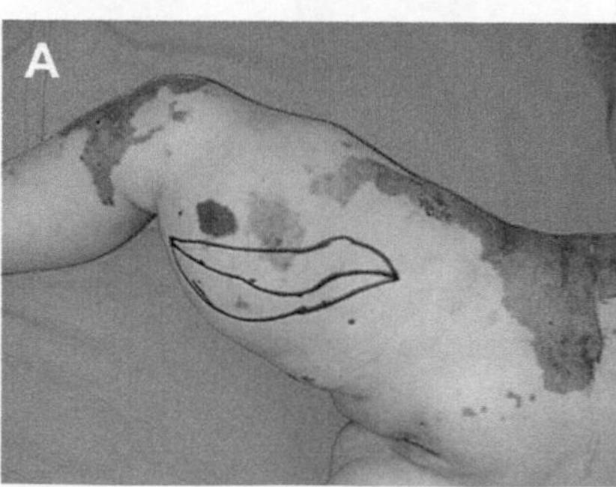

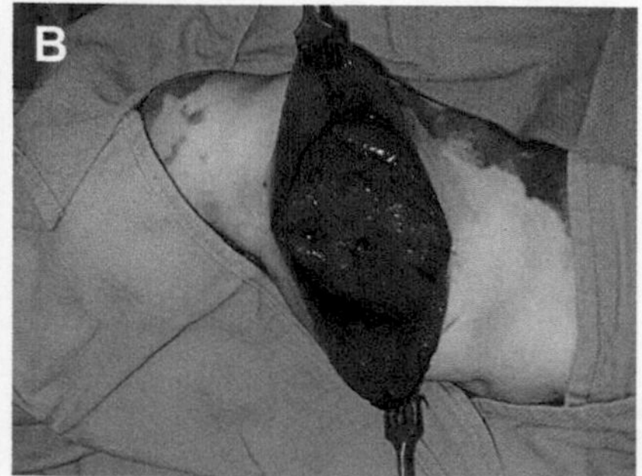

Fig. 6. CLVM with soft tissue hypertrophy of inner thigh. (*A*) Lenticular excision is marked for debulking. (*B*) Well-vascularized flaps mobilized in both directions to remove maximum amount of soft tissue.

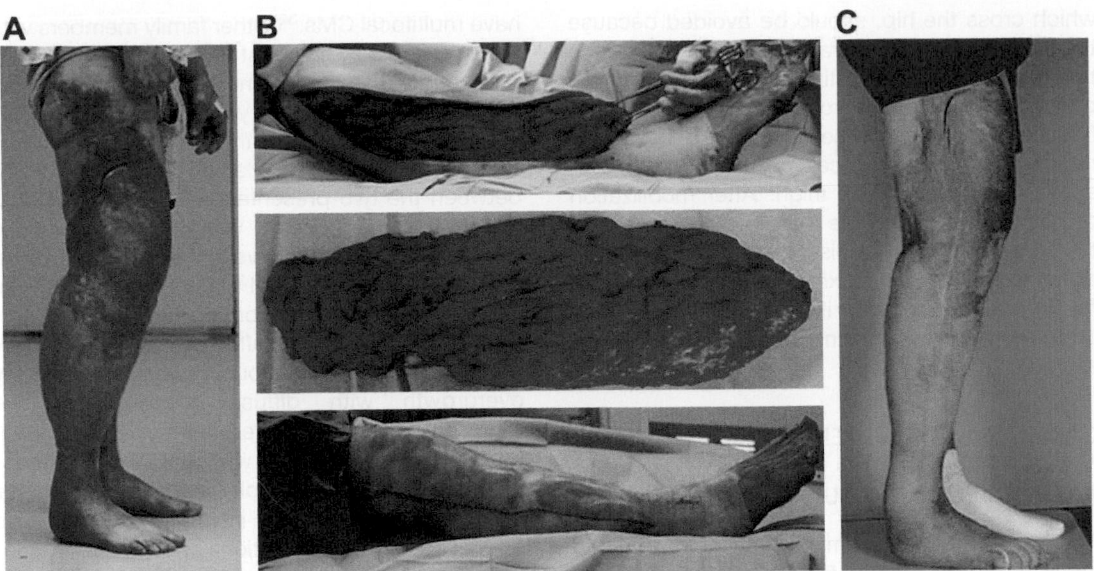

Fig. 7. Lower extremity debulking procedure for CLVM. (*A*) Preoperative appearance. (*B*) Skin flaps have been raised 90° in each direction (*top*). Soft tissue specimen (*middle*). Linear wound closure with moderate tension (*bottom*). (*C*) Four years postoperation.

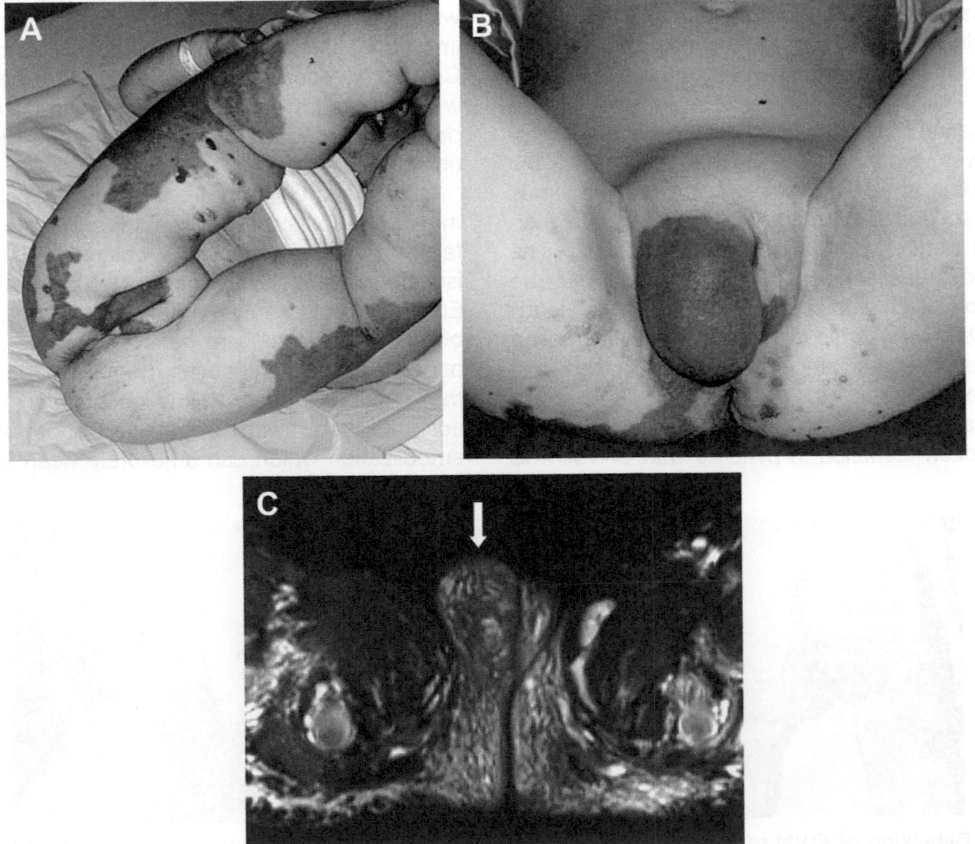

Fig. 8. Progression of CLVM of genitalia. (*A*) Mild hypertrophy of labia majora at 14 months of age. (*B*) By 9 years of age, the right labium majus has increased in size. (*C*) MRI at age 9 years of age shows microcystic LM (*arrow*).

which cross the hip, should be avoided because the scar effaces the infragluteal fold. Adherence to these principles optimizes buttock contour postoperatively. A superomedially based buttock flap can extend above the iliac crest to the lumbar region. An inferior flap can be mobilized to gain access to the posterior thigh. After mobilization of both flaps beyond the margin of malformation to be removed, the dissection is carried out down to the gluteus maximus fascia (**Fig. 9**). The fascia may be removed if the LM permeates the underlying muscle, but the muscle should not be excised.

CAPILLARY-ARTERIOVENOUS MALFORMATION AND CAPILLARY-ARTERIOVENOUS FISTULAS

Capillary-arteriovenous malformation (CAVM) and capillary-arteriovenous fistulas (CAVFs) correspond to the old eponym Parkes Weber syndrome. This syndrome is characterized by the presence of a confluent or patchy CM with underlying multiple microarteriovenous fistulas in association with soft tissue and skeletal hypertrophy of the affected limb (**Fig. 10**).[7,34] There is often an associated lymphatic component. Like other vascular malformations, the diagnosis may be suspected antenatally but cannot be confirmed until birth. The infant usually presents with diffuse enlargement of the involved limb, most commonly a lower extremity. In some instances, the syndrome is not obvious at birth and becomes apparent during infancy and childhood.[27] The ipsilateral buttock or trunk may be involved.[35] The stained areas are usually warm; a thrill may be palpable. Auscultation may detect a bruit. Handheld Doppler examination often reveals increased flow and low-resistance runoff when placed over the stained areas.

Mutations in RASA1, either de novo or inherited, have been identified in patients with CAVM who have multifocal CMs.[35] Other family members with the mutation may have just CMs, sometimes barely perceptible. The genetic mutation in those patients without multifocal CMs is yet to be elucidated. The CMs in patients without the RASA1 mutation are less hypertrophic and darker.[35] The distinction between the two presentations is clinically useful because some patients with RASA1 mutations were also found to have vein of Galen aneurysmal malformations and neural tumors strikingly similar to those seen in neurofibromatosis types 1 and 2.[35]

Radiographically, the affected extremity usually has fusiform, subcutaneous, muscular, and bony overgrowth with diffuse microfistulas (see **Fig. 10**). The bony overgrowth can result in a LLD, which is followed with plain films. Ultrasonography and color Doppler evaluation of arterial flow may be performed in infancy. Generalized arterial and venous dilatations are seen on angiography and venography. Angiography demonstrates discrete arteriovenous shunts, particularly around joint structures.[36] A soft tissue blush is observed involving muscles and subcutaneous fat (see **Fig. 10**). Contrast-enhanced T2-weighted MRI sequences reveal vascular flow voids.

CAVM is frequently misdiagnosed as either CM with overgrowth or CLVM, but the distinction is important. As many as 30% of patients with CAVM have cardiac overload which is generally well tolerated.[35] Occasionally, cardiac failure can develop secondary to shunting through the arteriovenous fistulas.

Infants and children are followed annually with monitoring for axial overgrowth, signs of cardiac failure, and cutaneous problems related to ischemia. Treatment is predicated on symptoms. Epiphysiodesis can improve LLDs. Surgical debulking procedures are generally not performed because the microfistulas frequently permeate the entire extremity. Flow reduction may be accomplished with repetitive superselective embolization which can ameliorate heart failure.[1]

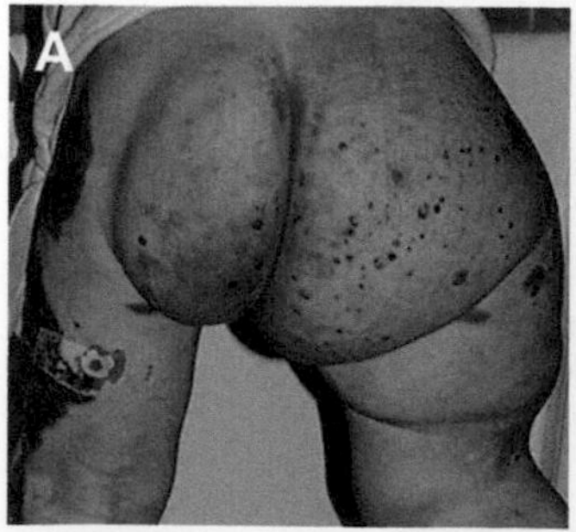

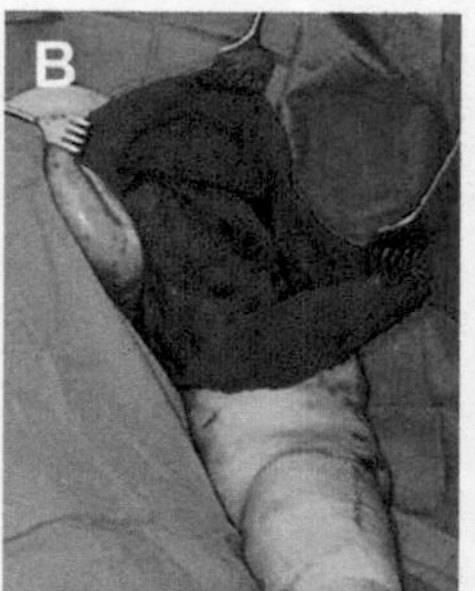

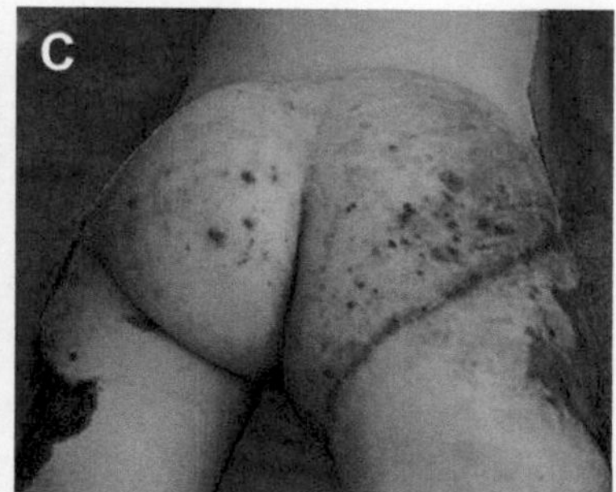

Fig. 9. Debulking of CLVM of the buttock. (*A*) Preoperative appearance of soft tissue overgrowth of bilateral buttocks. (*B*) Incision made in the anticipated infragluteal fold. Flaps are raised, and the soft tissue component was then excised. (*C*) Six months postoperation.

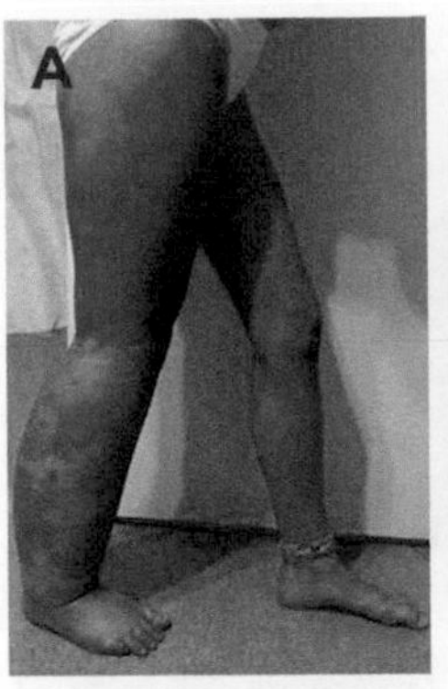

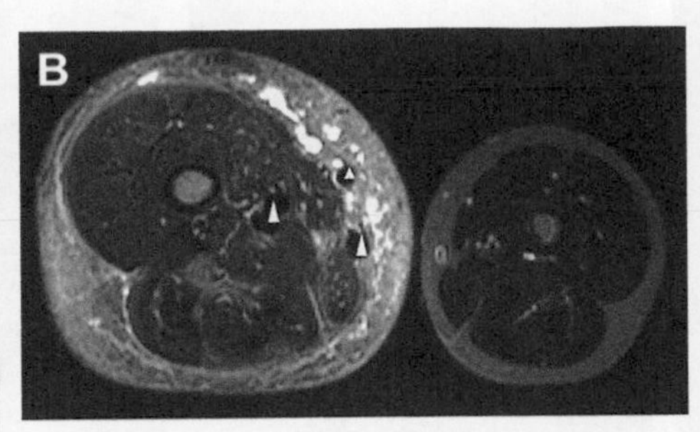

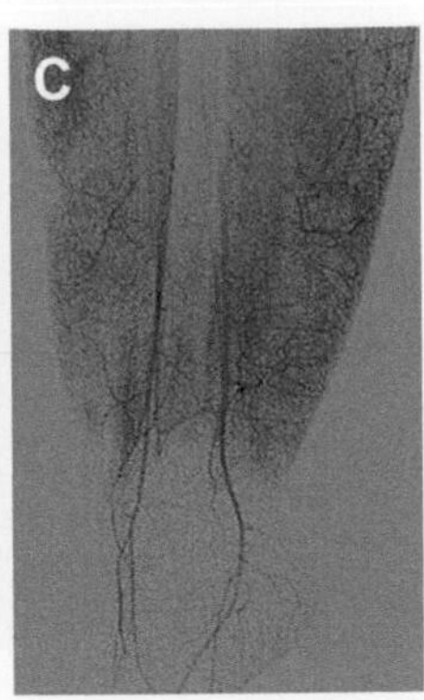

Fig. 10. CAVM of the extremity. (*A*) CAVM of the right lower extremity with soft tissue hypertrophy. (*B*) MRI demonstrates soft tissue and muscle overgrowth. Large draining veins are also present (*arrowheads*). (*C*) Typical angiographic appearance showing a diffuse soft tissue blush involving the skin, subcutis, and muscle representing microfistulas.

For recalcitrant disease, amputation may be required.

CLOVES SYNDROME

Congenital lipomatous overgrowth, vascular malformations, epidermal nevi, and skeletal anomalies (CLOVES) syndrome is a newly recognized syndrome.[37,38] Its main features are truncal lipomatous masses, vascular malformations, and acral/musculoskeletal anomalies (**Fig. 11**). Not all features must be present to make the diagnosis of CLOVES syndrome. Until recently, many patients with this syndrome were misdiagnosed as either having CLVM or Proteus syndrome. Like CLVM and Parkes Weber syndrome, CLOVES syndrome may be suspected antenatally because many of the abnormalities can be seen on prenatal ultrasonography. The pathogenesis of the disease is unknown.

The key feature is the presence of a truncal lipomatous mass that is usually noted at birth. The lesion is often mistaken for an LM, especially when located on the chest wall. The lesion may be located adjacent to a large LM. The fatty growths are often large, disfiguring, and painful. The lipomatous masses are hypervascular and exhibit rapid post-resection recurrence. These masses are also infiltrative and frequently extend from the trunk into adjacent areas such as the retroperitoneum, mediastinum, and thoracic cavity (see **Fig. 11**). Many of the lipomatous growths involve the spinal column and extend into the epidural space; compression of the cord, thecal sac, and nerve roots may occur.

Vascular malformations are also a distinguishing characteristic of CLOVES syndrome. All 25 of the reported cases have had slow-flow vascular malformations.[37,38] CMs can be seen on the trunk. LMs and lymphatic vesicles are frequently present within and around the truncal lipomatous masses. VMs, in the form of phlebectasia, can course over or around the truncal lesions. Ectatic veins may thrombose, causing DVT or PE, especially

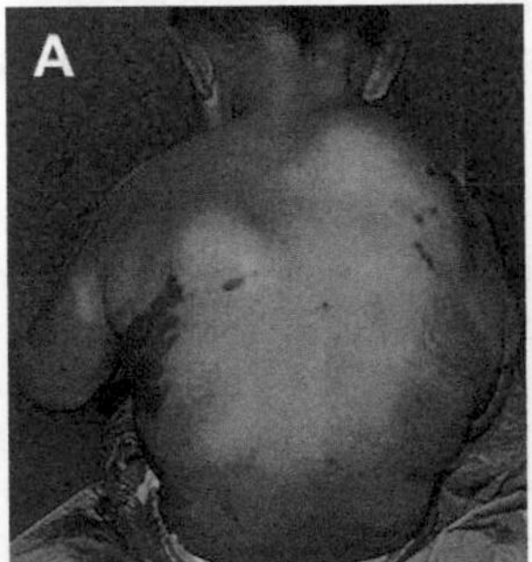

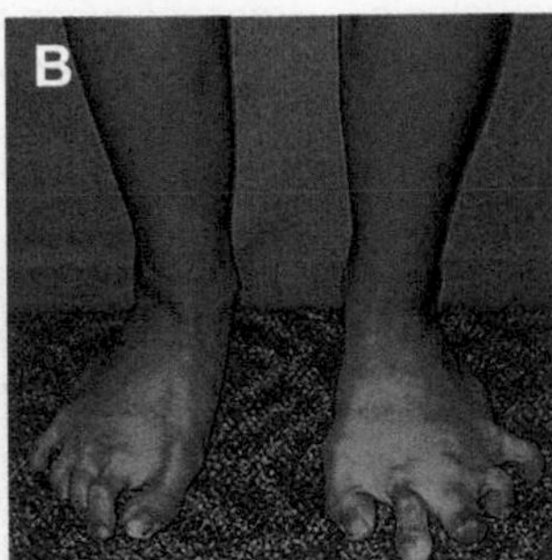

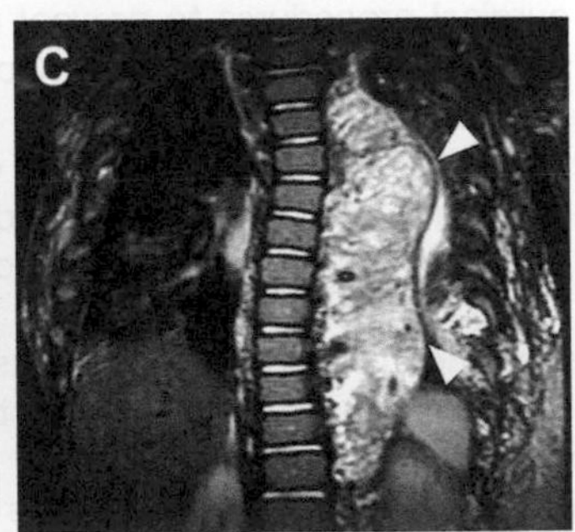

Fig. 11. Physical findings of the CLOVES syndrome. (*A*) Child with characteristic bilateral truncal lipomatous masses with a CM overlying the mass on the left. (*B*) A common acral skeletal anomaly showing widened triangular feet with increased first interdigital web space. (*C*) MRI depicting a truncal lipomatous mass with a lymphatic component (*arrowheads*). Scoliosis of the thoracic spine is also apparent.

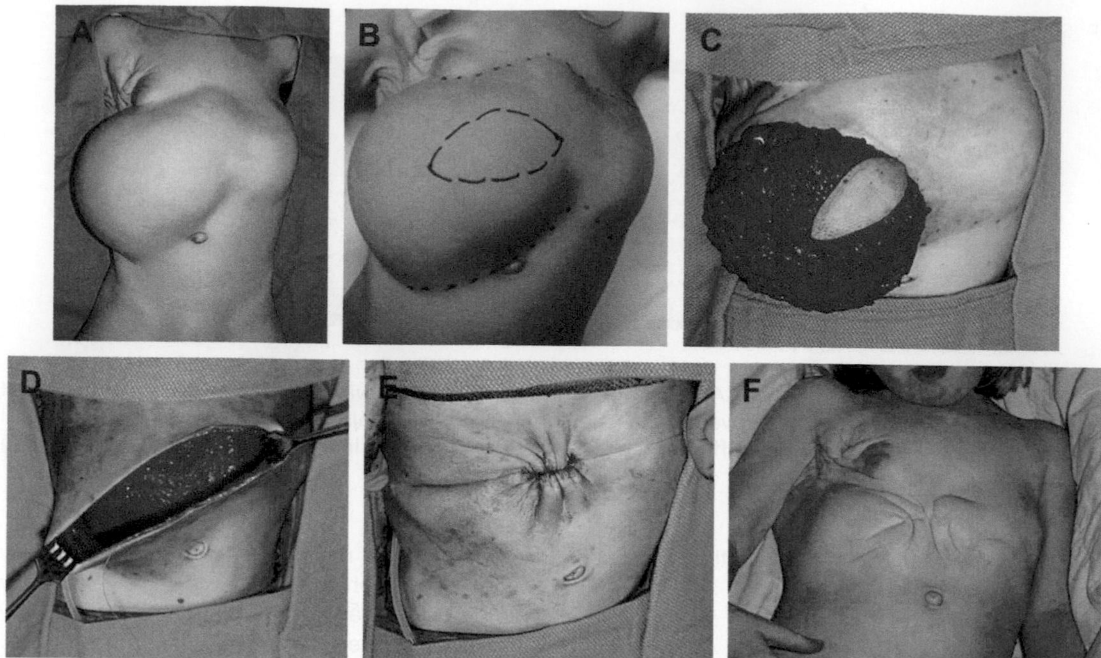

Fig. 12. Surgical debulking of a truncal lipomatous mass in CLOVES syndrome. (*A*) Preoperative image. (*B*) Lenticular excision is planned to minimize scar, operative time, and blood loss. (*C*) Mass is mobilized from the overlying dermis and is brought through the incision. (*D*) The cavity is inspected and a drain is placed. (*E*) The incision is closed in a purse-string fashion to decrease the size of the scar. (*F*) One year postresection.

perioperatively. MRI/MRV can further delineate the drainage patterns of these veins.

Fast-flow malformations are also common in CLOVES syndrome. In the larger of the two published series, 28% of patients were found to have perispinal fast-flow malformations.[37] AVMs, which occur in and around the lipomatous masses, contribute to the morbidity of this syndrome; paresis and spasticity have been observed in several of our patients. We recommend obtaining an MRI with venous and arterial sequences early in life to determine the presence, location, and extent of these fast-flow lesions. Patients require neurologic monitoring and may need interventional and/or surgical procedures to prevent neurologic morbidity. Embolization may be necessary to manage the fast-flow malformations.

Musculoskeletal abnormalities most commonly involve the feet and hands. Acral deformities include large, wide feet and hands, macrodactyly, and a wide sandal gap. Scoliosis has been observed in nearly half of the patients which is followed with plain films. Skeletal stabilization may be required.

Surgical principles for debulking the slow-flow malformations and lipomatous masses in CLOVES syndrome are similar to those for CLVM. Prior to any intervention, imaging should be carefully reviewed because the muscles are frequently involved or replaced by fatty tissue which may preclude resection. Preoperative counseling must include discussions regarding the recurrence of the lipomatous masses and risk of DVT and PE, particularly in the presence of phlebectatic veins. We recommend considering the use of LMWH and/or retrievable IVC filters and potentially superior vena caval filters in the perioperative period. In general, we do not recommend removal of asymptomatic malformations or lipomatous masses in the mediastinum, thorax, abdomen, or retroperitoneum. Macrocystic LMs may be treated with sclerotherapy and/or surgical excision. We surgically debulk disfiguring malformations and lipomatous masses when possible to improve mobility, reduce pain, and for psychosocial reasons (**Fig. 12**).

SUMMARY

Proper diagnosis of patients affected by complex combined vascular malformations is essential. These patients benefit from an interdisciplinary approach involving many medical and surgical specialists. Interventions must be tailored to the specific needs and symptoms of the patient. Outcomes are optimized with careful preoperative planning, identification of comorbidities, and realistic expectations on behalf of both the patient and surgeon.

REFERENCES

1. Mulliken JB, Fishman SJ, Burrows PE. Vascular anomalies. Curr Probl Surg 2000;37:517–84.
2. Hilaire GS. Histoire generale et particuliere des anomalies de l'organisation chez l'homme et les animaux. Paris: Tome I; 1832. p. 328–33.
3. Trelat U, Monod A. De l'hypertrophie unilaterale partielle ou totale du corps. Arch Gen Med 1869;13: 536–8 [in French].
4. Klippel M, Trénaunay P. Memoires originaux: du noevus variquex osteo-hypertrophique. Arch Gen Med 1900;185:641–72 [in French].
5. Oduber CE, van der Horst CM, Hennekam RC. Klippel-Trenaunay syndrome: diagnostic criteria and hypothesis on etiology. Ann Plast Surg 2008;60: 217–23.
6. Weber FP. Angioma formation in connection with hypertrophy of limbs and hemi-hypertrophy. Br J Dermatol 1907;19:231–5.
7. Weber FP. Hemangiectatic hypertrophy of limbs: congenital phlebarteriectasias and so-called congenital varicose veins. Br J Child Dis 1918;15: 13–7.
8. Fan C, Ouyang P, Timur AA, et al. Novel roles of GATA1 in regulation of angiogenic factor AGGF1 and endothelial cell function. J Biol Chem 2009; 284:23331–43.
9. Hu Y, Li L, Seidelmann SB, et al. Identification of association of common AGGF1 variants with susceptibility for Klippel-Trenaunay syndrome using the structure association program. Ann Hum Genet 2008;72:636–43.
10. Jacob AG, Driscoll DJ, Shaughnessy WJ, et al. Klippel-Trenaunay syndrome: spectrum and management. Mayo Clin Proc 1998;73:28–36.
11. Greene AK, Kieran M, Burrows PE, et al. Wilms tumor screening is unnecessary in Klippel-Trenaunay syndrome. Pediatrics 2004;113:e326–9.
12. Gloviczki P, Stanson AW, Stickler GB, et al. Klippel-Trenaunay syndrome: the risks and benefits of vascular interventions. Surgery 1991;110:469–79.
13. Fishman SJ, Shamberger RC, Fox VL, et al. Endorectal pull-through abates gastrointestinal hemorrhage from colorectal venous malformations. J Pediatr Surg 2000;35:982–4.
14. Kulungowski AM, Fox VL, Burrows PE, et al. Portomesenteric venous thrombosis associated with rectal venous malformation. J Pediatr Surg 2010; 45:1221–7.
15. Baskerville PA, Ackroyd JS, Lea Thomas M, et al. The Klippel-Trenaunay syndrome: clinical, radiological and haemodynamic features and management. Br J Surg 1985;72:232–6.
16. Gloviczki P, Hollier LH, Telander RL, et al. Surgical implications of Klippel-Trenaunay syndrome. Ann Surg 1983;197:353–62.
17. Mattassi R, Vaghi M. Management of the marginal vein: current issues. Phlebology 2007;22:283–6.
18. Gloviczki P, Driscoll DJ. Klippel-Trenaunay syndrome: current management. Phlebology 2007; 22:291–8.
19. Rojas Martinez R, Puech-Leao P, Guimaraes PM, et al. Persistence of the embryonic lateral marginal vein: report of two cases. Rev Hosp Clin Fac Med Sao Paulo 2001;56:159–62.
20. Cherry KJ, Gloviczki P, Stanson AW. Persistent sciatic vein: diagnosis and treatment of a rare condition. J Vasc Surg 1996;23:490–7.
21. Laor T, Burrows PE, Hoffer FA. Magnetic resonance venography of congenital vascular malformations of the extremities. Pediatr Radiol 1996;26:371–80.
22. Thomas ML. Radiologic assessment of vascular malformations. In: Mulliken JB, Young AE, editors. Vascular birthmarks. Philadelphia: Saunders; 1988. p. 141–59.
23. Samuel M, Spitz L. Klippel-Trenaunay syndrome: clinical features, complications and management in children. Br J Surg 1995;82:757–61.
24. Enjolras O, Ciabrini D, Mazoyer E, et al. Extensive pure venous malformations in the upper or lower limb: a review of 27 cases. J Am Acad Dermatol 1997;36:219–25.
25. Lee A, Driscoll D, Gloviczki P, et al. Evaluation and management of pain in patients with Klippel-Trenaunay syndrome: a review. Pediatrics 2005; 115:744–9.
26. Smithers CJ, Fishman SJ. Vascular anomalies. In: Ashcraft KW, Holcomb GW, Murphy JP, editors. Pediatric surgery. 4th edition. Philadelphia: Elsevier Saunders; 2004. p. 1038–53.
27. Enjolras O, Chapot R, Merland JJ. Vascular anomalies and the growth of limbs: a review. J Pediatr Orthop B 2004;13:349–57.
28. Cabrera J, Cabrera J Jr, Garcia-Olmedo MA, et al. Treatment of venous malformations with sclerosant in microfoam form. Arch Dermatol 2003;139:1409–16.
29. Eckmann DM. Polidocanol for endovenous microfoam sclerosant therapy. Expert Opin Investig Drugs 2009;18:1919–27.
30. Nitecki S, Bass A. Ultrasound-guided foam sclerotherapy in patients with Klippel-Trenaunay syndrome. Isr Med Assoc J 2007;9:72–5.
31. Redondo P, Bastarrika G, Sierra A, et al. Efficacy and safety of microfoam sclerotherapy in a patient with Klippel-Trenaunay syndrome and a patent foramen ovale. Arch Dermatol 2009;145:1147–51.
32. Gonzalez-Zeh R, Armisen R, Barahona S. Endovenous laser and echo-guided foam ablation in great saphenous vein reflux: one-year follow-up results. J Vasc Surg 2008;48:940–6.
33. Belov S, Loose DA, Muller E. Angeborene Gefabfehler (congenital vascular defects). Reinbeck (IA): Einhorn-Presse Verlag; 1989.

34. Mulliken JB, Young AE. Vascular birthmarks: hemangiomas and malformations. Philadelphia: Saunders; 1988.
35. Revencu N, Boon LM, Mulliken JB, et al. Parkes Weber syndrome, vein of Galen aneurysmal malformation, and other fast-flow vascular anomalies are caused by RASA1 mutations. Hum Mutat 2008;29: 959–65.
36. Marler JJ, Mulliken JB. Vascular anomalies. In: Mathes SJ, Hentz VR, editors. Plastic surgery. 2nd edition. Philadelphia: Elsevier; 2009. p. 19–68.
37. Alomari AI. Characterization of a distinct syndrome that associates complex truncal overgrowth, vascular, and acral anomalies: a descriptive study of 18 cases of CLOVES syndrome. Clin Dysmorphol 2009;18:1–7.
38. Sapp JC, Turner JT, van de Kamp JM, et al. Newly delineated syndrome of congenital lipomatous overgrowth, vascular malformations, and epidermal nevi (CLOVE syndrome) in seven patients. Am J Med Genet A 2007;143A: 2944–58.

Special Considerations in Vascular Anomalies: Airway Management

Ian N. Jacobs, MD[a,*], Anne Marie Cahill, MD[b]

KEYWORDS

- Vascular anomalies • Airway management • Airway imaging
- Endoscopy

Vascular anomalies are disorders of abnormal vasculogenesis or lymphogenesis.[1,2] Vascular malformations are labeled according to the vessel type including venous malformations, lymphatic malformations, capillary malformations, arteriovenous malformations, and mixed types (lymphaticovenous malformations). Vascular malformations may also be divided into low flow and high flow lesions. Low flow lesions include most vascular malformations, including capillary (port wine), venous malformations, lymphatic malformations, and combined lesions. High flow lesions include arteriovenous malformations (AVMs), arteriovenous fistula (AVFs), or aneurysms, which all have a high flow arterial pedicle. Venous malformations, lymphatic malformations, and AVMs are the most common vascular malformations to affect the aerodigestive tract, but are less common overall than hemangiomas. All types of vascular anomalies may involve the airway, causing varying degrees of upper airway obstruction as well as dysphagia and bleeding.

Certain signs and symptoms may implicate airway involvement with a hemangioma or vascular malformation. The most common pathology to affect the airway is a hemangioma and usually one with segmental distribution. The most common symptoms include biphasic stridor, recurrent croup, and retractions. Flexible laryngoscopy performed in the outpatient setting may show vascular staining of the endolarynx and may reveal a subglottic mass, but it may be difficult to appreciate small subglottic or tracheal hemangiomas on awake flexible laryngoscopy. It is necessary to distinguish a vascular anomaly from other airway lesions such as a congenital cyst. This is accomplished with imaging and endoscopy.

AIRWAY IMAGING

At the initial presentation of a child with stridor, plain films of the airway will show a tapered subglottic airway and a subglottic mass with a subglottic hemangioma and are very useful for assessing the subglottis (**Fig. 1**). This is to be differentiated from subglottic stenosis or subglottic cysts. With these two pathologies, there is usually a history of intubation except with congenital subglottic stenosis, which is quite rare.

Sonography may be useful for defining vascular anomalies, but has limited resolution. Both contrast-enhanced CT/CT angiography (CTA) and MRI/MR angiography (MRA) are the most precise at defining vascular lesions and their extent of involvement in the aerodigestive tract. The injection of an arterial phase contrast agent is most important for demonstrating the vascular

[a] Division of Otolaryngology, The Center for Pediatric Airway Disorders, The Children's Hospital of Philadelphia, University of Pennsylvania School of Medicine, 34th Street and Civic Center Boulevard, 1 Wood, Philadelphia, PA 19104, USA
[b] Interventional Radiology Division, Department of Radiology, The Children's Hospital of Philadelphia, 34th Street and Civic Center Boulevard, 3 Main, Philadelphia, PA 19104, USA
* Corresponding author.
E-mail address: jacobsi@email.chop.edu

Clin Plastic Surg 38 (2011) 121–131
doi:10.1016/j.cps.2010.08.008
0094-1298/11/$ – see front matter

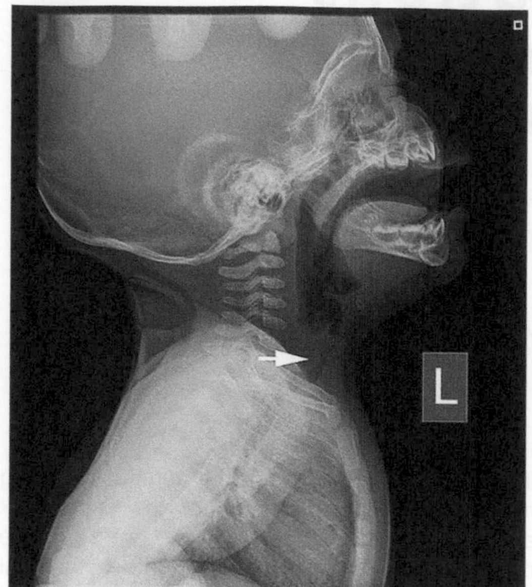

Fig. 1. Plain film of the airway revealing posteriorly based subglottic hemangioma.

nature of the lesions and the extent of disease in the neck. However, one may have a limited view of the actual airway. MRI is most helpful for defining lymphatic malformations and determining microcystic versus macrocystic disease. Angiography is useful for determining the structure and blood supply of AVM, AVF, and aneurysm and allows for embolization before definitive surgery.

OPERATIVE ENDOSCOPY

Microlaryngoscopy and bronchoscopy (MLB) is an essential technique for confirming a diagnosis of an airway vascular anomaly such as a subglottic hemangioma. The technique is performed under general anesthesia with spontaneous ventilation. This allows for the most accurate assessment of the airway. First, flexible laryngoscopy is performed to study the dynamic characteristics of the larynx such as vocal cord mobility and epiglottic position, glossoptosis, and laryngomalacia. A flexible scope with side port suction is used to do this.

Microlaryngoscopy is performed with a rigid anterior commissure-type laryngoscope such as a Benjamin or Parsons placed in the vallecula (**Fig. 2**) and used to expose the endolarynx and subglottic airway. This will reveal a subglottic hemangioma just below the vocal cords (**Fig. 3**). Magnification from a Storz Hopkins telescope is used to visualize the subglottic airway and the scope can be passed down to the level of the carina. It is important to carefully look at

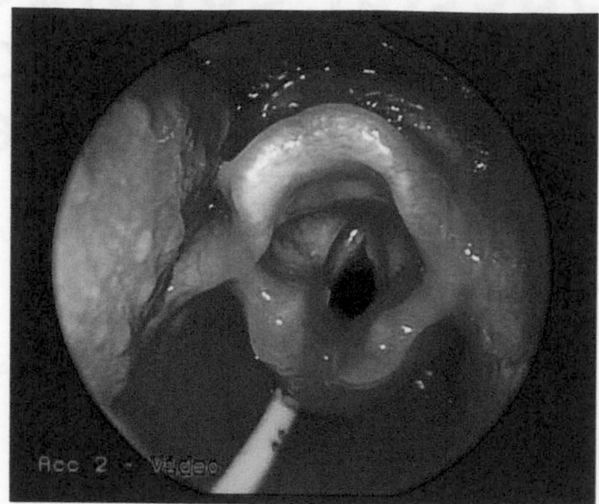

Fig. 2. Exposure of the endolarynx by placing the laryngoscope in the vallecula of the pharynx.

the trachealis muscle in the back wall of the trachea for staining, fullness, and signs of vascular disease (**Fig. 4**). Tracheal hemangioma may be subtle and its treatment is challenging.

MANAGEMENT OF HEMANGIOMAS AFFECTING THE AIRWAY

Hemangiomas are often seen in infants in the head and neck region and may involve the upper aerodigestive tract and airway. Involvement of the airway may result in varying degrees of upper airway obstruction as well as dysphagia and bleeding. Based on the distribution of the hemangioma, one may subclassify hemangiomas into focal, multifocal, or segmental based on the distribution characteristics. Focal implies a solitary lesion, whereas multifocal implies multiple. Segmental lesions occupy a dermatomal distribution. Most

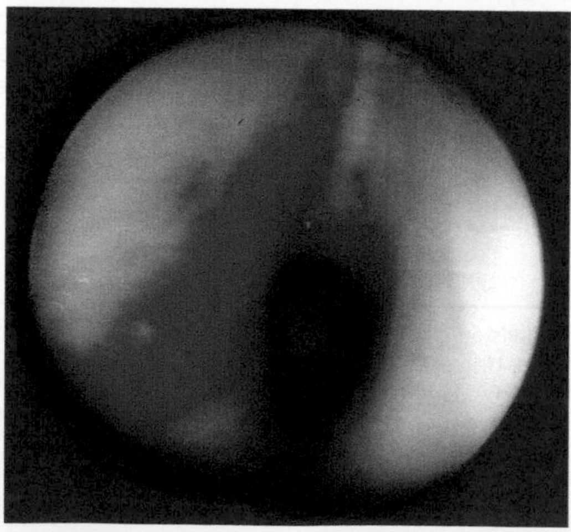

Fig. 3. Subglottic hemangioma.

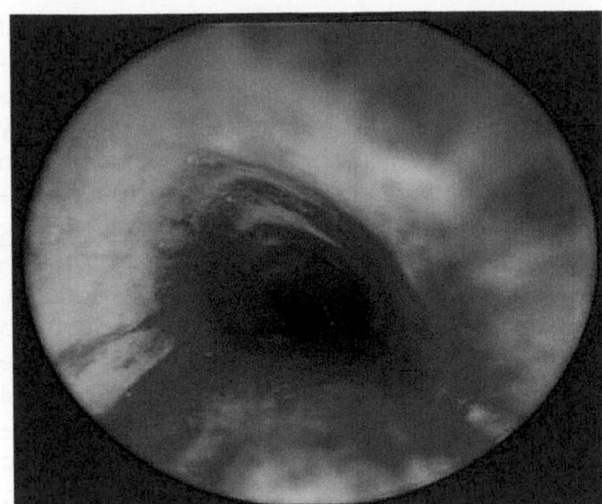

Fig. 4. Hemangioma staining of the posterior trachealis muscle.

hemangiomas are solitary; however, the distribution may have an impact on the prognosis and the potential for airway involvement. Segmental hemangiomas are more likely to have involvement of the aerodigestive tract relative to solitary lesions, and multifocal lesions are more likely to simultaneously involve the liver or other areas of the gastrointestinal system.

When there is involvement of the airway, the symptoms are often stridor, croup, and respiratory distress. It is important to characterize the severity of the respiratory distress and the characteristics of the stridor. An infant with no history of intubation with a croupy (barky) cough and biphasic stridor localizes the lesion to the subglottic larynx. In the case of an infant with skin hemangiomas, the airway lesion would likely be a subglottic hemangioma. Following physical examination, it is necessary to proceed to imaging and endoscopy to confirm a diagnosis.

Hemangiomas may be classified by thickness as superficial, deep, or compound, as well as by distribution as localized, multifocal, or segmental. A localized hemangioma would involve a solitary lesion in the skin or airway, whereas multifocal includes 6 or more, and segmental involves a distribution in a known anatomic region such as V3 segment of the fifth nerve. Generally, airway symptoms are more common with segmental hemangiomas, and the so-called "beard distribution" in V3 is associated with a 20% to 30% involvement of the upper airway. The classic and most common finding is subglottic hemangioma, which is most often laterally based or less commonly posterior.

Less common sites affecting the airway include postcricoid, tracheal, mediastinal, thoracic, and esophageal. They may stain the posterior trachealis muscle (see **Fig. 4**). Airway symptoms include biphasic stridor and recurrent croup. Diagnosis may be suggested by history and lack of another cause of subglottic stenosis, such as prolonged intubation. Plain neck films may suggest the diagnosis.

Treatment of airway hemangioma depends greatly on the severity of symptoms, degree of airway obstruction, and the position of involvement in the airway. The treatment options for infantile hemangiomas of the airway are as follows:

- Observation
- Steroids
- Interferon: Historic – spastic diplegia[3]
- Laser: CO_2, KTP, Candela
- Tracheotomy: Discuss risk
- Open resection with or without cartilage augmentation
- Propranolol.

For mild cases with minimal or no symptoms, observation is all that is necessary. The size of a small hemangioma may not cause turbulent airflow or may involve nonendoluminal sites, such as the postcricoid region, which will cause no major airway symptoms. In such cases, no treatment is necessary, but close observation with flexible laryngoscopies in the ambulatory setting every 3 to 4 months is needed. However, it is important to understand that the symptoms may initially worsen as the hemangioma proliferates. Bilateral hemangiomas may impact the airway the most (**Fig. 5**).

Mild cases or those that present with sudden acute airway symptoms may benefit from a short course of corticosteroids. This may be helpful during acute exacerbations, such as with upper respiratory infections. In addition, aerosolized

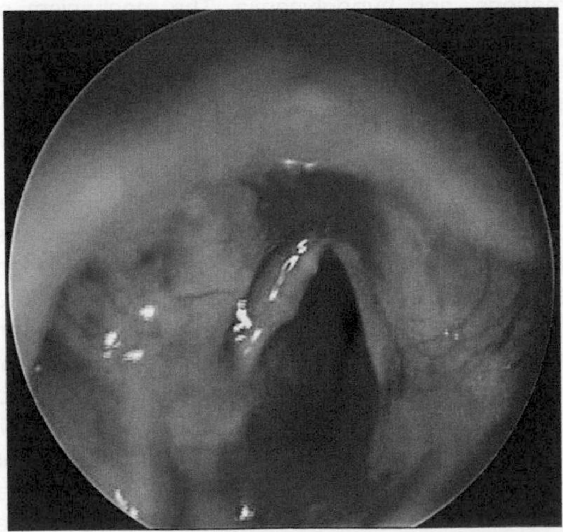

Fig. 5. Bilateral subglottic hemangioma with total airway obstruction.

racemic epinephrine may be used during acute exacerbations that can also occur with upper respiratory infections. Although racemic epinephrine can prevent an airway crisis, it may have rebound and is not a definitive treatment for airway hemangiomas. Corticosteroids decrease endothelial cell proliferation during the proliferative phase and hence they should be continued for most of this phase or there may be significant rebound. The typical treatment protocol would involve oral prednisone at a dosage of approximately 2 to 3 mg/kg/d for 4 to 6 months with a slow taper. Temporary side effects may include Cushingnoid appearance, behavior and mood changes, and rebound after discontinuation of steroids. Corticosteroids can also be administered intralesionally into lesions affecting the airway and may have more direct effects with less systemic side effects. Complications include bleeding and swelling after injection.

Recently, propranolol has been used to treat problematic airway hemangiomas. Before starting propranolol, one needs to get an MRI with gadolinium to rule out cerebrovascular disease and to avoid intracranial bleeds from rebound effects. Then an electrocardiogram is done to rule out arrhythmias and a fasting glucose is used to screen for hypoglycemia before starting and after the first 2 dosages. One should start at 0.5 mg/kg/d orally and work up to 2 mg/kg/d divided every 8 hours, but it can also be dosed every 12 hours. At the Children's Hospital of Philadelphia (CHOP), we start propranolol as an inpatient, but with close monitoring, outpatient start is feasible as well. The drug is quite safe, as there appear to be few side effects. In our experience, the most common reported side effect is sleepiness or hypoglycemia. Exclusion criteria include arrhythmias, intracranial vascular malformations, and hypoglycemia. The mechanism of action of propranolol, a nonselective beta-blocker, appears to be capillary vasoconstriction, decreased expression of vascular endothelial growth factor (VEGF) and basic fibroblast growth factor (bFGF), as well as apoptosis of capillary endothelial cells.[4] Denoyelle and colleagues[5] in Paris, France, described 2 infants with subglottic hemangiomas who responded very rapidly to propranolol with no side effects. Both the subglottic regions responded right away to propranolol and avoided open surgery. Messner,[6] at the 2009 Annual Meeting of the American Academy of Otolaryngology-Head and Neck Surgery, reported 6 responders of 7 patients tried on propranolol. The nonresponder was glucose transporter (GLUT)-1 negative. We have had 6 infants on treatment with 4 definite responders with no significant side effects. Our 2 nonresponders are GLUT-1 positive.

When pharmacologic means are not sufficient alone, lasers, such as CO_2 or potassium-titanyl-phosphate (KTP), can be used to treat surface hemangiomas in the airway.[7] The CO_2 laser may work very well against small exophytic lesions in the subglottic airway. In the 1980s and 1990s, it remained a workhorse for subglottic hemangiomas; however, experience has shown that the recurrence rate with this technique is high. In addition, the laser may need to be used multiple times to achieve a stable airway because it treats only the surface and may not be effective at all for bilateral or circumferential disease. In addition, overaggressive use of the laser may result in subglottic stenosis.[8] In the same way, the microdebrider, as demonstrated by Pransky and Canto,[9] may be useful for focal lesions amenable to laser ablation. Although this technique has some of the same limitations as the laser, it is easier to set up than the laser and has less chance of injury from its use.

Open resection and cartilage graft augmentation has been reported as an effective treatment for subglottic hemangiomas unresponsive to more conservative treatments.[10–14] The indication is a posterior or laterally based subglottic hemangioma that has failed steroids or propranolol. The procedure starts with a microlaryngoscopy, where the airway is assessed and secured with a small endotracheal tube orally. At this point, the patient may be given a course of intravenous steroids that may decrease bleeding during the resection.

The patient is positioned with the neck hyperextended and a transverse incision is made in the neck at about the level of the cricoid cartilage. A superior and inferior subplatymal flap is elevated to expose the laryngotracheal complex and the thyroid notch. This may expose extralaryngeal hemangioma in the neck (**Fig. 6**). Stay sutures are placed on the cricoids, which is opened in

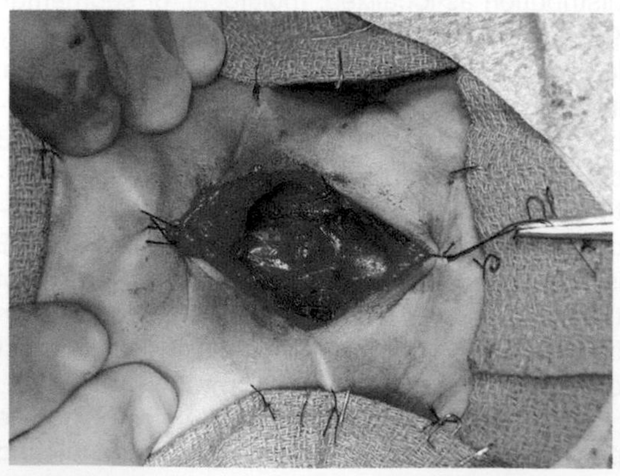

Fig. 6. Subplatysmal flaps with hemangioma on the outside of thyroid cartilage.

the midline. The incision is performed with a Beaver blade and extended up to just under the anterior commissure. It is important to avoid violating the AC unless necessary. Posterior-based lesions are incised in the direct midline and the lesion is carefully dissected off the cartilage plate of the posterior cricoid (**Fig. 7**) using otologic instruments such as the round knife, Rosen needle, and microtabe knife. An operating microscope may be prepped and used to facilitate visualization. Laterally based lesions may be approached by elevating a submucosal flap off the hemangioma from the laryngofissure down. When the lesion is resected completely, the flaps are sutured back into position using small vicryl. At this point, the airway is often stenotic and a small thyroid alar graft is harvested and used to augment the size of the subglottic airway (**Fig. 8**). The graft is harvested from the thyroid alar and usually measures no more than 5 to 6 mm in length and 2 to 3 mm in width in a small infant, but this is enough to offset the stenosis.

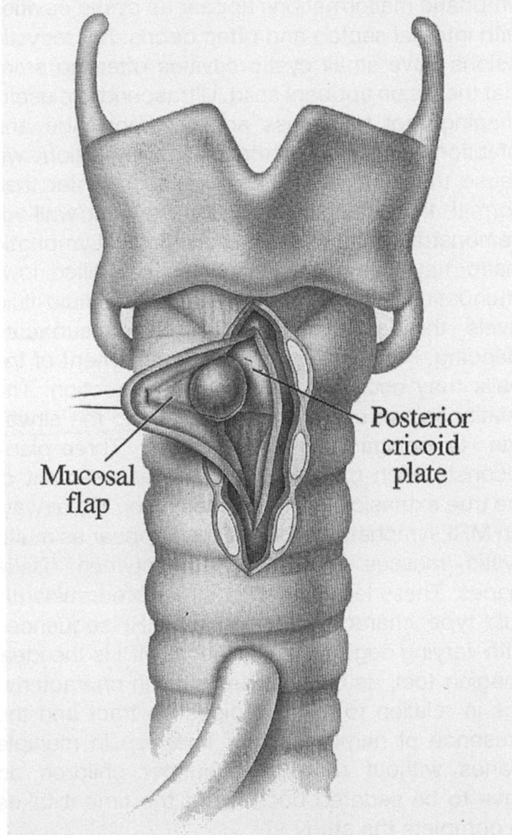

Fig. 7. Posterior mucosal cut on the surface of hemangioma to allow resection. (*From* Hartnick CJ, Cotton RT. Open excision of subglottic hemangioma. Oper Tech Otolaryngol Head Neck Surg 2002;13(1):55; with permission.)

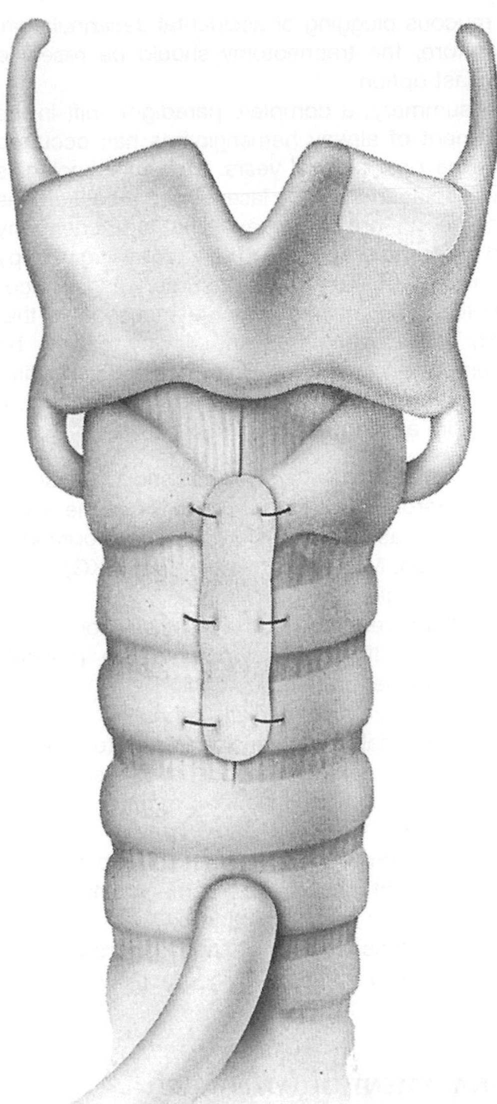

Fig. 8. Thyroid alar graft used to enlarge the subglottic airway. (*From* Hartnick CJ, Cotton RT. Open excision of subglottic hemangioma. Oper Tech Otolaryngol Head Neck Surg 2002;13(1):55; with permission.)

The wound is closed and the infant is kept nasally intubated for 5 to 7 days and then undergoes a microlaryngoscopy and bronchoscopy to evaluate the airway. If everything looks satisfactory, the patient is extubated the following day in the ICU. At CHOP, we have had 12 patients undergo this surgery, all with a remarkable resolution of their symptoms.

For life-threatening lesions that do not respond to any therapy, tracheotomy is a treatment option.[15] Although this is usually a temporary measure, as hemangiomas will involute over time, it carries the risk of speech delays and complications related to the tracheotomy such as mucous plugging or accidental decannulation. Therefore, the tracheotomy should be reserved as a last option.

In summary, a complete paradigm shift in the treatment of airway hemangiomas has occurred over the past several years. Newer technologies have replaced the CO_2 laser. Open resection has become an option for avoiding a tracheotomy and propranolol appears to be a promising therapy and may eventually supplant surgery and corticosteroids. The main take-home message is that many hemangiomas of the airway cannot be assumed to fully involute and many require definitive therapy. We recommend our treatment algorithm as follows:

- Initial airway symptoms: short course of steroids and then rapid taper at the same time as workup before starting propranolol (MLB, MRI, electrocardiogram [EKG], brain MRI, glucose).
- If no rebound, follow clinically for symptoms. If airway symptoms are present, consider trial of propranolol.
- If there is immediate rebound, consider early trial of propranolol. Get up to 2 mg/kg for 2 weeks and re-scope. If response is seen, then continue for 6 months and then taper.
- If no change on propranolol and focal or bilateral subglottic hemangioma, then consider open resection.
- If diffuse and no change on propranolol, consider tracheotomy and/or laser ablation.

MANAGEMENT OF LYMPHATIC MALFORMATIONS AFFECTING THE AIRWAY

Lymphatic malformations can vary from small isolated neck masses to extensive cervico-facial processes that infiltrate into large tissue planes. There is a staging system proposed by deSerres and colleagues[16] that may be used to predict outcome. Stage I includes unilateral infrahyoid disease. Stage II is unilateral suprahyoid disease. Stage III is unilateral suprahyoid and infrahyoid disease. Stage IV is bilateral suprahyoid disease and stage V is bilateral suprahyoid and infrahyoid disease.

For treatment purposes, lymphatic malformations may also be subdivided into macrocystic and microcystic. By definition, macrocysts are larger than 2 cm[16] and were formerly referred to as "cystic hygromas" and microcystic lesions were referred to as "lymphangiomas." The stage and cystic structure of the lymphatic malformations is crucial in determining the ideal surgical approach.

Lymphatic malformations are often noted at birth and may be detected by prenatal 2-dimensional ultrasound.[3] They occur most often in the cervicofascial region and they may be seen in the axilla, chest, and mediastinum as well. The cystic lesions can become infected and flare up during upper respiratory infections. Antibiotics and steroids may treat such flare-ups. Lymphatic malformations that infiltrate into the supraglottic portion of the larynx will cause severe airway obstruction. Extensive cervicofascial lesions will also secondarily involve the supraglottic larynx or regions of the pharynx causing airway compression. This may prevent safe extubation and lead to tracheotomy dependency.

Lymphatic malformations can be easily visualized by ultrasound, MRI, or CT scanning. In the interest of radiation reduction, CT should be reserved for acute lesion presentations such as airway compression or acute hemorrhage/infection of the lesion. On ultrasound, macrocystic lymphatic malformations appear as cystic cavities with internal septae and often debris. Microcystic lesions have small cystic cavities often so small that the lesion appears solid. Ultrasound is a useful imaging tool to assess acute hemorrhage and infection. Both hemorrhage and infection will cause the cyst contents to appear brighter than normal. In addition, in infection the cyst wall will demonstrate increased blood flow. Lymphatic malformations on CT appear as fluid-filled low-attenuation lesions, occasionally with fluid-fluid levels that can represent acute or subacute bleeding. Peripheral contrast enhancement of the walls may occur with bleeding or infection. The relationship of cervico-facial lesions to the airway can be elegantly demonstrated. Three-plane reconstruction can also enhance assessment of the true extrinsic effect of the lesion on the airway. On MRI, lymphatic malformations appear as multicystic masses that insinuate between tissue planes. These lesions demonstrate predominantly fluid-type characteristics on all MRI sequences with varying degrees of septation. MRI is the ideal imaging tool, as it can assess lesion characteristics in relation to the aerodigestive tract and the presence of hemorrhage or infection in multiple planes without radiation. Younger children do have to be sedated because of the time it takes to complete the study.

As previously mentioned, staging, extent of disease, age, associated symptoms, time to diagnosis, and completeness of excision strongly influence prognosis.[17] The histologic pattern and length of time to treatment did not influence prognosis. The most important factor is the ability to perform complete surgical excision without significant morbidity. The best results are for those lesions that can be cleanly resected with minimal morbidity. These are most often those lesions that are isolated to the infrahyoid or posterior triangle position of the neck. More extensive lesions that infiltrate into vital structures may require staged resections that are quite challenging or other treatments such as sclerotherapy or laser ablation. Treatment options for lymphatic malformations include observation for small lesions, early stage I with no cosmetic or functional compromise. They may persist, but cause no problems and may be watched for expansion. The decision to operate would be based on age of the patients and concerns about future symptoms.

1. Surgical excision: For focal lesions (stages I to III) involving the neck, parotid, or mediastinum, show neck lesions that are well circumscribed and can be completely resected to reduce the risk of recurrence. More extensive lesions (III to V) and microcystic disease that is not amenable to sclerotherapy may be resected in staged fashion.[3]
2. Laser ablation for compressed lesions, especially those that appear on mucosal surfaces, such as tongue lymphatic malformations. The CO_2 or neodymium:yttrium aluminum garnate (Nd:YAG) laser may be used to ablate compressed tongue lymphatic malformations (**Fig. 9**).[18]
3. Radiofrequency ablation may be used for the same type of microcystic lesions of the tongue and supraglottic larynx. The advantage is the avoidance of thermal energy and complications associated with laser use.[19]
4. Microdebrider excision may be useful for the large supraglottic lesions and debulk lesions causing supraglottic airway obstruction. We have used it in piecemeal fashion to reduce supraglottic obstructive lesions (**Fig. 10**).

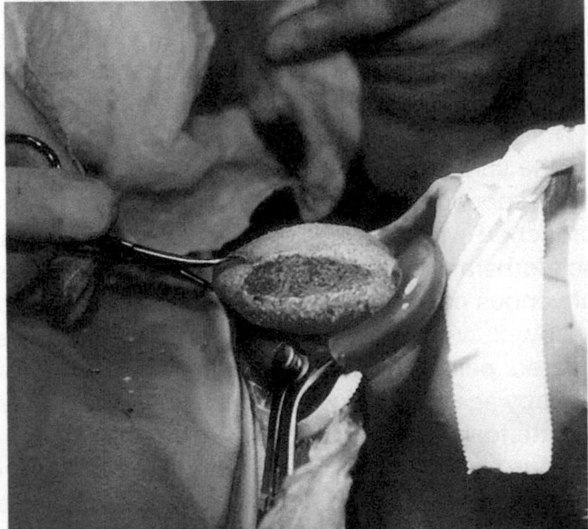

Fig. 9. Microcystic lymphatic malformation of the tongue requiring Nd:YAG laser ablation.

Sclerotherapy with a variety of sclerosing agents is the treatment of choice for more extensive macrocystic lesions that are not amenable to complete surgical excision. This would include large cervicofascial lesions or lesions that extend to regions that are not easily exposed such as skull base or parapharyngeal space (**Fig. 11**).[20] All have been shown to be effective with respect to treatment of lymphatic malformations with success rates ranging between 92% and 100% for macrocystic and 20% and 64% for microcystic lesions. Microcystic lesions tend to require more sessions than the macrocystic because of the presence of numerous small cysts. Different sclerosing agents have been used effectively for the treatment of lymphatic malformations, including doxycycline, ethibloc, absolute alcohol, sodium tetradecyl foam, bleomycin, and OK432.[21–28] Sclerotherapy of lymphatic malformations is generally performed with ultrasound guidance.

In our institution, for large cervico-facial lesions, we use doxycycline via catheter instillation and 3 consecutive treatments are performed at 24-hour intervals. The doxycycline is removed after 6 hours. The children are intubated and monitored in the ICU setting for the duration of the treatment (3–4 days). Preextubation MR imaging is performed to evaluate the residual extent of the lesion, inflammation, and airway status. The total dose of doxycycline used in our practice ranges from 150 to 200 mg per instillation in neonates to

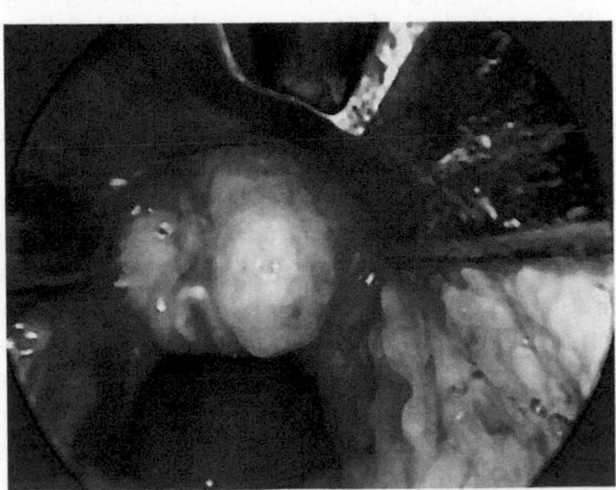

Fig. 10. Supraglottic lymphatic malformation.

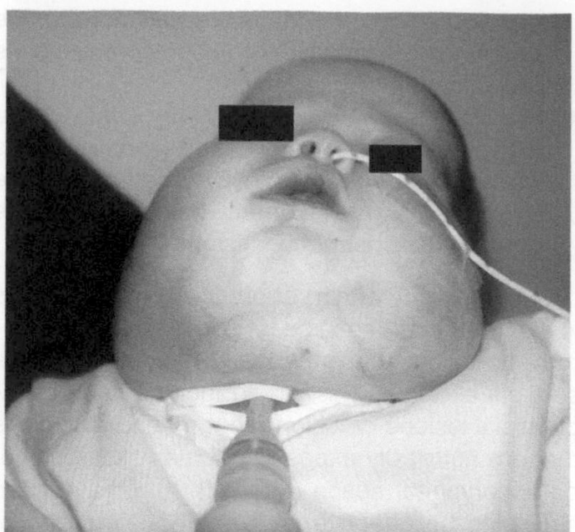

Fig. 11. Massive cervicofacial lymphatic malformation with tracheotomy.

a maximum of 1 g in older children. Neonates receiving more than 200 mg are more likely to experience side effects such as hypoglycemia, metabolic acidosis, and hemolytic anemia. Because of the high incidence of spontaneous infection together with an increased risk upon accessing the lesion, prophylactic antibiotics have been recommended immediately before sclerotherapy of lymphatic malformations.[21–23]

Tracheotomy may be necessary to secure the airway with lymphatic malformations that cause severe upper airway obstruction from involvement of the supraglottic larynx or massive cervicofascial lymphatic malformations. The tracheotomy may need to be placed in early infancy.

The EXIT procedure, or ex utero intrapartum treatment procedure, may be required to secure the airway during delivery for massive cervicofacial disease that presents on delivery making the securing of the airway difficult. Three-dimensional ultrasonography and fetal MRI can accurately diagnosis prenatal lymphangiomas with a great deal of accuracy and predict delivery problems. Those lesions that completely obstruct the oropharynx may require an emergent airway at delivery and a planned EXIT procedure may be necessary.[3]

The EXIT is an extension of a standard caesarian section, where an incision is made in midline of the uterus. The baby is delivered on the placental circulation, and a fetal/airway team then establishes an airway either through endotracheal intubation or emergency tracheotomy. Once the airway is secured, the placental artery and vein can be ligated. Large lymphatic malformations that obstruct the oropharynx may make intubation difficult or impossible. In such cases, the EXIT procedure permits time to establish a safe airway. Because only a few centers in the United States and the world perform this highly specialized procedure, any baby with an obstructing mass discovered on ultrasound should be referred to such a center for evaluation.

MANAGEMENT OF VENOUS MALFORMATIONS AFFECTING THE AIRWAY

Venous malformations may involve a number of sites in the upper airway and may be quite extensive, like their counterpart the lymphatic malformations. They can involve the base of the tongue, pharynx, supraglottic larynx, and trachea. They most commonly occur in the supraglottic larynx followed by the trachea. In these locations, they can cause varying degrees of airway obstruction. The association with smooth and skeletal muscle may lead to compression of these lesions. Many lesions may remain small and require no treatment. Laryngotracheal involvement is rare. Large lesions may cause airway obstruction, voice change, and bleeding and hence require active intervention.

Venous malformations can be imaged with ultrasound, CT scanning, or MRI. Ultrasound with Doppler imaging provides information on the patency of the vessels, compressibility, and any areas of thrombus. Ultrasound is limited in regions adjacent to the airway. MRI with contrast provides 3-plane information regarding the spatial relationships of the lesion to the aerodigestive tract. On flow-sensitive sequences, areas of thrombosis can be identified. The relationship of the lesion to normal or abnormal outflow veins can be mapped.

These lesions usually do not have a distinct capsule and therefore complete surgical excision is usually not possible. The mainstay of surgical treatment for lesions affecting the airway involves a combination of laser photocoagulation with the laser including the CO_2,[29] Nd:YAG,[30] or the KTP.[24,31] The laser is used in a noncontact fashion on the surface of the lesion and can be combined with sequential sclerotherapy.[32] Most are approached with endoscopic exposure. Sequential sclerotherapy creates inflammation and sclerosis of venous channels with subsequent involution.

Low-flow venous malformations can also be treated percutaneously with a variety of sclerotherapy agents such as ethanol, sodium tetradecyl sulfate foam, ethibloc and polidocanol, and endovenous laser therapy.[22,33–41] Sclerotherapy is performed with a combination of ultrasound and fluoroscopic guidance. Ultrasound provides good visualization of the lesion during needle access and fluoroscopy is used to monitor the sclerosant injection to decrease the risk of extravasation or undesired egress into normal veins. Sclerotherapy of lesions in the cervico-facial region should be performed with general anesthesia for airway protection. In addition, the injection of the sclerosant is painful and postprocedure edema may compromise the airway.

In our institution, the sclerotherapy agent of choice is sodium tetradecyl foam, the foam being created by adding a combination of oily contrast medium (ethiodol) and air. The foam consistency creates increased surface tension enabling greater contact with the vessel wall for a longer period than more liquid agents.

Ethanol is commonly used as an alternative agent in many centers. The recommended ethanol dosing is 1 mg/mL to a maximum of 50 mL, which in children should be conservatively limited to 0.5 mg/kg if possible. Serum ethanol levels in children have been recorded after sclerotherapy to levels significant for the risk of respiratory depression, cardiac arrhythmias, seizures, rhabdomyolysis, and hypoglycemia.[42] In addition, coagulation disorders have also been described with the use of ethanol for sclerotherapy.[43]

In general, on completion of the procedure edema will be present. The swelling will maximize over 1 to 2 days. Swelling and induration of the skin have been shown to predict both therapeutic effect and prolonged recovery in low-flow vascular malformations.[22]

MANAGEMENT OF ARTERIOVENOUS MALFORMATIONS AFFECTING THE AIRWAY

These high flow vascular malformations can occur anywhere in the head and neck region and rarely affect the upper airway. Although they may occur in the trachea, bronchi, or larynx, they most commonly occur in the lung parenchyma. Pulmonary arteriovenous malformations are commonly associated with hereditary hemorrhagic telangiectasia and may be a source of hemoptysis. Diagnosis is performed through diagnostic angiography and treatments can be performed by embolization at the time of angiography. They can be followed by contrast-enhanced CT of the chest. Embolization can also precede surgical excision as a means for minimizing bleeding. In rare circumstances, surgical resection may be considered after preoperative embolization.[44]

Arterial malformations are the most problematic and symptomatic of the vascular malformation group. Because of their size and location, most arterial malformations are inoperable or require extensive, potentially disfiguring resection. Transcatheter and percutanous nidal embolization is now often the first therapeutic option and is an effective approach that can be used as a palliative procedure or as an adjunct to a surgical resection.

Arteriovenous malformations can be embolized either by direct percutaneous puncture into the nidus or by using an endovascular approach or a combination of both. Several agents have been used, including absolute alcohol, onyx, and adhesive glue. These are the most penetrating agents if the lesion is to be embolized for potential "cure." If the embolization is preoperative, additional agents such as coils and polyvinyl alcohol particles are used to reduce lesional blood flow.[45–48]

SUMMARY AND FUTURE DEVELOPMENTS

The opportunities for treatment of vascular anomalies of the airway will change dramatically as advances in new technologies emerge. We expect to see a major evolution in the care of patients with vascular malformations of the airway. Improvements in treatment will include newer surgical techniques, such as radiofrequency ablation or improved lasers, and new treatment modalities, such as new vasoactive drugs and highly selective beta blockade. In addition, earlier prenatal diagnosis with widespread use of 3-dimensional ultrasound is likely to lead to earlier interventions. In addition, early detection of novel molecular signals to determine aggressiveness and predict clinical behavior is likely to influence treatment.[1] Last, interventional radiologists will continue to make advances in minimally invasive techniques. Open surgical techniques that we use today may become obsolete in the future.

REFERENCES

1. Blei F. Basic and clinical aspects of vascular anomalies. Curr Opin Pediatr 2005;17:501–9.
2. Tasnadi G. Epidemiology and etiology of congenital vascular malformations. Semin Vasc Surg 1993;6: 200.
3. Eivazi B, Sierra-Zuleta F, Ermisch S, et al. Therapy for prenatally diagnosed lymphangioma-multimodal procedure and interdisciplinary challenge. Z Geburtshilfe Neonatol 2009;213(4):155–60.
4. Leaute-Labreze C, Dumas de la Roque E, Hubiche T, et al. Propranolol for severe hemangiomas of infancy. N Engl J Med 2008;358(24): 2649–51.
5. Denoyelle F, Leboulanger N, Enjolras O, et al. Role of propranolol in the therapeutic strategy of infantile laryngotracheal hemangioma. Int J Pediatr Otorhinolaryngol 2009;73(8):1168–72.

6. Messner A. Abstracts of the American Academy of Otolaryngology Head and Neck Surgery. San Diego (CA), October 4–7, 2009. Alexandria (VA): The American Academy of Otolaryngology-Head and Neck Surgery; 2009.
7. Sie KC, McGill T, Healy GB. Subglottic hemangioma: ten years experience with the carbon dioxide laser. Ann Otol Rhinol Laryngol 1994;103:167–72.
8. Cotton RT, Tewfik T. Laryngeal stenosis following carbon dioxide laser in the subglottic hemangioma. Ann Otol Rhinol Laryngol 1985;94:494–7.
9. Pransky S, Canto C. Management of subglottic hemangiomas. Curr Opin Otolaryngol Head Neck Surg 2004;12:509–12.
10. Wiatrak BJ, Reilly JS, Seid AD, et al. Open surgical resection of subglottic hemangioma in children. Int J Pediatr Otorhinolaryngol 1996;34(1–2):191–206.
11. Van Den Abbeele T, Triglia JM, Lesanne E, et al. Surgical removal of subglottic hemangioma in children. Laryngoscope 1999;109:1281–6.
12. Javia L, Zur K, Jacobs IN. Abstracts of the American Academy of Pediatric Otolaryngology, Las Vegas (NV), April, 2010.
13. O-Lee T, Messner A. Open surgical resection of subglottic hemangioma with microscopic dissection. Int J Pediatr Otorhinolaryngol 2007;71(9):1371–6.
14. Vijayasekaren S, White DR, Hartley BE, et al. Open excision of subglottic hemangioma to avoid a tracheotomy. Arch Otolaryngol Head Neck Surg 2006; 132(2):159–63.
15. Feurstein SS. Subglottic hemangioma in infants. Laryngoscope 1973;83:466–75.
16. DeSerres LM, Sie KC, Richardson MA. Lymphatic malformations of the head and neck. Arch Otolaryngol Head Neck Surg 1995;121(5):577–82.
17. Raveh E, de Jong AL, Taylor GP, et al. Prognostic factors in the treatment of lymphatic malformations. Arch Otolaryngol Head Neck Surg 1997;123(10): 1061–5.
18. Wiegand S, Zimmerman AP, Neff A, et al. Microcystic lymphatic malformations of the tongue: diagnosis, classification and treatment. Arch Otolaryngol Head Neck Surg 2009;135(10):976–83.
19. Roy S, Reyes S, Smith LP. Bipolar radiofrequency plasma ablation (coblation) of lymphatic malformations of the tongue. Int J Pediatr Otorhinolaryngol 2009;73(2):289–93.
20. Burrows PE, Mitri RK, Alomari A, et al. Percutaneous sclerotherapy of lymphatic malformations with doxycycline. Lymphat Res Biol 2008;6(3–4):209–16.
21. Burrows PE, Mason KP. Percutaneous treatment of low flow vascular malformations. J Vasc Interv Radiol 2004;15(5):431–45.
22. Legiehn GM, Heran MK. Classification, diagnosis, and interventional radiologic management of vascular malformations. Orthop Clin North Am 2006;37:435–74.
23. Shiels WE 2nd, Kenney BD, Caniano DA, et al. Definitive percutaneous treatment of lymphatic malformations of the trunk and extremities. J Pediatr Surg 2008;43:136–9 [discussion: 140].
24. Shiels WE 2nd, Kang DR, Murakami JW, et al. Percutaneous treatment of lymphatic malformations. Otolaryngol Head Neck Surg 2009;141:219–24.
25. Okazaki T, Iwatani S, Yanai T, et al. Treatment of lymphangioma in children: our experience of 128 cases. J Pediatr Surg 2007;42:386–9.
26. Dubois J, Garel L, Abela A, et al. Lymphangiomas in children: percutaneous sclerotherapy with an alcoholic solution of zein. Radiology 1997;204:651–4.
27. Alomari AI, Karian VE, Lord DJ, et al. Percutaneous sclerotherapy for lymphatic malformations: a retrospective analysis of patient-evaluated improvement. J Vasc Interv Radiol 2006;17:1639–48.
28. Simpson GT, Healy GB, McGill T, et al. Benign tumors and lesions of the larynx in children: surgical excision with the CO_2 laser. Ann Otol Rhinol Laryngol 1979;88: 479–85.
29. Cholewa D, Waldschmidt J. Laser treatment of hemangiomas of the larynx and trachea. Lasers Surg Med 1998;23:221–32.
30. Rebiez E, April MM, Bohigian RK, et al. Nd:YAG laser treatment of venous malformations of the head and neck: an update. Otolaryngol Head Neck Surg 1991;105:655–61.
31. Madgy D, Ahsan SF, Kest D, et al. The application of the potassium-titanyl-phosphate (KTP) laser in the management of subglottic hemangioma. Arch Otolaryngol Head Neck Surg 2001;127:47–50.
32. Ohlms LA, Forsen J, Burrows PE. Venous malformations of the pediatric airway. Int J Pediatr Otorhinolaryngol 1996;37(2):99–114.
33. Dubois JM, Sebag GH, De Prost Y, et al. Soft-tissue venous malformations in children: percutaneous sclerotherapy with Ethibloc. Radiology 1991;180: 195–8.
34. Lee BB. New approaches to the treatment of congenital vascular malformations (CVMs)—a single centre experience. Eur J Vasc Endovasc Surg 2005; 30:184–97.
35. O'Donovan JC, Donaldson JS, Morello FP, et al. Symptomatic hemangiomas and venous malformations in infants, children, and young adults: treatment with percutaneous injection of sodium tetradecyl sulfate. AJR Am J Roentgenol 1997;169: 723–9.
36. Mimura H, Fujiwara H, Hiraki T, et al. Polidocanol sclerotherapy for painful venous malformations: evaluation of safety and efficacy in pain relief. Eur Radiol 2009;19(10):2474–80.
37. Lee IH, Kim KH, Jeon P, et al. Ethanol sclerotherapy for the management of craniofacial venous malformations: the interim results. Korean J Radiol 2009; 10(3):269–76.

38. Liu Y, Liu D, Wang Y, et al. Clinical study of sclerotherapy of maxillofacial venous malformation using absolute ethanol and pingyangmycin. J Oral Maxillofac Surg 2009;67(1):98–104.
39. Lee CH, Chen SG. Direct percutaneous ethanol instillation for treatment of venous malformation in the face and neck. Br J Plast Surg 2005;58(8):1073–8.
40. Sidhu MK, Perkins JA, Shaw DW, et al. Ultrasound-guided endovenous diode laser in the treatment of congenital venous malformations: preliminary experience. J Vasc Interv Radiol 2005;16(6):879–84.
41. Mason KP, Michna E, Zurakowski D, et al. Serum ethanol levels in children and adults after ethanol embolization or sclerotherapy for vascular anomalies. Radiology. 2000;217(1):127–32.
42. Mason KP, Neufeld EJ, Karian VE, et al. Coagulation abnormalities in pediatric and adult patients after sclerotherapy or embolization of vascular anomalies. AJR Am J Roentgenol. 2001;177(6):1359–63.
43. Iqbal M, Rossoff LJ, Marzouk KA, et al. Pulmonary arteriovenous malformations: a clinical review. Postgrad Med J 2000;76(897):390–4.
44. Starke RM, Komotar RJ, Otten ML, et al. Adjuvant embolization with N-butyl cyanoacrylate in the treatment of cerebral arteriovenous malformations: outcomes, complications, and predictors of neurologic deficits. Stroke 2009;40:2783–90.
45. Do YS, Yakes WF, Shin SW, et al. Ethanol embolization of arteriovenous malformations: interim results. Radiology 2005;235:674–82.
46. Hamada J, Kai Y, Morioka M, et al. A nonadhesive liquid embolic agent composed of ethylene vinyl alcohol copolymer and ethanol mixture for the treatment of cerebral arteriovenous malformations: experimental study. J Neurosurg 2002;97:889–95.
47. Panagiotopoulos V, Gizewski E, Asgari S, et al. Embolization of intracranial arteriovenous malformations with ethylene-vinyl alcohol copolymer (Onyx). AJNR Am J Neuroradiol 2009;30:99–106.
48. Rennert J, Herold T, Schreyer AG, et al. Evaluation of a liquid embolization agent (Onyx) for transcatheter embolization for renal vascular lesions. Rofo 2009;181:996–1001.

Special Considerations in Vascular Anomalies: Operative Management of Craniofacial Osseous Lesions

Renee M. Burke, MD[a], Robert J. Morin, MD[a], Chad A. Perlyn, MD, PhD[b], Boris Laure, MD[c], S. Anthony Wolfe, MD[a,*]

KEYWORDS

- Craniofacial • Skeletal • Vascular • Anomalies
- Management

The treatment of vascular anomalies of the head and neck typically focuses on restoration of abnormal structures of the soft tissues. However, vascular anomalies can affect the craniofacial skeleton, and osseous reconstruction may be indicated. Osseous involvement occurs as either a primary or secondary phenomenon. In primary osseous involvement, the vascular anomaly expands the bone from within. Secondary osseous involvement occurs when bony hypertrophy develops because of increased blood flow to the lymphatic tissue. This article focuses on the management of the osseous deformities associated with vascular anomalies.

VENOUS MALFORMATIONS

Venous malformations (VMs) of the bone are extremely rare, accounting for less than 1% of all osseous lesions. The diagnosis is confounded by antiquated clinical and pathologic terminology. Historically, these types of lesions were referred to as intraosseous hemangioma. However, pathologic and molecular evaluations have shown these lesions to be caused by VMs.[1] Most commonly, these VMs affect the zygoma, mandible, maxillary sinus, and the frontal, parietal, and nasal bones.[2]

Patients typically present with distortion of the facial skeleton, which may be associated with hypertrophy of soft tissues and vascular staining of the overlying skin. When no skin changes are present, these patients are often initially presumed to have fibrous dysplasia, particularly when the lesion affects the zygoma or frontal bone.

Evaluation of these patients is performed with a computed tomographic (CT) scan with coronal, sagittal, and 3-dimensional (3D) reconstruction. Radiographic findings that suggest this diagnosis include circumscribed, osteolytic, hivelike lesions with trabeculations.[3] Angiography may be performed to further document the extent of the lesion and better characterize the vascular inflow and outflow.

Patients with VMs of the facial bones often require surgical resection of the lesion. Although reports of sclerotherapy and embolization have been documented, they do not address the expanded abnormal bone and restoration of the facial skeleton. Therefore, wide resection of the lesion is recommended. After resection of these malformations,

[a] Division of Plastic Surgery, Miami Children's Hospital, Miami, FL, USA
[b] Florida International University College of Medicine, Miami Children's Hospital, 13400 SW 120th Street, Miami, FL 33186, USA
[c] Department of Maxillofacial Surgery, Trousseau Hospital, Tours, France
* Corresponding author. 3100 Southwest 62nd Avenue, Suite 2230 Miami, FL 33155-3009.
E-mail address: Anthony.Wolfe@mch.com

Clin Plastic Surg 38 (2011) 133–142
doi:10.1016/j.cps.2010.08.013

significant defects in the facial skeleton may occur and should be corrected during the initial surgery, if possible. Depending on the size of the defect, bone grafting or vascularized bone transfer best achieves reconstruction of vital craniofacial bony structures. Three-dimensional models may be useful in anticipating the defect and planning the reconstruction. The ultimate goal is to restore the facial skeleton to make the patient both functionally and aesthetically normal.[4]

Case 1: VM of Bone

A 4-year-old boy presented with an expanding mass on the left side of his face (**Fig. 1**A). On physical examination, he was found to have a prominent left facial skeleton, soft tissue hypertrophy, and a capillary malformation of the left cheek. A CT scan showed a calcified spiculated mass in the left zygoma (see **Fig. 1**B). The mass was excised with adequate margins through coronal and intraoral incisions (see **Fig. 1**C). Immediate reconstruction of the left orbit and zygoma with calvarial bone grafts was performed. A lead template was used to create an anatomically correct bone graft that fit perfectly into the orbital and zygomatic defect (see **Fig. 1**D, E). The final pathology report found the mass to be a VM of the bone. A postoperative CT scan showed complete excision of the malformation and near-anatomic reconstruction of the left orbitozygomatic complex (see **Fig. 1**F). A picture sent by the patient's family 2 years after surgery displays persistent soft tissue hypertrophy (see **Fig. 1**G).

Case 2: VM of Bone

A 27-year-old man presented with what was thought to be a sebaceous cyst close to the temporal hairline on the left forehead (**Fig. 2**A). This lesion was scheduled to be removed as an office procedure, but at the time of excision, the lesion was firm and the cranial bone seemed to be involved. An incisional biopsy was performed, and the pathology report showed VM of the bone. A CT scan showed a left frontal bone lesion extending to the inner table. After 1 month, a resection of the full-thickness calvarial lesion and a split-thickness cranial bone cranioplasty reconstruction was performed (see **Fig. 2**B–D). **Fig. 2**E shows the patient with a normal forehead contour 6 months after surgery.

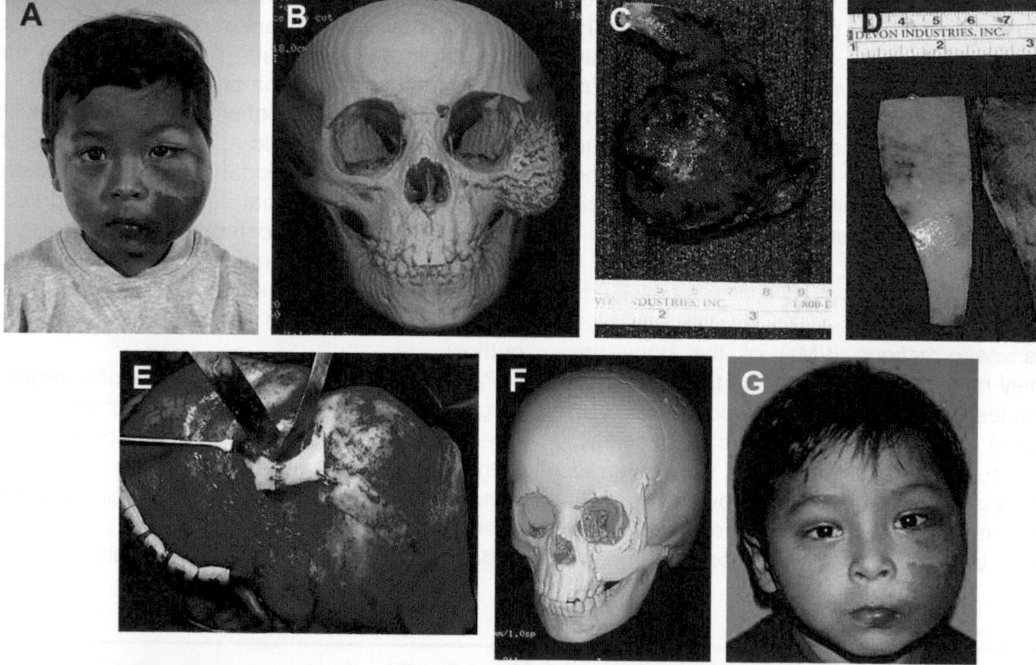

Fig. 1. (*A*) A 4-year-old boy with a left zygomatic intraosseous VM, overlying soft tissue thickening, and capillary malformation of the left cheek. (*B*) Three-dimensional reconstruction demonstrating a large calcified sclerotic and spiculated lesion involving the left zygoma extending into the lateral wall of the orbit and the zygomatic arch. (*C*) Surgical specimen at the time of resection, later determined to be an intraosseous VM on pathologic evaluation. (*D*) Lead template and split calvarial bone graft used to reconstruct the left lateral wall and zygoma. (*E*) Calvarial bone grafts in place. (*F*) Postoperative 3D CT scan demonstrating a reconstructed zygoma, lateral orbital wall, and zygomatic arch. (*G*) A 2-year postoperative picture sent by his family in South America.

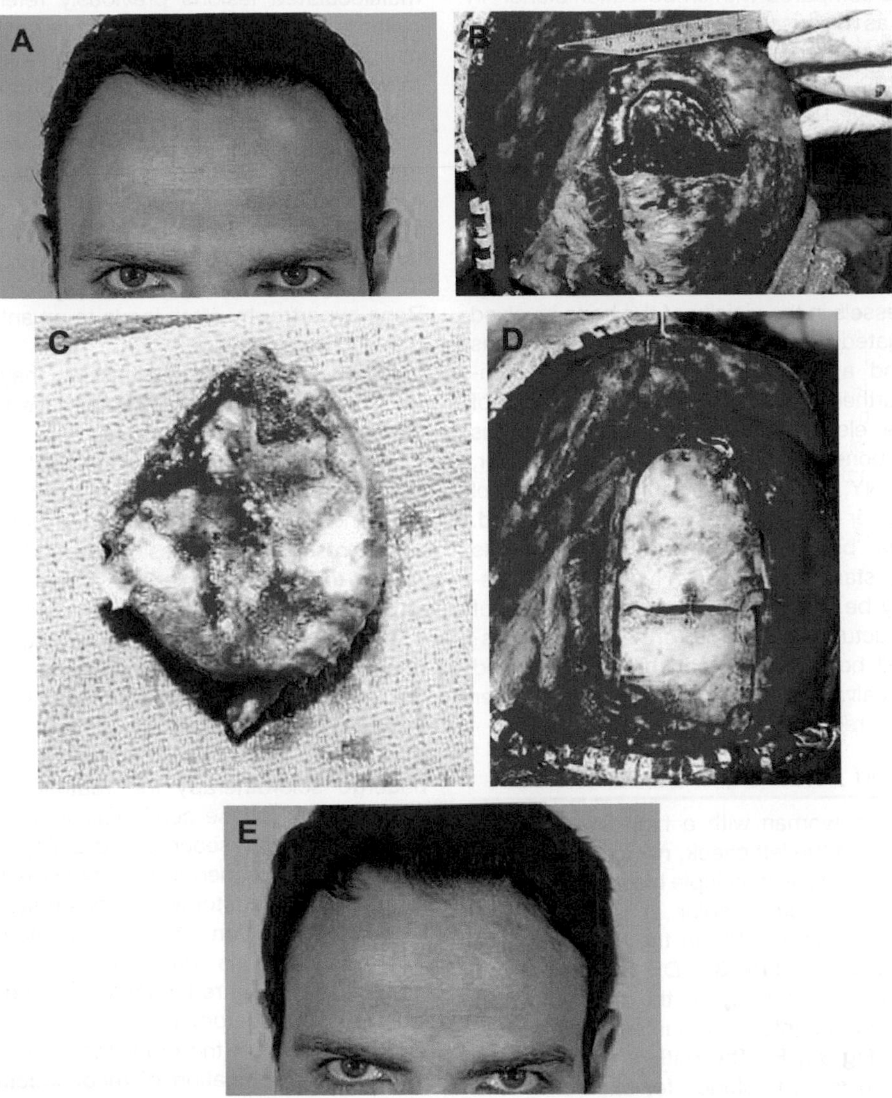

Fig. 2. (*A*) Left forehead mass near temporal hairline. (*B*) Full-thickness calvarial defect after resection. (*C*) Resected specimen determined by pathology to be a VM of the bone. (*D*) Split-thickness cranioplasty reconstruction. (*E*) Normal forehead contour 6 months postoperation.

ARTERIOVENOUS MALFORMATIONS

Arteriovenous malformations (AVMs) are high-flow lesions that can occur in the head and neck region, with the mandible, maxilla, and tongue most frequently involved. These lesions may involve the facial skeleton, and when they do, they may be associated with life-threatening bleeding, particularly after simple procedures such as dental extractions. Intraosseous lesions tend to expand the bone to a point where radiolucency is seen on radiographic examination.[3,4] Patients may complain of swelling in the jaw, toothache, or acute hemorrhage. A classic finding is periodontal bone loss. The workup of suspected AVMs in the head and neck should include both magnetic resonance imaging and imaging of both the common carotids. Imaging can be done using magnetic resonance angiography, magnetic resonance venography, or conventional angiography. Careful evaluation of these examinations demonstrate the extent of the lesion and the nature of the vascular supply. Suspected bony involvement is best evaluated with CT.

Treatment of soft tissue AVMs usually includes selective embolization followed by surgical resection within 12 to 24 hours. Surgical resection (with or without embolization) has been shown to have a lower recurrence rate and longer time to recurrence compared with embolization alone.[5] In addition, as discussed with VMs, embolization alone does not recontour the abnormal skeleton. Before performing a resection, it is important to share with the patient that the lesion may reexpand after treatment but that the technique offers the best chance for a favorable and sustained outcome.[6] Lesions affecting the bone require wide dissection and resection. Temporary clamping of the external carotids is helpful in controlling what could otherwise be significant bleeding. Smaller vessels in the vicinity of the bone involved can be ligated before resection. Some surgeons recommend a supraperiosteal dissection technique to further limit blood loss. A combination of aggressive electrocoagulation and a generous amount of bone wax or powdered Gelfoam (Pfizer, New York, NY, USA) is usually sufficient to control bleeding after the bony resection is performed. Blood must be available in adequate amounts before the start of the case. Hypotensive anesthesia may be helpful as well. Reconstruction of skeletal structures must be performed when necessary. Small bony defects can be reconstructed easily with calvarial or iliac crest bone grafts. Larger defects may require free tissue transfer.

Case 3: AVM

A 20-year-old woman with a high-flow vascular malformation of the left cheek, neck, and lips presented with a history of multiple bleeding episodes from a left mandibular molar. A CT angiogram demonstrated a large AVM in the left cheek and buccal space (see **Fig. 3**A–D). Expansion and sclerosis of the left body of the mandible with destruction of the anterior and inferior cortex was noted (see **Fig 3**E, F). The patient was taken to the operating room in stages for excision of the AVM, reduction of the mandible, and resection of the left third molar. In order to control bleeding during one surgery, her external carotid was temporarily ligated; the left third mandibular molar was extracted, and the socket packed firmly with Surgice (Ethicon, West Somerville, NJ, USA), which was secured by a tie-over bolster fashion with 0 silk suture. Postoperative pictures reveal improved facial contour (see **Fig. 3**G, H).

LYMPHATIC MALFORMATIONS

Lymphatic malformations (LMs) are slow-growing lesions that result from dilated and malformed lymphatic channels that fail to connect with or drain into the venous system. As the retained secretions build up, cystic components develop within these channels. The cysts range in severity from tiny superficial cysts to large, deep, multiloculated lesions previously referred to as cystic hygromas. LMs tend to enlarge proportionally with the growth of the child, although sudden rapid expansion is possible. LMs commonly affect the cervicofacial region and present as a painless, soft, slowly enlarging mass. They are most frequently encountered in the anterior and posterior triangles of the neck, although they may involve the orbit, lips, and tongue. About 80% of cervicofacial LMs cause bone hypertrophy, most frequently seen in the maxillary or mandible. Bone hypertrophy often leads to an anterior open bite and prognathism.[7]

Although LMs are benign lesions, they can reach massive sizes and may be life-threatening secondary to infection, bleeding, and airway compromise. Diffuse cervicofacial LMs may compress vital neurovascular structures in the face and neck, including the mediastinum in 2% of patients. This compression can lead to compression of the trachea, esophagus, and pharynx and ultimately death from airway compromise.[8]

Treatment of LMs varies depending on both the condition of the patient and the characteristics of the malformation at the time of presentation. Patients with localized disease and no compromise of the airway or other vital structures may undergo sclerotherapy for treatment. However, patients with diffuse cervicofacial LMs must first have their airway secured and ability to feed assessed. Many patients with massive LMs often require a tracheostomy and gastrostomy before further intervention. Surgical management of diffuse disease is often a lifelong debulking process, including reduction of macroglossia and closure of macrostomia.

Management of the craniofacial skeleton often requires a combination of reconstructive procedures. Osteotomies are used to reduce the bony hypertrophy seen in patients with diffuse LMs. In addition, orthognathic procedures, such as mandibular setbacks, are frequently required for the malocclusion resulting from the bony hypertrophy. In the senior author's (S.A.W.) experience, these huge LMs are one of the most difficult and frustrating conditions to manage.

Case 4: LM

This 5-year-old boy had a massive cervicofacial LM requiring a tracheostomy at birth for airway obstruction. He presented with macrostomia, oral incompetence, lower facial palsy, and obvious mandibular hypertrophy (**Fig. 4**A). During the next 4 years, he underwent multiple soft tissue debulking procedures, during which no evidence of discernable nerves were encountered between

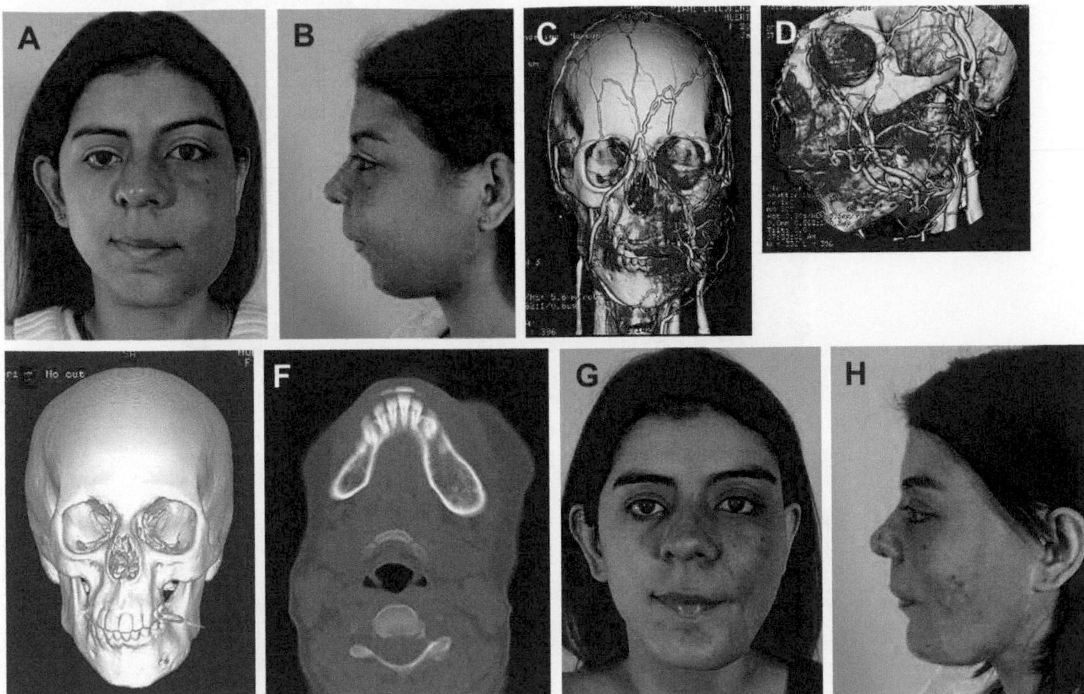

Fig. 3. (*A, B*) Large AVM in the left cheek and buccal space. (*C*) CT angiogram (CTA) of AVM originating from the left facial, lingual, and internal maxillary artery. (*D*) CTA of the AVM originating from the left facial, lingual, and internal maxillary artery. (*E, F*) Expansion and sclerosis of the left aspect of the body of the mandible, with destruction of the anterior and inferior cortex. (*G, H*) Postoperative result after excision of the AVM and left mandibular third molar, genioplasty, and correction of macrostomia.

the skin and periosteum. Bilateral commissuroplasties and placement of a fascia lata sling to the lower lip, in an attempt to improve his severe lip incompetence, were also performed. The patient was not followed up until 15 years of age, at which time treatment of the mandibular hypertrophy and anterior open bite was discussed (see **Fig. 4**B). Mandibular resection is planned and requires a stereoligthographic model, because orthodontic treatment is impossible for this patient (see **Fig. 4**C).

Case 5: LM

A 5-month-old girl has a massive cervicofacial LM that required tracheostomy placement at age 1 month as well as a giant LM of the tongue (**Fig. 5**A). She underwent a tongue reduction at age 10 months for repeated episodes of bleeding. At age 3 years, she underwent further reduction of the tongue and debulking of the LM from the soft tissue (**Fig. 5**B). Bilateral mandibular ramal osteotomies and coronoidectomies were also performed to close the anterior open bite and set back her mandible in an attempt to obtain proper occlusion. She underwent repeat osteotomies of the mandibular rami at age 8 years for correction of the massive overgrowth of her mandible and recurrent anterior open bite. However, she returned at age 10 years with the lower third of her face having hypertrophied tremendously, requiring further bony and soft tissue reduction of her face and mandible (**Fig. 5**C). At age 12 years, a CT scan (**Fig. 5**D) shows results of repeat mandibular osteotomy and reduction of chin.

Case 6: LM

This patient was diagnosed in utero as having a massive LM involving both the cervicofacial region and mediastinum (**Fig. 6**A). He was delivered via a cruciate cesarean section because of the size of the lesion. He underwent a tracheostomy, gastrostomy, and multiple debulking procedures, including a median sternotomy for resection of the mediastinal portion of the tumor. The LM continued to increase in size, and intralesional OK-432 (picibanil) injection was attempted at 8 months of age, with little success (see **Fig. 6**B). However, the lesion progressed (see **Fig. 6**C), and the patient died at 3 years of age from progressive bronchopulmonary compression.

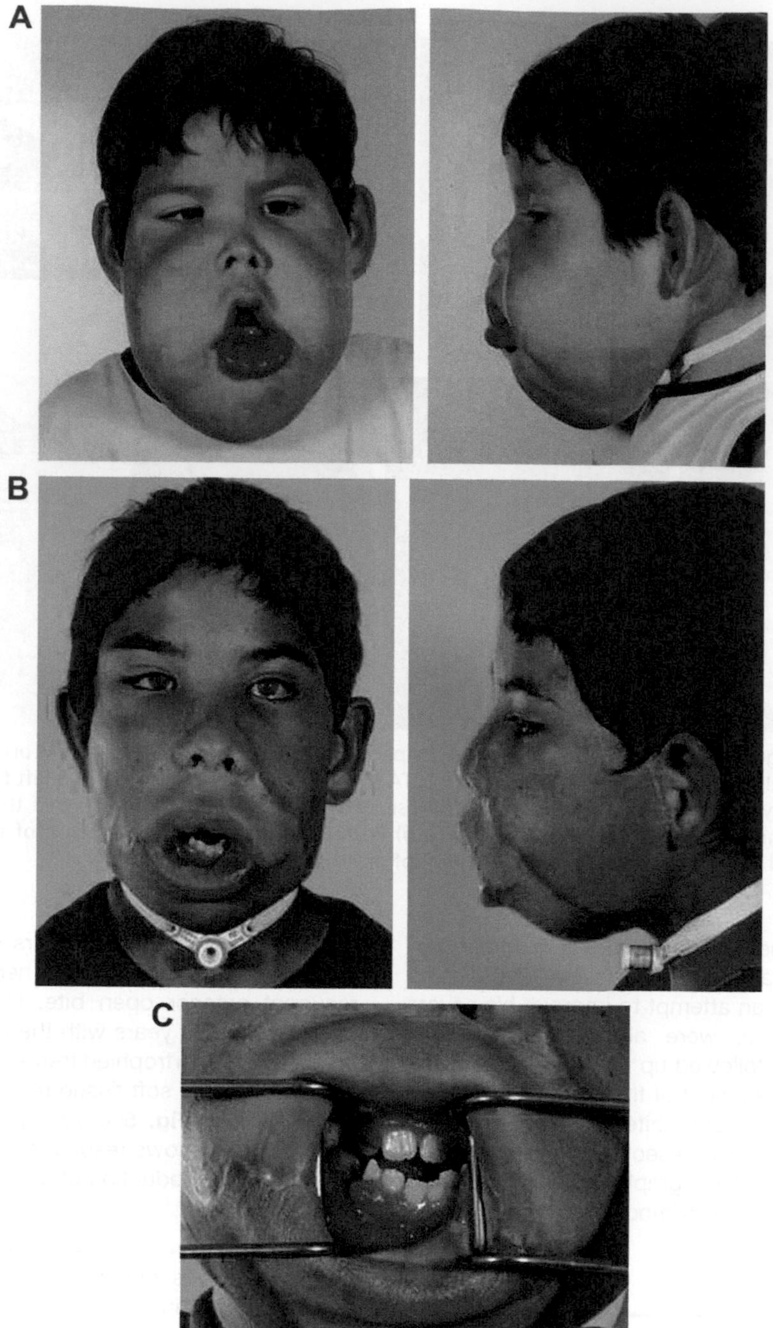

Fig. 4. (*A*) A 5-year-old boy with massive cervicofacial LM with secondary mandibular hypertrophy, oral incompetence, and lower facial palsy. (*B, C*) Patient at 15 years of age, after multiple debulking procedures, bilateral commissuroplasties, and fascia lata sling to lower lip. The patient has an anterior open bite and mandibular hypertrophy that require further treatment.

OTHER CONDITIONS: JUVENILE ANGIOFIBROMA

Although not classified as a vascular anomaly, juvenile angiofibromas (JAs) are benign tumors that develop most commonly in the nasopharynx of adolescent boys. Also referred to as nasopharyngeal angiofibromas, they have a firm rubbery texture and develop adjacent to the sphenopalatine foramen. As the tumors increase in size, they displace the nasopharyngeal mucosa anteriorly

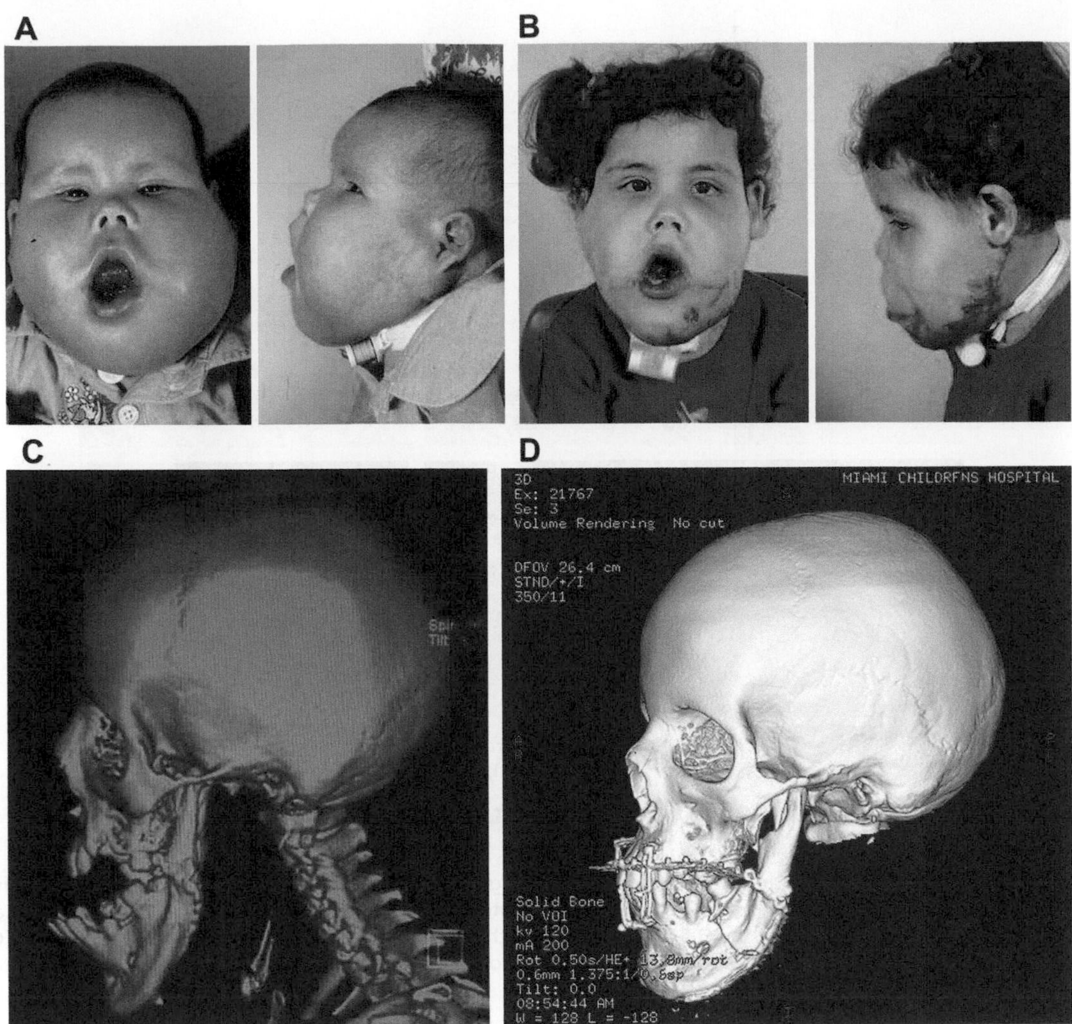

Fig. 5. (*A*) A 5-month-old girl with massive cervicofacial LM requiring a tracheostomy at 1 month of age. This patient displays significant mandibular overgrowth and anterior open bite that are frequently seen in these patients. (*B*) The patient at 3 years of age, after reduction of the tongue, debulking of the tumor in the soft tissues, and closure of the oral commissures. She continues to show significant mandibular hypertrophy and a significant anterior open bite. (*C*) CT scan of the patient at age 10 years. She had previously undergone osteotomies from just anterior to the gonial angle superiorly to the sigmoid notch. Also, bilateral coronoidectomies were performed to obtain proper occlusion. (*D*) CT scan of the patient at age 12 years after repeat mandibular osteotomy and reduction of chin.

and inferiorly, filling the nasal cavity and deviating the septum to the contralateral side. JAs also have a propensity to bleed because of an inability of the vessels to vasoconstrict or form a platelet plug, making these tumors life-threatening, given their location. Because of this complication, the treatment paradigm is similar to that of the AVMs, and they are included in this article for completeness.

The most common presenting complaints in most patients with JAs are unilateral nasal obstruction and recurrent severe episodes of epistaxis. Invasion of the eustachian tubes, maxillary sinus, and orbit can result in otitis media, sinusitis, orbital ptosis, and visual changes. A nasal speculum examination may identify a pink-purple polypoid mass, and a CT scan must be

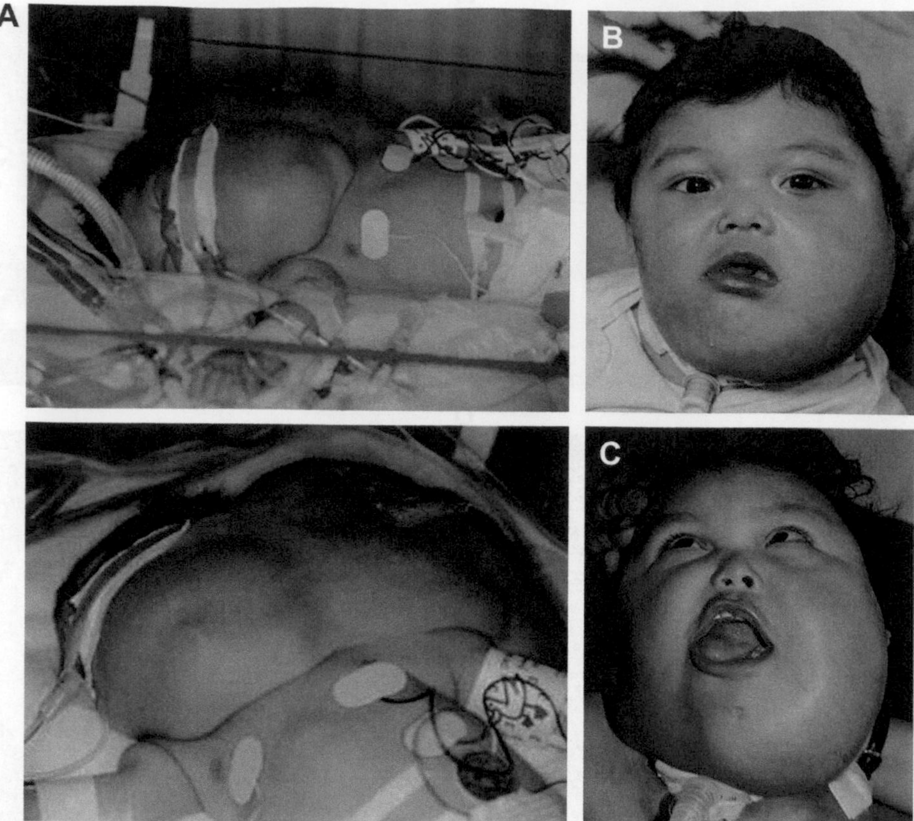

Fig. 6. (*A*) Patient at 3 days of age, with massive LM requiring debulking from both an external approach for the cervicofacial portion of the lesion as well as a median sternotomy for the mediastinal involvement. (*B*) Patient at 1 year of age, after completion of the OK-432 injections, with continued progressive enlargement of the LM. (*C*) Patient at 2 years of age, with increased size of the lesion. However, the patient died of progressive bronchopulmonary compression.

ordered if JA is clinically suspected. Biopsies are not indicated in these patients because of the highly vascular nature of the lesion.[9]

Treatment of JAs requires complete excision of the lesion. As with AVMs, patients undergo arterial embolization of the tumor 24 to 72 hours before the surgery to decrease the risk of intraoperative hemorrhage. Surgical access is best approached through a Le Fort I osteotomy, which can be combined with an infratemporal fossa approach for tumors with intracranial extension.[10,11] Recurrence rates with this approach are now less than 10%. Historically, radiation has been used to treat JAs; however, this treatment is reserved for patients who are unable to undergo surgery because of high recurrence rates and risk of malignant transformation of the tumor.[12]

Case 7: JA

A 13-year-old boy presented with recurrent epistaxis, loss of all but light perception in the left eye, and decreasing vision in the right eye (**Fig. 7**A). He was given a presumptive diagnosis of JA, and a CT scan displayed a large mass occupying the entire cranial base, nasal cavity, and area beneath the left maxillary sinus (see **Fig. 7**B). He underwent embolization of the left internal maxillary artery feeding the tumor before surgery (see **Fig. 7**C). The tumor was approached via a coronal incision and facial bipartition, which made possible the easy removal of the tumor to the floor of the palate (see **Fig. 7**D–G). Bone grafts were placed in the nasal dorsum and cranial base (see **Fig. 7**H). He displayed good facial proportions

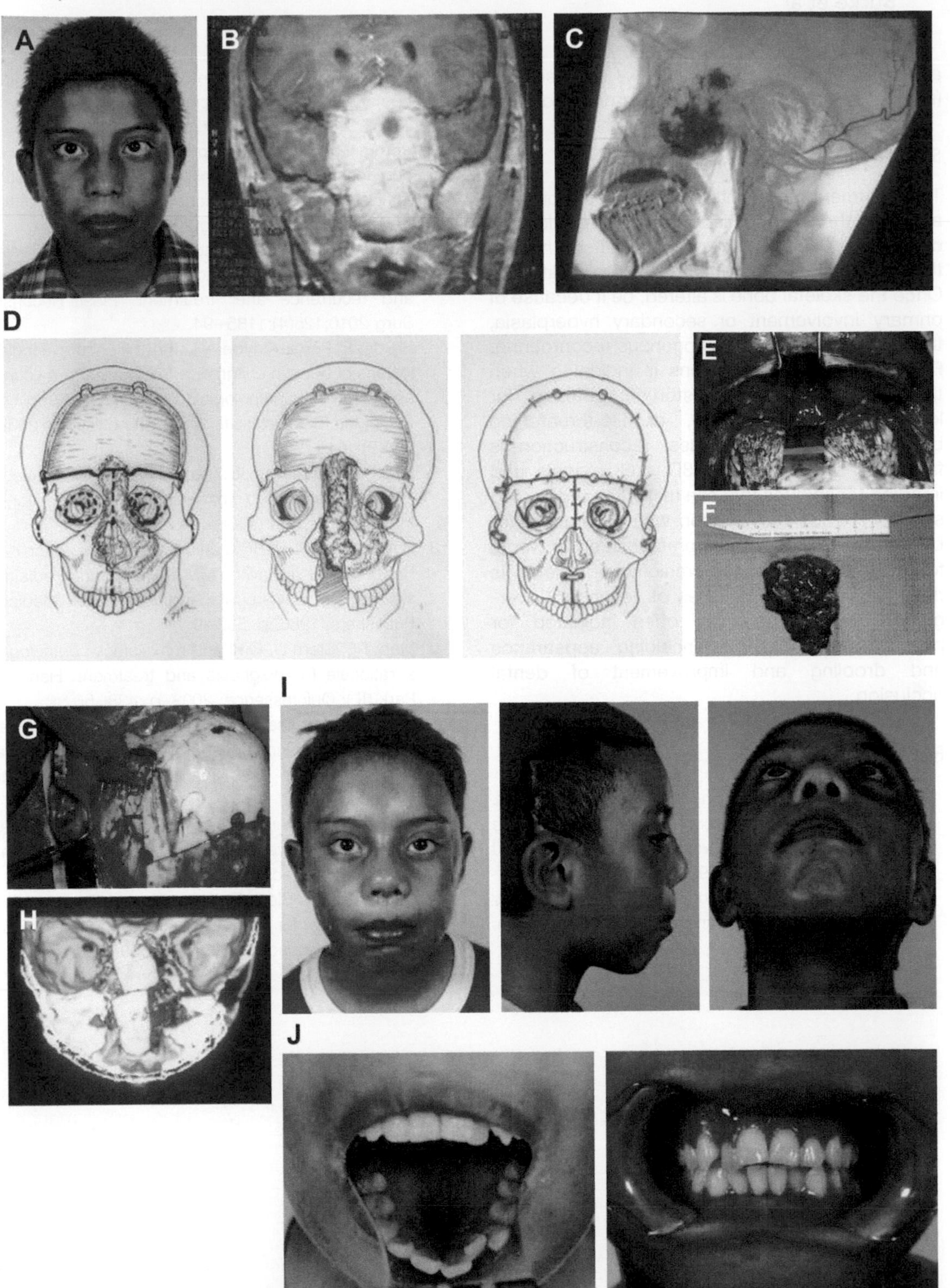

Fig. 7. (*A*) A 13-year-old boy who presented with recurrent nose bleeds, loss of all but light perception in the left eye, and decreasing vision in the right eye. (*B*) CT scan showing a mass extending and occupying the entire cranial base. (*C*) Mass involving the entire left maxillary sinus during preoperative angiographic embolization of the left internal maxillary artery. (*D*) Proposed approach to facial bipartition for resection of tumor. (*E*) Intracranial exposure of the JA. (*F*) Resected tumor specimen, later confirmed by pathology to be JA. (*G*) Closure of facial bipartition and coronal incision with resuspension of temporalis muscle. (*H*) Postoperative CT scan demonstrating bone grafts to the cranial base. (*I*) Patient 1 week after surgery, with good facial proportions and well-healed coronal and nasal incisions. (*J*) Mirror displaying a well-healed palate at 3 weeks after surgery and normal occlusion.

and a well-healed palate 3 weeks after surgery (see **Fig. 7**I–J) and returned to his home country.

SUMMARY

The treatment of patients with vascular anomalies affecting the craniofacial skeleton is particularly challenging. Unlike the lesions that affect the soft tissue, there is little role for nonsurgical treatment. Once the skeletal bone is altered, be it because of primary involvement or secondary hyperplasia, there is little chance of autogenous recontouring. Resection of primary lesions is indicated when there is gross skeletal distortion, potential for loss of critical function, or life-threatening bleeding. In complex cases, reconstruction is facilitated by the use of 3D skull models and imaging techniques that can mirror the unaffected side to provide the surgeon with a template for bone grafting. The use of prefabricated implants for reconstruction of the craniofacial skeleton is not recommended. In cases of secondary overgrowth, surgery is most often indicated for psychosocial concerns, including appearance and drooling and improvement of dental occlusion.

REFERENCES

1. Srinivasan B, Ethunandan M, Van der Horst C, et al. Intraosseous 'haemangioma' of the zygoma: more appropriately termed a venous malformation. Int J Oral Maxillofac Surg 2009;38(10):1066–70.
2. Valentini V, Nicolai G, Lore B, et al. Intraosseous hemangiomas. J Cranifac Surg 2008;19(6): 1459–64.
3. Cheng NC, Lai DM, Hsie MH, et al. Intraosseous hemangiomas of the facial bone. Plast Reconstr Surg 2006;117(7):2366–72.
4. Perugini M, Renzi G, Gasparini G, et al. Intraosseoul hemangioma of the maxillofacial district: clinical analysis and surgical treatment in 10 consecutive patients. J Craniofac Surg 2004;15(6):980–5.
5. Liu AS, Mulliken JB, Zurakowski D, et al. Extracranial arteriovenous malformations: natural progression and recurrence after treatment. Plast Reconstr Surg 2010;125(4):1185–94.
6. Bruder E, Perez-Atayde AR, Jundt G, et al. Vascular lesions of bone in children, adolescents, and young adults: A clinicopathologic reappraisal and application of the ISSVA classification. Virchows Arch 2009; 454(2):161–79.
7. Boyd JB, Mulliken JB, Kaban LB, et al. Skeletal changes associated with vascular malformations. Plast Reconstr Surg 1984;74:789.
8. Ravitch MM, Rush BF. Cystic hygroma. In: Welch KJ, Randolph JG Jr, Ravitch MM, et al, editors. Pediatric surgery. 4th edition. Chicago: Year Book Medical Publishers; 1986. p. 533–9.
9. Marx RE, Stern D. Oral and maxillofacial pathology: a rationale for diagnosis and treatment. Hanover Park (IL): Quintessence; 2003. p. 438–56.
10. Margalit N, Wasserzug O, De-Row A, et al. Surgical treatment of juvenile nasopharyngeal angiofibroma with intracranial extension. J Neurosurg Pediatr 2009;4(2):113–7.
11. Cansiz H, Guvenc MG, Sekercioglu N. Surgical approaches to juvenile nasopharyngeal angiofibroma. J Craniomaxillofac Surg 2006;34(1):3–8.
12. Cummings BJ, Blend R, Keane T, et al. Primary radiation therapy for juvenile nasopharyngeal angiofibroma. Laryngoscope 1984;94:1599–605.

Special Considerations in Vascular Anomalies: Operative Management of Upper Extremity Lesions

Joseph Upton, MD, Amir Taghinia, MD*

KEYWORDS

• Vascular anomalies • Upper extremity • Surgery
• Fast-flow lesion • Venous malformations
• Lymphatic malformations • Mixed lesions

The past 3 decades has seen a steady, almost exponential, increase in knowledge of vascular anomalies. A useful biologic classification system has evolved. A careful physical examination augmented with refined imaging will yield an accurate diagnosis and set the stage for treatment. A multidisciplinary team can offer treatment options with some degree of predictability. One option is surgery, which can be fraught with numerous complications. This article focuses on surgical principles and technical pearls in the treatment of these unique problems involving the upper limb. If incorporated into routine management, these suggestions will improve surgical outcomes.

GENERAL CONSIDERATIONS

Surgical treatment of vascular anomalies is neither for the timid nor the arrogant. A well-balanced approach that incorporates calculated risk and cautious execution is necessary; one that can only be cultivated with experience. The surgeon who devotes a practice to the treatment of these lesions is obligated to document meticulously and analyze critically; habits that will serve one well for life-long learning.

At the outset, it should be stressed that unless one amputates a limb, these lesions can never be absolutely eradicated. Persistence of the vascular anomaly is the rule, despite significant extirpative operations. This fact is important to consider during preoperative planning and future interventions.

The diagnosis and treatment of vascular anomalies is rapidly changing. Parents and patients must be kept informed about the natural history of the particular malformation, options for treatment, and new types of surgical, pharmacologic, and minimally-invasive interventions. Many children with significant venous malformations (VMs) are treated conservatively during childhood and present as teenagers requesting surgery. These decisions can be difficult, because both functional and aesthetic considerations must be considered. The authors have noted that both lymphatic malformations (LMs) and VMs tend to become more symptomatic in adolescent girls than boys. Contrasted are fast-flow lesions that are slow-growing, indolent, and insidious. Surgeons must provide a clear explanation of all potential complications and expected short- and long-term outcomes before any surgical treatment.[1]

The surgeon who has the courage to treat difficult fast-flow lesions should also be prepared to amputate a symptomatic nonfunctional or painful digit or limb after unsuccessful attempts at palliation. Patients with severe pain will often request amputation of the affected part. Others may wish

Department of Plastic Surgery, Children's Hospital, 300 Longwood Avenue, Boston, MA 02115, USA
* Corresponding author.
E-mail address: amir.taghinia@childrens.harvard.edu

Clin Plastic Surg 38 (2011) 143–151
doi:10.1016/j.cps.2010.08.011

to persist despite a functionless parasitic limb or digit. The most difficult decisions are in young children who do not verbalize their pain, and some teenagers who have minimal tolerance to pain and have not adapted well to their limb malformation. In difficult lesions, amputation should be considered and discussed preoperatively. The reconstructive surgeon need not view amputation as a failure.

Although a comprehensive review of surgical complications is beyond the scope of this article, these include compartment syndrome, bleeding, wound dehiscence, infection, devascularization of a limb or digit, secondary contracture, tendon adherence, and pain secondary to nerve injury. Adherence to basic surgical principles as outlined in this article will minimize these potential problems.[1,2] Large vascular anomalies involving any portion of the upper limb are not impossible problems. Surgical treatment is often the best remedy and should not be viewed as the last-resort option.

Box 1
Principles and technical pearls in the treatment of vascular anomalies of the upper limb

Plan carefully before the operation

Place incisions strategically

Operate in a blood-less field

Use fine surgical instruments

Identify and tag important structures

Dissect discreetly, rapidly, and confidently

Avoid intraneural dissection

Close meticulously

Immobilize the extremity postoperatively

Follow the patient regularly

PRINCIPLES

Surgical principles gain acceptance with time and must be periodically reassessed and refined, particularly in this rapidly advancing field. Principles should not be confused with surgical techniques that change frequently, and are modulated to a great extent by technology. Many of the following principles have evolved from the early operative experience with vascular malformations (especially the fast-flow types), which was punctuated with complications.[1–7] These principles are briefly outlined in **Box 1**.

Preoperative Planning

Preoperative planning is the cardinal principle of surgical treatment. Most poor outcomes can be avoided by adhering to this principle alone. Planning should include correlation of the size, extent, and involvement of structures with physical examination and imaging. Imaging modalities include plain radiographs, ultrasound, MRI, and angiography. Before surgery on complex fast-flow lesions, a step-by-step plan of resection, including the approach and extent, must be determined and followed. Serial studies of growing children are often invaluable in showing the true extent of involvement of the extremity. However, the absolute extension of a VM, lymphaticovenous malformation (LVM), or arteriovenous malformation (AVM) may not be completely delineated by these studies, and intraoperative decision-making may be required once the true extent becomes visible. Despite this, it is critical for surgeons to abide (as much as possible) by the initial plan; straying from the plan may lead to a violation of uninvolved areas, an inadvertent injury to neurovascular structures, a waste of precious tourniquet time, and an incomplete excision.

For complex lesions, the authors have found it helpful to print the angiogram and label the nidus, shunts, and all large branches within that portion of the lesion to be excised. These scans should be displayed in the operating room for easy reference during the procedure. Other preparatory steps for fast-flow lesions include central venous and peripheral arterial monitoring, availability of fast-flow warmers and blood products for transfusion, and intensive care unit monitoring postoperatively.

Placement of Incisions

Placement of incisions is important, particularly in children. When planning an incision, surgeons should consider exposure, blood supply, function, aesthetics, and future surgery. Incisions should be long enough to provide full exposure of the entire lesion (**Figs. 1**A and **2**). Small incisions provide no surgical advantage, and risk injury to important structures. In the digits, a high mid-axial incision is preferred because it provides excellent exposure dorsally and volarly, can be used again, and is typically well hidden. Dorsal longitudinal hand and digital incisions are avoided if possible because they provide less exposure and are more conspicuous. Palmar incisions can lead to contracture if poorly planned; zig-zag incisions and those using normal skin creases are recommended.

Ironically, vascular insufficiency can exist in the presence of a vascular anomaly, especially fast-flow types; thus, blood supply should be

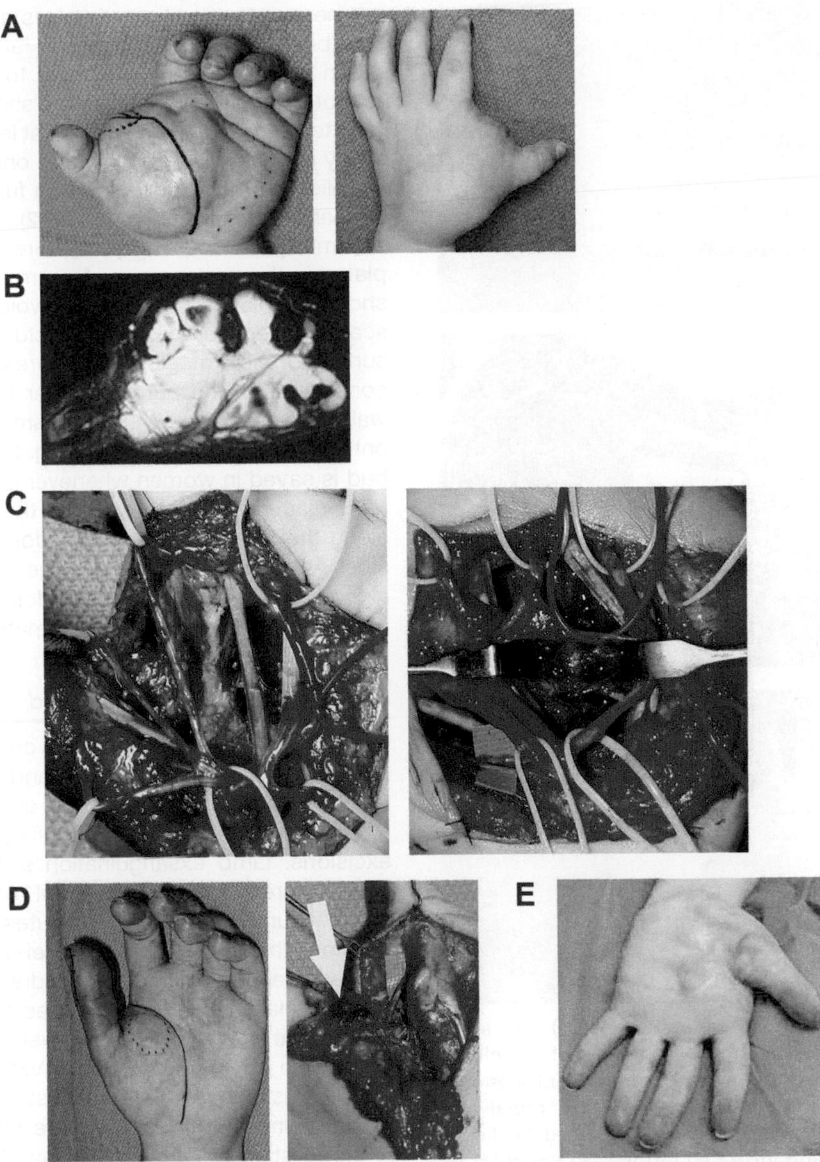

Fig. 1. Massive venous malformation (VM) of hand. (*A*) This 4-year-old child with a painful and bulky VM presented after unsuccessful sclerotherapy and partial excision. She was beginning to neglect her hand. The generous incision was placed in the thenar flexion crease and was large enough to excise the entire lesion. The dotted line over the hypothenar eminence marks the planned extent of the lesion and dissection. (*B*) MRI showed a multiloculated through-and-through lesion. (*C*) Vessel loops encircle the sensory nerves and the palmar arch. Note the similar appearance of nerves (*yellow*) and arteries (*red*) once the field is blood-stained. Deep in the field is the transversely oriented deep motor branch of the ulnar nerve (*right*). Microscopic dissection was used. (*D*) Four years later, persistent VM with thromboses and adipose tissue were excised from the thumb and first web space. The scarred ulnar digital nerve to the thumb beneath the background was redissected. The inset shows intralesional thromboses (*arrow*). Note the abundance of adipose tissue within the malformation. (*E*) During her teenage years, new masses appeared along the periphery of the original excision. The involved regions are soft and she remains asymptomatic.

considered during planning of incisions. The dorsum of the hand has an axial blood supply above the overlying fascia, whereas the palm of the hand receives intermittent perforators from palmar arterial branches. Thus, large flaps can be developed safely in the dorsum, but similar flaps are prone to ischemia in the palm. To avoid digital vascular compromise, only one half of a digit

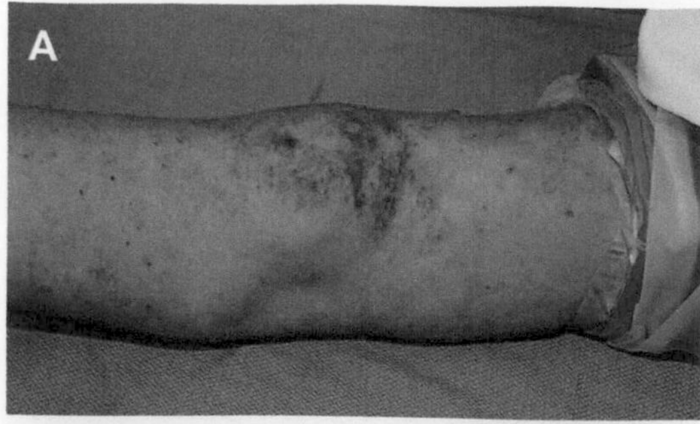

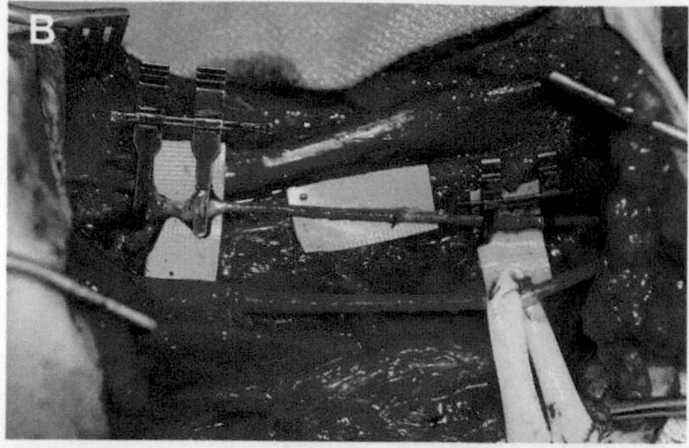

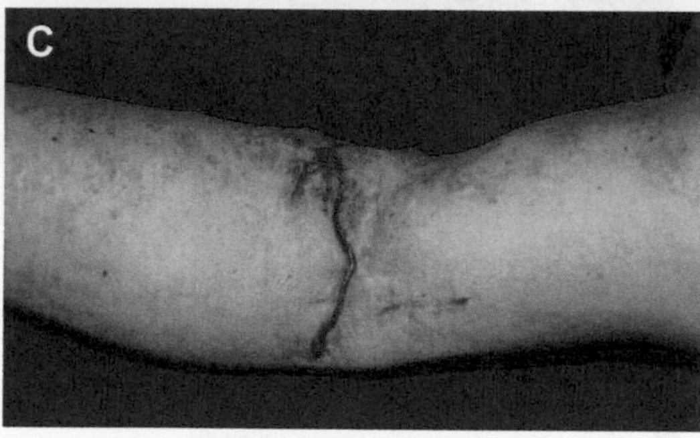

Fig. 2. Glomovenous malformation. (*A*) An adult woman presented with a painful mass of the elbow after a previous excision complicated by intralesional bleeding. Although her hand was pink, radial and ulnar pulses were absent; she complained of diminished strength and increased fatigue. (*B*) Her old scars were excised and the symptomatic clusters of thrombosed veins were removed through a generous incision. Revascularization of the resected brachial artery was performed with an autogenous graft. The median nerve is retracted by the Penrose drain. (*C*) The atrophic involved skin took longer to heal than normal. Limited early extension of the elbow was performed with a hand therapist to prevent a flexion contracture. She regained full motion and function within 3 months.

should be dissected at a time. If possible, at least one or two large dorsal veins per finger should be preserved to enhance venous drainage, especially when excising a diffuse lymphatic lesion in the hand or foot. The superficial venous system should not be resected or ligated unless a deep system has been identified along the arterial system. When a critical arterial segment to a digit, hand, or foot is removed, this segment should be reconstructed with a vein graft so that at least one digital artery is preserved per digit and one major artery supplies the hand or foot with a functional intact palmar or plantar arch (see **Fig. 2**).

If multiple debulking procedures are contemplated in the upper arm or forearm, each incision should be planned carefully to avoid unnecessary scarring over neurovascular structures. The medial surface of the arm, elbow, and forearm is the least conspicuous. The authors prefer to place chest wall incisions along the inframammary fold and onto the anterior axillary line (**Fig. 3**D). The breast bud is saved in women whenever possible. In the foot, placement of incisions in the medial arch, along the borders, and on the dorsal surfaces is safe. As in the hand, scars in the web spaces or along eponychial or paronychial folds will contract and are likely to become problematic.

Dissection in a Blood-less Field

Dissection in a blood-less field is critical for identification of important structures and delineation of the vascular lesion. To this end, use of the pneumatic tourniquet is essential for all but the simplest excisions. Limb exsanguination should be thorough before tourniquet inflation; if bleeding occurs in the wound within 5 to 10 minutes of tourniquet inflation, the arm should be re-elevated and the process repeated. In small children the authors use the elastic Esmarch wrap as the tourniquet secured at the mid-humeral level (see **Fig. 3**C). Dissection of VMs, LVMs, and AVMs with arteriovenous fistulas (AVFs) is most vulnerable to blood-staining, whereas LMs are more forgiving. A blood-stained field within any dissection will decrease visibility, obliterate fascial planes, and set the stage for potential injury to important structures.

With chest wall LM and capillary-lymphati covenous malformation (CLVM) excisions or brachial plexus explorations, the tourniquet cannot be used. During these long procedures blood loss can be insidious, especially in small children. A premium is thus placed on meticulous hemostasis—best accomplished by careful dissection and preemptive ligation or clipping of vessels before they are cut.

To further minimize surgical blood-loss and blood-staining, three types of cautery devices are used selectively: the monopolar cautery, the bipolar microsurgical cautery, and the battery-operated hand-held ophthalmic cautery. Each device has

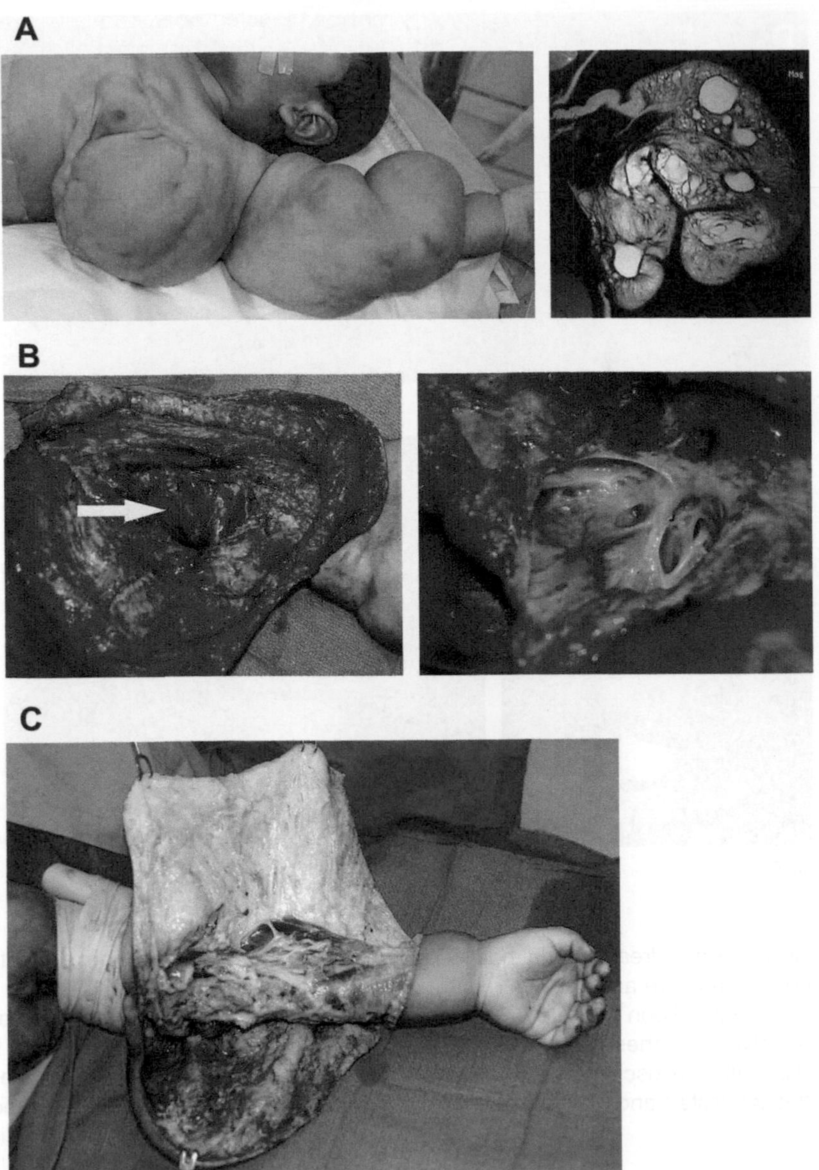

Fig. 3. Lymphatic malformation (LM) of chest wall and extremity. (*A*) This 18-month-old boy presented with a large LM involving the chest, axilla, and ipsilateral arm with sparing of the hand. MRI showed large macrocysts in the proximal portions of the lesion and a large amount of mesenchymal tissue and adipose within the subcutaneous tissue planes. Distal to the elbow the cysts were predominantly microcystic. (*B*) A large incision was used to expose the chest wall and axilla. The arrow is on the serratus anterior muscle flanked by the pectoralis major and minor (*above*) and the latissimus dorsi (*lateral*). The long thoracic nerve has been preserved. Large, interconnecting macrocysts permeate the brachial plexus, which should not be skeletonized during these dissections. (*C*) The forearm has been exposed through a posteromedial incision. Upward traction is essential for exposure of the areolar tissue planes for dissection. This LM extended beyond the subcutaneous space along tissue planes between muscle groups. Sensory nerves to retained portions of skin are preserved if possible. Large and small subcutaneous veins are sacrificed. (*D*) A subcuticular closure was used for all incisions and a drain placed in the upper portion of the incision. (*E*) Preoperative and 3-month postoperative views after a two-staged excision. His shoulder abduction posturing corrected spontaneously.

a specific use. The monopolar cautery is for subcutaneous dissection, the bipolar cautery is for small vessels, and the ophthalmic cautery is used for developing surgical planes, especially within muscles that tend to fasciculate with the monopolar cautery. Tissue sealants have been a useful adjunct at the end of a procedure once the tourniquet is deflated. Excision of fast-flow lesions

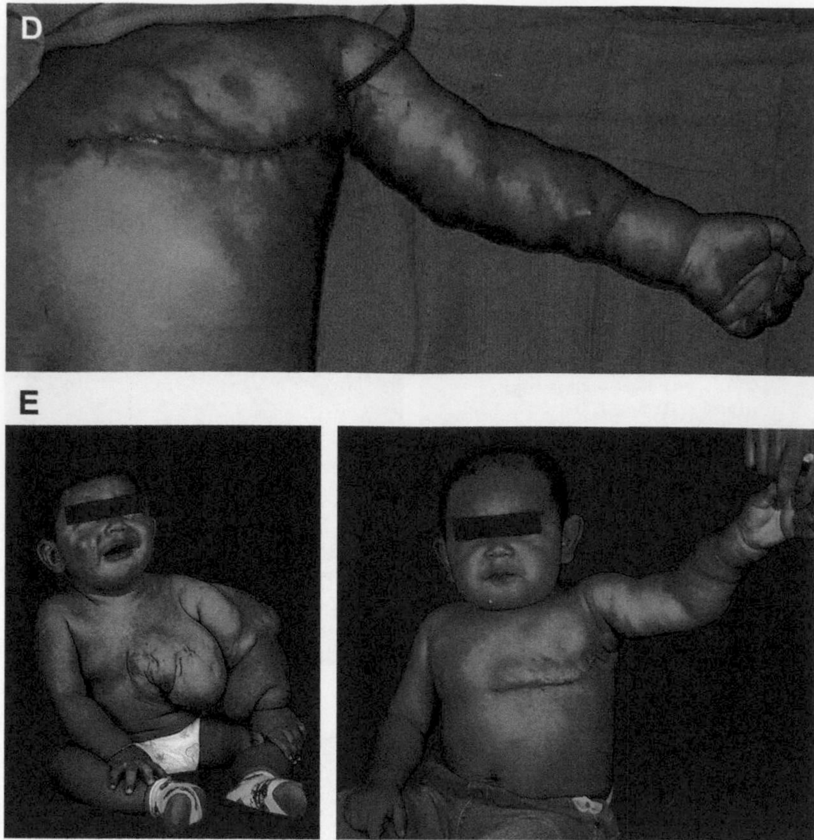

Fig. 3. (*continued*)

of the chest and axilla are dreaded (but not impossible) procedures, and are accomplished with the aid of intra-arterial balloon catheters, hypothermia, hypotensive anesthesia, cell savers, adequate blood and fluid resuscitation, and experienced anesthesiologists and cardiovascular surgeons.

Use of Fine Surgical Tools

Use of fine surgical tools is critical. Magnification, either loupe or microscope, makes a tremendous difference in the identification and preservation of normal neurovascular structures. Small vessels, such as vincular pedicles to the flexor tendons, nutrient vessels to the digital joints and carpal bones, and dorsal sensory nerves, should be preserved if possible (**Fig. 1**C). Vascular anomalies will usually displace, but not invade, neighboring soft tissues. Therefore, they are likened to digitopalmar Dupuytren's cords, which distort normal structures but do not obliterate them. Despite the anatomic distortion, an areolar connective tissue plane is usually preserved along the epineural surface of nerves and the adventitial plane of normal arteries and veins.

The trick to surgical isolation is upward traction of the adjacent soft tissue and blunt scissor dissection directly along the surface of the vessel or nerve (see **Fig. 3**C). These dissections cannot be performed without the use of delicate, undamaged, top-quality scissors and fine-toothed forceps. Our surgical kits contain at least six different pairs of scissors for this purpose. Colored vessel loops are used to encircle veins (blue), arteries (red), nerves (yellow), and tendons (white) for both retraction during resection and easier identification once the tourniquet has been released. Large vessels needed for subsequent reconstruction are always marked; two clips for veins and one clip for arteries.

An experienced surgical assistant is an invaluable asset. For the academic surgeon, a senior resident or fellow is preferred; for the private practitioner, these lesions are usually not handled alone unless they are simple. Nothing eases a tedious dissection better than a pair of experienced hands to provide retraction, countertraction, and control of unwanted bleeding.

Strength and endurance of one assistant becomes important in the treatment of large, diffuse LMs, VMs, and LVMs and any fast-flow lesion involving the chest wall, axilla, arm, and elbow regions, where the maintenance of traction and countertraction of surgical planes is essential. These procedures can be long and excruciating for any assistant.

Identification and Tagging of Normal Structures

Identify and tag normal structures first. Despite considerable distortion by the vascular malformation, the normal limb anatomy remains constant. Thus, intimate knowledge of anatomy is critical to avoid complications. Anatomic anomalies always exist but are the exception rather than the rule, even in vascular anomalies.

Dorsal veins are marked on the skin before exsanguination. Nerves are recognized by the omnipresent perineural fat, even in vascular malformations and densely scarred regions. The palmer dissection illustrated in **Fig. 1** presents a difficult undertaking. In the hand, compulsive identification of the sensory nerves and palmer arch was performed in proximal normal regions of the hand and then dissected distally using the loops for retraction. The entire palmer arch and all branches of the median and ulnar nerves were completed during the first tourniquet run. The distal portion of the lesion and extension into the first web space were dissected during the second. This approach of identifying the surrounding normal structures, aptly termed *circling the wagons*, is critical in preventing complications. This identification may be confusing and tedious in LMs, VMs, and mixed lesions because of the presence of abundant amounts of adipose tissue, which usually has a darker hue than the subcutaneous fat seen in normal portions of the same extremity (see **Figs. 1**A and **3**C). Nevertheless, it is crucial to persevere with dissection of the normal structures before diving into excision.

The first 90 minutes of the operation is the best time to complete this most difficult portion of the procedure, because the tissues have the least blood-staining and swelling (see **Fig. 1**C). The surgeon must move rapidly and confidently through the dissection. These lesions can be complicated and unforgiving; surgeons who stop frequently to teach, make probe, ponder, and procrastinate will soon find themselves operating within a heavily blood-stained field. Sterling Bunnell, a pioneer hand surgeon, aptly likened this experience to "…operating in the bottom of an inkwell."

Discreet But Thorough Excision

Discreet but thorough excision is advocated. The dissection should be limited to a specified area (hence discreet) but should be performed thoroughly so that subsequent reentry into a densely scarred bed will be unnecessary. Often, the malformation extends well beyond its anticipated limits (see **Fig. 1**D). In certain regions, limited staged excisions are better than one extensive and protracted dissection that leaves abnormal tissue behind (see **Fig. 3**). For example, the digits should be debulked in stages: first one side through a high mid-axial incision, then the other side in another stage. A single procedure is usually best for the dorsum or palm of the hand or wrist in a patient with a diffuse LM or VM. The axilla, brachial plexus, and anterior surfaces of elbow and wrist are preferably dissected in one operation when the neurovascular structures are undamaged. The palm of the hand can be approached more than once as long as a thorough dissection within each given region is performed and the tissues to be subsequently removed remain untouched. The palmar arches, intrinsic muscles, and all nerves (including the deep motor branch of the ulnar nerve) can be preserved (see **Fig. 1**C).

Avoidance of Intraneural Dissection

Avoid intraneural dissection whenever possible, despite gross involvement. The initial identification of a nerve or artery provides the best opportunity to place encircling loops, which may be helpful with retraction and isolation of adjacent structures. Excessive dissection or excessive manipulation of nerves, particularly within VMs, often leave in-continuity neuromas with partial or complete loss of distal sensory or motor function. These secondary symptoms are usually much worse than those associated with the vascular malformation.

Brachial plexus dissections are challenging in all cases and are performed in symptomatic patients with LMs, VMs, or mixed lesions. Interconnecting macro cysts typically permeate the plexus, which need not be skeletonized (see **Fig. 3**B). The case illustrated in **Fig. 3** is characteristic of a large, seemingly insurmountable LM. The entire chest wall and axillary dissection was completed in one stage and extended up into the involved brachial plexus. The large cysts were all decompressed, and as much of the lesion as possible was removed without injury to the individual neural cords or peripheral nerves, including the motor branches to chest wall and supporting scapular muscles (see **Fig. 3**B). In this patient the forearm excision was completed in two stages: one dorsal and one palmer a month later.

Partial dissections within large muscle groups should be avoided. VMs, LVMs, and other mixed lesions can involve the muscle; the decision to resect muscle and the amount to be removed must be made by the surgeon and can often be determined preoperatively. If a significant portion of the muscle is involved, removal of the entire involved muscle en bloc is preferred to avoid redissection in scar. Localized lesions within a muscle can be simply excised. VMs, mixed CLVMs, LVMs, and capillary-arteriovenous malformations (CAVM) are the most problematic lesions. Pure LMs do not characteristically penetrate deep to the muscular fascia; however, they may extend along fascial planes between muscle groups. It is easy to progress around and between muscle groups without realizing the depth of the dissection within the axilla, arm, or elbow (see **Fig. 3**C).

Meticulous and Thoughtful Closure

Meticulous and thoughtful closure is mandatory. Frequently, wound closure is considered the least important portion of the procedure, and is therefore relegated to the most junior member of the team. However, in complex cases, a poorly planned or executed closure can be a significant source of complications. It takes experienced eyes to identify poorly perfused skin and experienced hands to feel undue tension on flaps.

It is usually best to remove and replace skin that is heavily scarred from a previous procedure, chronically infected and ulcerated, severely atrophic, populated by coalesced lymphatic vesicles, or deprived by a proximal steal phenomenon. At the end of the operation, tissues with questionable viability can be excised and resurfaced or observed and resected later. Regions notorious for flap loss are those in the palm with large VMs and large areas of coalesced skin vesicles, and capillary staining in large LMs or mixed lesions.

Subcuticular closures with absorbable sutures are preferred in the arm, forearm, and dorsum of the hand (see **Fig. 3**D). Careful eversion of glabrous skin wounds is performed with absorbable chromic sutures in children and nonabsorbable sutures in adults. Despite meticulous technique, any incision of skin containing LM may become hypertrophic.

Drains should be used liberally, and delayed primary closure of the wound should be considered with excessive bleeding. Persistent postoperative bleeding is usually best treated with direct pressure, elevation, and immobilization, rather than with reexploration. Liberal use of tissue sealant products is encouraged and has been used to control oozing from unresected portions of the malformation.

Immobilization of the Operated Extremity

Postoperative management can be as important as preoperative planning and intraoperative execution, especially in children. In the treatment of children with vascular anomalies, the postoperative lack or loss of immobilization is the single most important cause of wound dehiscence, maceration, and chronic infection. Surgeons who have had children tend to appreciate this variable more than those who are childless.

The favorable aspect of operating on children, however, is that they do not develop stiffness or joint contractures. Thus, implementing postoperative rehabilitation is not as important in children as it is in the adult patient.

Follow-Up Evaluation

Follow-up evaluation should be performed compulsively at yearly intervals. These evaluations allow (1) tailoring of the treatment plan based on growth of the lesion, (2) continued learning for the parents and patients, and (3) continued learning for the surgeon, with increasing awareness of both surgical and nonsurgical cause and effect.

Early childhood, adolescence, and pregnancy are times when change may occur in vascular malformations from hormonal influences. Both slow- and fast-flow lesions may expand dramatically during pregnancy, with use of high-estrogen antiovulant medication, or after trauma. Large AVMs, LMs, or mixed lesions may be well tolerated by young children, only to become burdensome to teenagers because of their expansion, bulk, ulceration, and appearance or vascular steal symptoms. Scans and other studies need not be repeated unless they will influence treatment decisions.

These patients and parents often have questions that are not easily answered by their family physician because of the paucity of information available in the medical literature. For them, the surgeon is not only a treating physician but also a valuable resource of information. Similarly, patients are the surgeon's most cherished teachers. Only through careful documentation and critical long-term analysis of results can one improve surgical outcomes in this difficult field of surgery.

REFERENCES

1. Upton J, Coombs C, Mulliken JB, et al. Vascular malformations of the upper limb: a review of 270 patients. J Hand Surg Am 1999;24:1019.
2. Upton J, Marler JJ. Vascular anomalies of the upper extremity. In: Mathes S, editor. Plastic surgery, Volume VIII. Philadelphia: Saunders-Elsevier; 2006. p. 369–416.
3. deTakats G. Vascular anomalies of the extremities. Report of five cases. Surg Gynecol Obstet 1932;55:227.
4. Malan E, Puglionisi A. Congenital angiodysplasias of the extremities. (Note I: generalities and classifications: venous dysplasias). J Cardiovasc Surg (Torino) 1964;5:87.
5. Malan E, Puglionisi A. Congenital angiodysplasias of the extremities. (Note II: arterial, arterial and venous, haemolymphatic dysplasias). J Cardiovasc Surg (Torino) 1965;6:255.
6. Szilagyi DE, Smiith RF, Elliott JP, et al. Congenital arteriovenous anomalies of the limbs. Arch Surg 1976; 111:423.
7. Upton J, Mulliken JB, Murray JE. Classification and rationale for treatment of vascular anomalies in the upper extremity. J Hand Surg Am 1985; 10:970.

Special Considerations in Vascular Anomalies: Hematologic Management

Denise M. Adams, MD[a,b,*]

KEYWORDS

- Vascular anomalies • Hemangiomas
- Vascular malformations
- Kaposiform hemangioendothelioma • Coagulopathy

Proper care of the patient with a vascular anomaly requires the expertise of multiple specialists. Because of the need for an interdisciplinary approach, several vascular anomalies centers have now been developed across the world. A hematologist/oncologist provides clinical acumen in establishing a correct diagnosis and guiding the medical management of these patients. These patients can have complicated coagulopathies and need medical therapy. The hematologist/oncologist provides insights into the availability and suitability of enrollment into clinical trials or the use of novel experimental treatments for these complicated conditions. This article emphasizes the hematologic complications and management of these patients.

VASCULAR TUMORS

The most common vascular tumor is the hemangioma of infancy that can be simple or complex and may be associated with other anomalies.[1] Infantile hemangiomas are not associated with a thrombocytopenic coagulopathy, and the patients with infantile hemangiomas do not have signs of active coagulopathy. Infants with hemangiomas may have a slightly elevated platelet count, with minor increase in dimerized plasmin fragment D (D-dimer) levels, and slightly decreased fibrinogen levels, all of which are within the normal range of measurement.

Congenital hemangioma can be distinguished from infantile hemangioma because the former is fully developed at birth and can be diagnosed in utero. Congenital hemangioma has 2 subgroups: the rapidly involuting congenital hemangiomas (RICHs) and the noninvoluting congenital hemangiomas (NICHs).[2] The RICH lesions can appear violaceous at birth but rapidly regress during the first year of life. The NICH lesions are fully developed at birth and do not involute. There are distinguishing histochemical endothelial markers (such as Glut-1) that are present in infantile hemangiomas but not in the congenital hemangiomas.[3]

Congenital hemangiomas can be associated with coagulopathy (thrombocytopenia, low fibrinogen levels, and increased levels of fibrin degradation products and D dimers). The coagulopathy usually occurs in RICH and is distinguished from Kasabach-Merritt phenomenon (KMP) because it is self-limited and is usually not associated with bleeding complications.[4]

Hemangiomas and congenital hemangiomas should not be confused with the lesions known as kaposiform hemangioendotheliomas (KHEs) and tufted angiomas (TAs). KHEs and TAs were

[a] Division of Hematology/Oncology, Cincinnati Children's Hospital Medical Center, University of Cincinnati, MLC 7015, 3333 Burnet Avenue, Cincinnati, OH 45229, USA
[b] Hemangioma and Vascular Malformation Center, Cincinnati Children's Hospital Medical Center, 3333 Burnet Avenue, Cincinnati, OH 45229, USA
* Division of Hematology/Oncology, Cincinnati Children's Hospital Medical Center, University of Cincinnati, MLC 7015, 3333 Burnet Avenue, Cincinnati, OH 45229.
E-mail address: Denise.Adams@cchmc.org

Clin Plastic Surg 38 (2011) 153–160
doi:10.1016/j.cps.2010.08.002

first described in 1940 by Kasabach and Merritt[5] when they reported an infant with thrombocytopenic purpura caused by, what they thought was, a giant capillary hemangioma. Subsequently, the association of capillary hemangiomas with thrombocytopenia was referred to as Kasabach-Merritt Syndrome (KMS).

In 1997, 2 groups of investigators demonstrated that these lesions were not true hemangiomas but distinct vascular tumors diagnosed histologically as KHE or TA.[6,7] KHEs and TAs have a different clinical profile than hemangiomas, with a predilection for the upper trunk, extremities, thigh, sacrum, or retroperitoneum. They are warm, firm, indurated, purpuric lesions. Magnetic resonance imaging shows that these lesions invade the skin and subcutaneous fat and muscle. The lesions are usually focal, but some reports have described their spread in lymph nodes as well. These tumors can be associated with what is now called KMP, which includes an enlarging vascular lesion, profound thrombocytopenia, microangiopathic hemolytic anemia, and a mild consumptive coagulopathy. KMP has been associated with a mortality rate as high as 20% to 30%. KHE and TA are not always associated with KMP,[8] but the coagulopathy seen in KMP causes morbidity and mortality in patients with these lesions. The resulting profound thrombocytopenia and hypofibrinogenemia cause the most serious hemorrhagic complications. The primary cause of this coagulopathic abnormality is profound thrombocytopenia. Several theories have been proposed to explain this particular coagulopathy, such as trapping or consumption of platelets in the tumor, increased peripheral destruction of platelets outside the tumor, and decreased production of platelets in the bone marrow.[9,10]

Several therapies have been reported for the treatment of these lesions, but none has been uniformly effective. Therapies include the systemic use of corticosteroids, interferon, antifibrinolytic agents, and chemotherapy including the use of vincristine, cyclophosphamide, and actinomycin.[11–13] These lesions are challenging to manage because their clinical presentation and response to therapy can vary greatly. Platelet infusions should be limited because they can stimulate proliferation of the lesions, secondary to proangiogenic factors in platelet granules. Fibrinogen levels should thus be kept high (>100 mg/Dl). Clinical response can be subtle and may take months to occur. Some lesions can remain for years after resolution of the KMP, leading to other morbidities such as orthopedic anomalies and chronic pain. Cincinnati Children's Hospital Medical Center presently has a clinical registry open to prospectively investigate the clinical course of these lesions (http://www.cincinnatichildrens.org/svc/alpha/h/vascular). Coagulopathic abnormalities in vascular malformations (venous malformation [VM], lymphatic malformation, lymphaticovenous malformation [LVM], capillary-lymphaticovenous malformation [CLVM]) are likely caused by different mechanisms and should not be labeled as KMP (**Table 1**).

Another distinct vascular disorder cutaneovisceral angiomatosis with thrombocytopenia is a rare disorder presenting at birth with cutaneous and visceral lesions (in gastrointestinal tract, lung, spleen, bone, muscle). This disorder has a proliferative potential and thus can be classified as having elements of a malformation and tumor.[14] This condition has also been called multifocal lymphangioendotheliomatosis with thrombocytopenia because it was identified lymphatic histomorphologic features.[15] The associated thrombocytopenia is in the range of 10,000 to 70,000 cells/mm^3. The cause of the thrombocytopenia is unclear but perhaps is related to endothelial hyperplasia. Gastrointestinal tract bleeding with associated congenital, multifocal, discrete red/brown/blue macules and papules is the typical presentation. These patients have been treated with medical

Table 1
Abnormal coagulation in vascular anomalies

Features	KHE/TA	VM/LM/ LVM/CLVM
Hematologic Features		
Platelets	Very low	Low
Fibrinogen	Significantly decreased	Decreased
PT/aPTT	Normal or increased	Increased
D dimer	↑	↑↑
Pathogenesis	Platelet trapping Fibrinogen consumption	Stasis and thrombin activation on abnormal vasculature
Management	Pharmacologic treatment Avoid platelets No heparin	Sclerotherapy Resection LMWH Compression

Abbreviations: aPTT, activated partial prothrombin time; LM, lymphatic malformation; LMWH, low-molecular-weight heparin; PT, prothrombin time.

Data from Mulliken JB, Anupindi S, Ezekowitz RA. Case 13-2004: a newborn girl with a large cutaneous lesion, thrombocytopenia and anemia. N Engl J Med 2004; 350:1764.

management such as corticosteroid, interferon, and thalidomide, with mixed results.

VASCULAR MALFORMATIONS

Hematologists play a key role in the management of vascular malformations because the lesions can result in severe coagulopathies. Coagulopathic abnormalities can occur in almost all malformations but are most significant in diffuse and multifocal VMs, LVMs, and CLVMs. The coagulopathy is referred to as localized intravascular coagulopathy (LIC) and is characterized by low levels of plasma fibrinogen, factor V, factor VIII, factor XIII (prekallikrein), and antithrombin.[16] The levels of D dimers and fibrin split products are also elevated in LIC. Minor to moderate thrombocytopenia may also be observed. With surgical resection, sclerotherapy, embolization, trauma, infection, or drugs, LIC can sometimes progress to disseminated intravascular coagulation (DIC) that can be life threatening. Furthermore, this chronic consumptive coagulopathy can cause the formation of microthrombi, which calcify (forming phleboliths) and cause pain.

The pathogenesis of the coagulopathy in vascular malformations is probably multifactorial and best understood in relation to Virchow triad of abnormalities of the blood vessel wall, blood flow, and blood composition.[17] One hypothesis is that the endothelium lining these lesions may not be normal (structurally or functionally), leading to abnormal interactions with blood products that initiate coagulation. A second hypothesis relates to the size of the vessels and the velocity of blood flow. Flow abnormalities occur because of variation in channel size and structural abnormalities, resulting in local pooling of blood and stasis that can further damage the endothelium and activate the coagulation process.

Vascular endothelial cells play an important role in the regulation of coagulation.[18–20] These cells have both procoagulant and anticoagulant properties that can be activated or deactivated by endothelial damage. Blood flow has multiple influences on platelet and fluid-phase coagulations.[21,22] Local shear can occur secondary to blood flow. These factors can induce platelet aggregation and thrombus formation or interfere with platelet adhesion, causing an increased bleeding tendency.

VMs

There have been several descriptive investigations of coagulopathy in patients with VM. Enjolras and colleagues[23] reviewed 27 cases of extensive pure VM in the upper and lower limb and found that 88% of these patients had LIC. The coagulopathy was associated with very low levels of plasma fibrinogen and soluble complexes, increase in levels of fibrin split products, and a moderately low platelet count. This chronic consumptive coagulopathy caused episodes of thrombosis (leading to formation of phleboliths) or bleeding (hemarthrosis, hematomas, or intraoperative blood loss). The condition worsened after discontinuing the use of elastic stockings, after therapeutic intervention (embolization or surgical procedure), after spontaneous fracture of a bone in the area of VM, or during pregnancy or menses. The investigators subsequently confirmed their findings in a retrospective evaluation of 24 patients with extensive VM or venous anomalies.[24] Furthermore, they characterized the difference between LIC caused by these lesions and the coagulopathy that typifies KMP in certain vascular tumors. They also categorized the anomalies based on a severity scoring system (a point was given to each involved site) and found that higher VM severity scores were associated with more severe LIC. They concluded that the use of graded permanent elastic compression garments and low-molecular-weight heparin (LMWH) was an effective preventative measure. Coagulative disorders in patients with VM of the limbs and trunk were later characterized with the same findings.[25] The investigators underscored the high incidence of coagulopathy and pain in intramuscular VMs. Another important finding was a low von Willebrand Factor (vWF) level in 39% of patients a less than 50% vWF level in 12% of patients. vWF is a protein synthesized by endothelial cells and megakaryoctes. Low levels of vWF can lead to an increased risk of bleeding. Dompmartin and colleagues[26] reinforced the association of LIC with VMs and reported increased D-dimer levels in patients with trunk venous anomalies, diffuse and extensive lesions, and in the presence of phleboliths. Dompmartin and colleagues[27] demonstrated that the elevated D-dimer level was highly specific for VMs and suggested its use as a biomarker for the clinical evaluation of vascular anomalies. Maguiness and colleagues[28] reported that determination of D-dimer level would help diagnose certain vascular anomalies, such as VMs versus fast-flow lesions and VMs versus glomovenous malformations. They also recommended using this biomarker during therapy.

There are a few reports on the risks of coagulopathy during interventional radiologic procedures.[29] Mason and colleagues[30] analyzed coagulative abnormalities in patients undergoing embolization or sclerotherapy for vascular anomalies. They found an increased incidence of coagulopathy during injection with dehydrated alcohol or sodium tetradecyl sulfate. The coagulopathy consisted of a decrease in platelet count and fibrinogen level, an increase in prothrombin time, and a conversion from negative to positive D-dimer test result.

Klippel-Trénaunay Syndrome (CLVM)

Klippel-Trénaunay syndrome (KTS) is characterized by extensive CLVM in limbs, pelvis, and/or trunk, usually with overgrowth. Patients with this condition are prone to coagulative abnormalities, both hemorrhagic and thrombotic events, because of the extent of this combined slow-flow lesion, the abnormal venous anatomy, and the concurrent or associated lymphatic component. There are numerous reports in the literature documenting the increased incidence of coagulopathy in these patients.[31–44] However, there are no prospective data on the specific mechanisms for the coagulopathy in KTS, some of which are similar to that of VMs.

Patients with KTS seem to have a form of LIC that can progress to DIC after intervention, such as operation or sclerotherapy, and that can be aggravated by immobilization after these procedures. Another precipitating factor, well known to surgeons who operate on vascular anomalies in the limb, is the increased risk of bleeding with the use of a tourniquet for resection of a CLVM as well as capillary-lymphatic malformation and LVM. It is presumed that cessation of blood flow by the tourniquet causes changes in clotting factors, leading to bleeding and further DIC.[45,46] Aware of this transient coagulopathy, the surgeons know the importance of waiting and compressing the wound before closure. There are case reports of patients with slow-flow anomalies, documenting major hemorrhagic episodes that have responded to supportive therapy with fresh frozen plasma, heparin, and other antifibrinolytic agents such as tranexamic acid (TXA).[38,43] Thrombotic events, including potentially fatal pulmonary emboli, are common especially after an operation, trauma, and radiological procedures; however, they can also occur spontaneously. This spontaneous prothrombotic condition is poorly explained. Venous thromboembolism has been reported to occur in a frequency ranging from 8% to 22%. In a Mayo Clinic series of 252 patients with KTS and mean age of 11.5 years, 4% of patients had pulmonary embolism (PE), 4% had deep venous thrombosis, and 15% had superficial thrombosis. Postoperatively, of 49 patients, 4% had bleeding events, 1.5% had PE, and 1.5% had deep venous thrombosis (higher than the risk in the general population).[47] Oduber and colleagues[48] reported a series of 4 patients with chronic thromboembolic pulmonary hypertension that was thought to be caused by recurrent PE in vascular malformations. The investigators stressed the need for early detection in these patients. They also recommended the following considerations lifelong prophylactic anticoagulation in patients with proven thromboembolism, elastic compression and placement of a caval filter, and a multidisciplinary approach to these patients with a hematologist and a pulmonologist.

Large draining veins presumably increase the likelihood that if a venous thromboembolism is present, the resulting pulmonary embolus could be large. Furthermore, procedures such as sclerotherapy that intentionally cause vascular stasis may predispose to clot formation. There are no data on other associated prothrombophilic states increasing the thrombotic risk in these patients. Nevertheless, it is likely that the incidence of thrombosis in these patients is greater than the combined incidence of all known inherited thrombophilic states. These slow-flow combined anomalies are risk factors for thrombosis even without a family history of thromboembolic disease.

OVERGROWTH SYNDROMES

Overgrowth syndromes, such as Proteus syndrome, have associated risk for PE. Proteus syndrome is associated with disproportionate asymmetric overgrowth of body parts, cerebriform connective tissue nevi, epidermal nevi; vascular malformations; and dysregulated adipose tissue. The cause of this complication is unknown but that of the thromboembolism is thought to be enlarged veins.[49] Other overgrowth syndromes may have this embolic risk because of stagnant flow in dilated anomalous veins. An example is congenital lipomatous overgrowth, vascular malformations, epidermal nevi, and skeletal/scoliosis and spinal abnormalities (CLOVES) syndrome that includes ectatic thoracic and central veins. Patients with this complication are at high risk for sudden death, and some groups recommend prophylactic caval filters before interventional procedures.[50]

Lymphatic Malformations

Pure lymphatic malformations have been associated with minor thrombocytopenia and other more severe coagulopathies, such as DIC. Furthermore, the pathogenesis is not completely understood or well studied.

Genetic Thrombophilia

Several congenital or acquired thrombophilic conditions have been identified in the general population as risk factors for venous thromboembolism. These conditions include antithrombin, protein C, and protein S deficiency; factor V Leiden mutation; C677T MTHFR gene mutation; plasminogen activator inhibitor (PAI-1) 4G/G polymorphism; hyperhomocysteinemia; antiphospholipid antibodies; lupus anticoagulant; and G20210A prothrombin gene mutation.[51,52] There are other situations in which endothelial abnormalities increase the risk of thrombosis, such as sickle cell disease and malignancy.[53–54] In adults, genetic alterations have been shown to interact with other risk factors, such as use of oral contraceptives, trauma, immobilization, and surgical procedures, to increase the thrombotic risk. The overall risk in the presence of multiple risk factors can exceed the sum of the separate effects. There is no information about the prevalence of thrombophilic predispositions in patients with vascular anomalies. It is presumed that patients with a genetic predisposition toward thrombophilia have an increased risk for thrombosis and coagulopathy if they also have an extensive slow-flow vascular malformation, but studies of thrombophilia and vascular anomalies have not been published to date.

MANAGEMENT OF COAGULOPATHIES

It is important to discuss about patients with potential coagulopathy in an interdisciplinary manner. There are no prospective studies on medical management and thus evidence-based therapeutic regimens are lacking. Institutional treatment plans should be developed until prospective trials are initiated. All patients who are symptomatic with a high-risk vascular anomaly (VM, LVM, CLVM) that is diffuse or multifocal should have hematologic evaluation as a baseline and again before any surgical or interventional procedure and during pregnancy. Laboratory tests include a complete blood cell count; evaluation of prothrombin time, partial thromboplastin time, fibrinogen and D-dimer levels; and a prothrombotic assessment (ie, prothrombin gene mutation, PAI-1 polymorphism, and levels of protein C and S, thrombin-antithrombin complex, factor V Leiden, factor VIII, homocysteine, lupus anticoagulant, anticardiolipin antibody, and antithrombin III). Patients found to have abnormalities in this initial blood examination should have a hematologic consultation before an operation or interventional procedure or during pregnancy. At the authors' institution, those patients at high risk for complications are treated with LMWH (enoxaparin) for at least 2 weeks before and after an operation or radiologic intervention. Dosing is 0.5 mg/kg/dose (maximum of 60 mg/dose) once or twice a day subcutaneously (adults, 30 mg twice a day). Administering LMWH should be stopped 12 hours before the procedure and restarted 12 hours after the procedure. If LMWH is used for an extended period, heparin levels (antifactor Xa) should be determined 4 to 6 hours after subcutaneous injection. The target level of antifactor Xa should be less than 0.5 units/mL for prophylaxis.[55] A complete blood cell count should initially be done monthly, and dual-energy x-ray absorptiometry should be performed during long-term use of LMWH because of the risk of osteopenia. LMWH can be used daily to alleviate pain caused by inflammation, thrombosis, and formation of phleboliths in large VMs; the same dosing is used. Dosing during pregnancy may vary and should be determined by a hematologist and obstetrician specializing in maternal-fetal medicine.

Patients with KTS or an extensive VM, especially if there has been a documented prior thrombotic event (eg, PE), need anticoagulation therapy for an extended period, perhaps indefinitely. These patients can be treated short term with LMWH or heparin and then the treatment can be shifted to oral vitamin K antagonists, such as warfarin (Coumadin). Some patients respond better to LMWH and have a tendency to have recurrent thrombosis after treatment with vitamin K antagonists. A few patients with acute thromboembolic events may require the placement of an inferior or superior vena caval filter in addition to anticoagulant therapy.

Antifibrinolytic agents such as ϵ-aminocaproic acid (EACA) and TXA have been used to treat hemorrhagic coagulopathy caused by vascular anomalies.[56–58] Both the agents attach to the lysine-binding sites of plasminogen and plasmin, displacing plasminogen from its fibrin surface. TXA is more potent and has a longer half-life than EACA. Widespread use has been limited because of concerns of increased risk of thrombosis; however, there are no retrospective or prospective studies. Furthermore, antiplatelet agents such as aspirin, ticlopidine, and clopidogrel have been shown to have equivocal clinical benefit, but further studies are needed. Compression garments reduce the amount of blood trapping in these lesions and probably decrease LIC.

Other pharmacologic treatments, such as interferon, have been reported to be effective in improving the coagulopathy in vascular malformations. These reports are limited to personal communication and case studies. There have been no prospective studies showing efficacy.[59,60]

NOVEL APPROACHES

Vascular malformations are a challenging group of disorders for physicians. Treatment has mainly been surgical or through interventional procedures. Particular attention to new sclerosing agents and embolization techniques is important in improving the management of these patients. However, such agents need to address the pathophysiological differences in these malformations, because agents effective for arterial malformations may not be effective for lymphatic malformations or VMs.

As with vascular tumors, medical therapy needs to be targeted at the limited knowledge of the pathophysiology of these malformations. One exciting area with great potential is the recent discovery of genetic alterations within these lesions.[61] Some genetic alterations could serve as therapeutic targets and thus aid in treatment options. For example, the PTEN gene mutation has been identified in patients with extensive arteriovenous malformations and other anomalies.[62] Rapamycin or other mammalian target of rapamycin (mTOR) inhibitors are predicted to be effective in disorders in which the PTEN/mTOR/STAT3 pathway is affected.[62] New antithrombotic agents with similar effectiveness as LMWH need to be investigated because lifelong anticoagulation is needed after a significant thrombotic event has occurred. At present, clear and agreed-on medical management guidelines are lacking for these complications, highlighting the need for further research.

REFERENCES

1. Mulliken JB, Glowacki J. Hemangiomas and vascular malformations in infants and children: a classification based on endothelial characteristics. Plast Reconstr Surg 1982;69(3):412–22.
2. Mulliken JB, Enjoras O. Congenital hemangiomas and infantile hemangioma: missing links. J Am Acad Dermatol 2004;50(6):875–82.
3. North PE, Waner M, Mizeracki A, et al. GLUT 1: a newly discovered immunohistochemical marker for juvenile hemangiomas. Hum Pathol 2000;31(1): 11–22.
4. Baselga E, Cordisco M, Garzon M, et al. Congenital haemangioma associated with transient thrombocytopenia and coagulopathy: a case series. Br J Dermatol 2008;158:1363.
5. Kasabach H, Merritt K. Capillary hemangioma with extensive purpura: report of a case. Am J Dis Child 1940;59:1063–70.
6. Sarkar M, Mulliken JB, Kozakewich HP, et al. Thrombocytopenic coagulopathy (Kasabach-Merritt phenomenon) is associated with kaposiform hemangioendothelioma and not with common infantile hemangioma. Plast Reconstr Surg 1997;100(6): 1377–86.
7. Enjolras O, Wassef M, Mazoyer E, et al. Infants with Kasabach-Merritt syndrome do not have "true" hemangiomas. J Pediatr 1997;130(4):631–40.
8. Gruman A, Liang MG, Mulliken JB, et al. Kaposiform hemangioendothelioma without Kasabach-Merritt phenomenon. J Am Acad Dermatol 2005;52(4): 616–22.
9. Inceman S, Tangun Y. Chronic defibrination syndrome due to a giant hemangioma associated with microangiopathic hemolytic anemia. Am J Med 1969;46:997.
10. Staub PW, Kessler S, Schreiber A, et al. Chronic intravascular coagulation in the Kasabach-Merritt syndrome: preferential accumulation of fibrinogen 131 I in a giant hemangioma. Arch Intern Med 1972;129:475.
11. Haisley-Royster C, Enjolras O, Frieden IJ, et al. Kasabach-Merritt phenomenon: a retrospective study of treatment with vincristine. J Pediatr Hematol Oncol 2002;24(6):459–62.
12. Mulliken JB, Anupindi S, Ezekowitz RA, et al. Case 13-2004: a newborn girl with a large cutaneous lesion, thrombocytopenia, and anemia. N Engl J Med 2004;350:1764–75.
13. Hauer J, Graubner U, Konstantopoulos N, et al. Effective treatment of kaposiform hemangioendotheliomas associated with Kasabach-Merritt phenomenon using four-drug regimen. Pediatr Blood Cancer 2007;49(6):852–4.
14. Prasad V, Fishman SJ, Mulliken JB, et al. Cutaneovisceral angiomatosis with thrombocytopenia. Pediatr Dev Pathol 2005;8:407.
15. North PE, Kahn T, Cordsco MR, et al. Multifocal lymphangioendotheliomatosis with thrombocytopenia: a newly recognized clinicopathological entity. Arch Dermatol 2004;140:599.
16. Mulliken JB, Young AE, editors. Vascular birthmarks: hemangiomas and malformations. Philadelphia: WB Saunders; 1988. p. 320.
17. Wintrobe M. Blood, pure and eloquent. New York: McGraw Hill; 1980. p. 10.
18. Ware JA, Heistad DD. Platelet-endothelium interactions. N Engl J Med 1993;328:628.
19. Cines DB, Pollak ES, Buck CA, et al. Endothelial cells in physiology and in the pathophysiology of vascular disorders. Blood 1998;91:3527.
20. Nawroth P, Kisiel W, Stern D. The role of endothelium in the homeostatic balance of haemostasis. Clin Haematol 1985;14:531.
21. Turitto VT, Hall CL. Mechanical factors affecting hemostasis and thrombosis. Thromb Res 1998; 92:525.
22. Nemerson Y, Turitto VT. The effect of flow on hemostasis and thrombosis. Thromb Haemost 1991;66:272.
23. Enjolras O, Ciabrini D, Mazoyer E, et al. Extensive pure venous malformations in the upper or lower

limb: a review of 27 cases. J Am Acad Dermatol 1997;36:219.
24. Mazoyer E, Enjolras O, Laurian C, et al. Coagulation abnormalities associated with extensive venous malformations of the limbs: differentiation from Kasabach-Merritt syndrome. Clin Lab Haematol 2002;24:243.
25. Mazoyer E, Enjolras O, Bisdorff A, et al. Coagulation disorders in patients with venous malformation of the limbs and trunk. Arch Dermatol 2008;144:861.
26. Dompmartin A, Acher A, Thibon P, et al. Association of localized intravascular coagulopathy with venous malformations. Arch Dermatol 2008;144:873.
27. Dompmartin A, Ballieux F, Thibon P, et al. Elevated D-dimer level in the differential diagnosis of venous malformations. Arch Dermatol 2009;145:1239.
28. Maguiness S, Koerper M, Frieden I. Relevance of D-dimer testing in patients with venous malformations. Arch Dermatol 2009;145:1239.
29. Rhee CY, Spivack M, Al-Mondhiry H. Subacute consumption coagulopathy-an unusual complication of angiography. Am J Med Sci 1975;269:391.
30. Mason KP, Neufeld EJ, Karian VE, et al. Coagulation abnormalities in pediatric and adult patients after sclerotherapy or embolization of vascular anomalies. AJR Am J Roentgenol 2001;177:1359.
31. Endo Y, Takahashi K, Mamiya S, et al. Factor XIII deficiency associated with Klippel-Weber disease, platelet dysfunction and cryofibrinogenemia. Acta Haematol 1983;69:398.
32. Baskerville PA, Ackroyd JS, Lea Thomas M, et al. The Kippel-Trénaunay syndrome: clinical, radiological, and haemodynamic features and management. Br J Surg 1985;72:232.
33. Baskerville PA. [Thromboembolic disease and congenital venous abnormalities]. Phlebologie 1987;40:531 [in French].
34. Joshi M, Cole S, Knibbs MA, et al. Pulmonary abnormalities in Klippel-Trénaunay syndrome. Chest 1992; 102:1274.
35. Muluk SC, Ginns LC, Simigran MJ, et al. Klippel-Trénaunay syndrome with multiple pulmonary emboli- an unusual cause of progressive pulmonary dysfunction. J Vasc Surg 1995;21:696.
36. Yamamoto H, Muneta T, Asahina S, et al. Lower leg fracture with Parkes-Weber syndrome complicated by disseminated intravascular coagulation. J Orthop Trauma 1995;9:449.
37. Neubert AG, Golden MA, Rose NC. Kasabach-Merritt coagulopathy complicating Klippel-Trénaunay-Weber syndrome in pregnancy. Obstet Gynecol 1995;85:831.
38. Aronoff DM, Roshon M. Severe hemorrhage complicating the Klippel-Trénaunay-Weber syndrome. South Med J 1998;91:1073.
39. Jacob AG, Driscoll DJ, Shaughnessy WJ, et al. Klippel-Trénaunay syndrome: spectrum and management. Mayo Clin Proc 1998;73:28.
40. Dobbs P, Caunt A, Alderson TJ. Epidural analgesia in an obstetric patient with Klippel-Trénaunay syndrome. Br J Anaesth 1999;82:144–6.
41. Gianlupi A, Harper RW, Dwyre DM, et al. Recurrent pulmonary embolism associated with Klippel-Trénaunay-Weber syndrome. Chest 1999;115:1199.
42. Walder B, Kapelanski DP, Auger WR, et al. Successful pulmonary thromboendarterectomy in a patient with Klippel-Trénaunay syndrome. Chest 2000;117:1520.
43. Noel AA, Gloviszki P, Cherry KJ, et al. Surgical treatment of venous malformations in Klippel-Trénaunay syndrome. J Vasc Surg 2000;32:840.
44. Huiras E, Barnes C, Eichenfield L, et al. Pulmonary thromboembolism associated with Klippel-Trénaunay syndrome. Pediatrics 2005;116:e596.
45. Wilgis EF. Observations on the effects of tourniquet ischemia. J Bone Joint Surg Am 1971;53:1343.
46. Wilgis EF. Tourniquet in reconstructive surgery of the hand. Handchirurgie 1972;4:99.
47. Gloviczki P, Driscoll D. Klippel-Trénaunay syndrome: current management. Phlebology 2007;22:291–8.
48. Oduber C, Gerdes V, van der Horst CM, et al. Vascular malformations as underlying cause of chronic thromboembolism and pulmonary hypertension. J Plast Reconstr Aesthet Surg 2009;62:684.
49. Cohen MM. Proteus syndrome: an update. Am J Med Genet C Semin Med Genet 2005;15:137.
50. Alomari A. Characterization of a distinct syndrome that associates complex truncal overgrowth, vascular, and acral anomalies: a descriptive study of 18 cases of CLOVES syndrome. Clin Dysmorphol 2009;18:1–7.
51. Nowak-Gottl U, Junker R, Kreuz W, et al. Risk of recurrent venous thrombosis in children with combined prothrombotic risk factors. Blood 2001;97:858.
52. Tormene D, Simioni P, Prandoni P, et al. The incidence of venous thromboembolism in thrombophilic children: a prospective cohort study. Blood 2002; 100:2403.
53. Austin H, Key NS, Benson JM, et al. Sickle cell trait and the risk of venous thromboembolism among blacks. Blood 2007;110(3):908–12.
54. Decousus H, Moulin N, Quenet S, et al. Thrombophilia and risk of venous thrombosis in patients with cancer. Thromb Res 2007;120(Suppl 2): S51–61.
55. Weitz JI. Low-molecular-weight heparin. N Engl J Med 1997;337:688.
56. Warrell RP, Kempin SJ. Treatment of severe coagulopathy in the Kasabach-Merritt syndrome with aminocaproic acid and cryoprecipitate. N Engl J Med 1985;313:309.
57. Morad AB, McClain KL, Ogden AK. The role of tranexamic acid in the treatment of giant hemangiomas in newborns. Am J Pediatr Hematol Oncol 1993;15:383.

58. Katsaros D, Grundfest-Broniatowski S. Successful management of visceral Klippel-Trénaunay-Weber syndrome with the antifibrinolytic agent tranexamic acid (cycolcapron): a case report. Am Surg 1998; 64:302.
59. Enjolras O. Vascular tumors and vascular malformations: are we at the dawn of a better knowledge. Pediatr Dermatol 1991;16:238.
60. Apak H, Celkan T, Oskan A, et al. Blued rubber bleb nevus syndrome associated with consumptive coagulopathy: treatment with interferon. Dermatology 2004;208:345.
61. Tan WH, Baris HN, Burrows PE, et al. The spectrum of vascular anomalies in patients with PTEN mutations: implications for diagnosis and management. J Med Genet 2007;44(9):594–602, 62.
62. O'Reilly KE, Rojo F, She QB, et al. mTOR inhibition induces upstream receptor tyrosine kinase signaling and activates Akt. Cancer Res 2006; 66(3):1500–8.

Index

Note: Page numbers of article titles are in **boldface** type.

Clin Plastic Surg 38 (2011) 161–163
doi:10.1016/S0094-1298(10)00145-8

Moving?

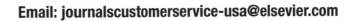

Make sure your subscription moves with you!

To notify us of your new address, find your **Clinics Account Number** (located on your mailing label above your name), and contact customer service at:

Email: journalscustomerservice-usa@elsevier.com

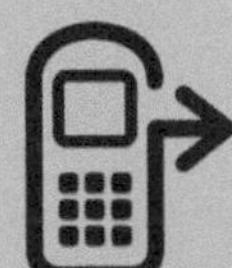

800-654-2452 (subscribers in the U.S. & Canada)
314-447-8871 (subscribers outside of the U.S. & Canada)

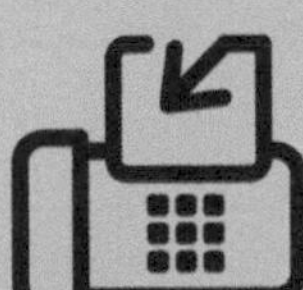

Fax number: 314-447-8029

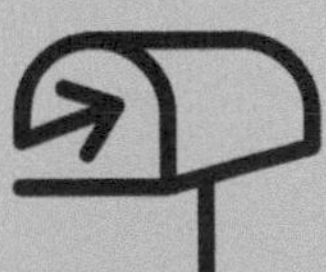

Elsevier Health Sciences Division
Subscription Customer Service
3251 Riverport Lane
Maryland Heights, MO 63043

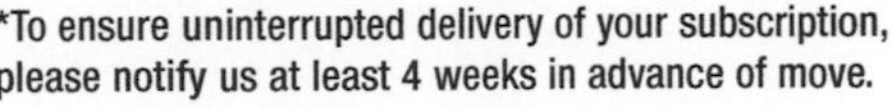

*To ensure uninterrupted delivery of your subscription,
please notify us at least 4 weeks in advance of move.

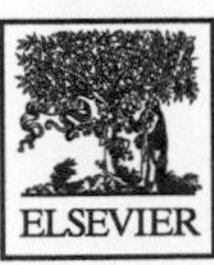

Printed and bound by CPI Group (UK) Ltd, Croydon, CR0 4YY
03/10/2024
01040358-0008